FOR THEIR OWN GOOD

The Transformation of
English Working-Class Health Culture,
1880–1970

LUCINDA McRAY BEIER

The Ohio State University Press
Columbus

Library of Congress Cataloging-in-Publication Data
Beier, Lucinda McCray.
For their own good : the transformation of English working-class health culture, 1880–1970
/ Lucinda McCray Beier.
p. ; cm.
Includes bibliographical references and index.
ISBN 978-0-8142-1094-9 (cloth : alk. paper)
1. Working class—Medical care—Great Britain—History—20th century. 2. Working class—
Medical care—Great Britain—History—19th century. 3. Public health—Great Britain—
History—20th century. 4. Public health—Great Britain—History—19th century. I. Title.
[DNLM: 1. Urban Health Services—history—England. 2. Attitude to Health—England.
3. Health Knowledge, Attitudes, Practice—England. 4. History, 19th Century—England.
5. History, 20th Century—England. 6. Social Class—England. 7. Social Medicine—history—
England. WA 11 FE5 B422f 2008]
RA418.3.G7B45 2008
362.10941—dc22
2008023683
This book is available in the following editions:
Cloth (ISBN 978-0-8142-1094-9)
CD-ROM (ISBN 978-0-8142-9174-0)

Front cover photo courtesy of Lancashire County Library and Information Service.
http://lanternimages.lancashire.gov.uk link.
Cover design by Melissa Ryan.
Type set in ITC New Baskerville.
Printed by Thomson-Shore, Inc.

♾ The paper used in this publication meets the minimum requirements of the American
National Standard for Information Sciences—Permanence of Paper for Printed Library
Materials. ANSI Z39.48–1992.

9 8 7 6 5 4 3 2 1

To Elizabeth A. M. Roberts
without whose vision, guidance, hard work, and loving spirit
this book would not have been written

Contents

Acknowledgments

❧

It is my pleasure and honor to acknowledge the many individuals and institutions without whom this project could not have been completed. First, I must recognize the 239 oral history informants whose memories first made it clear that there was a book to be written. Their good humor, strength, and collective reconstitution of a world that might otherwise be forgotten taught me far more about both the human condition and working-class Lancashire than this study can ever express. I owe them my deepest gratitude—as well as apologies for any inadvertent misinterpretations of their life experiences.

Thanks to the Centre for North-West Regional Studies, the History Department, and the Library at Lancaster University—especially Jean Turnbull, Christine Wilkinson, Jacqueline Whiteside, Kenneth Harrison, and Angus Winchester—for their generous support and hospitality, particularly during my research visit in 2004. Thanks also to research assistance from Tom Dixon and to staff members of the National Library of Medicine, the North West Film Archive, the British Film Institute, and the British Library Newspaper Reading Room.

I am grateful for the National Library of Medicine Publication Grant (5 G13 LM 008353) that enabled me to spend two years completing research and writing. Similarly, thanks are due to Illinois State University for the sabbatical, internal research grant, and travel funding that helped me complete this project. I also want to acknowledge the expert assistance of Interlibrary Loan and subject matter librarians at Illinois State University's Milner Library—especially Vanette Schwartz, for whom nothing is impossible. In addition, I must thank Cindy Caldwell for photocopying above and beyond the call of duty.

Thanks to Sandy Crooms and Maggie Diehl, of The Ohio State University Press, for shepherding the manuscript to publication. I also want to acknowledge the recommendations of Graham Mooney, Elizabeth Roberts, Lee Beier, and two anonymous reviewers, which have much improved the final product. I owe a great debt to Jeffrey Richards for taking the time to talk to me about the history of film. In addition, I am grateful to my colleagues in the Social Science History Association and the American Asso-

ix

ciation for the History of Medicine, who over the past decade have listened to and constructively critiqued various iterations of the arguments appearing in this book: you know who you are.

Thanks to the *Bulletin of the History of Medicine* and the *Social History of Medicine* for permission to reprint substantial portions of articles.

Finally, I want to express my affectionate gratitude to those who nurtured the writer—and therefore the project—during its long evolution. For making me feel at home, thanks to Judith and Roger Addison, Katy and Thomas Woods, and Elizabeth and Hugh Roberts. Thanks to Hollis Webster and Alice Berry for letting me explain. Thanks to my dog-girl, Scout, and the blue bike for balance, harmony, inspiration, and problem solving. And, as always, my loving gratitude to Lee for listening and caring, as well as to Joe, Jesse, Jake, and Zach, my wonderful Lancashire lads.

Chapter One

~

Introduction

ORIGINS

Most books are autobiographical—at least in the sense that they reflect the author's interests and emerge from some important insight or experience. This book is more autobiographical than many. It would not have been written had I not in 1978, as a new bride and a graduate student of the social history of health and medicine, moved from the American Midwest to northern England and begun participant observation of a medical culture that was quite different from my own. While the biomedical theories and therapies were similar to those I grew up with in the United States, care environments, personnel, and a range of expectations (from routine infant care to financial obligations) were very foreign to me and specific to my new home.[1] White-uniformed midwives delivered my babies in a hospital that had a tea lady but no billing department; our general practitioner made house calls or saw us in a "surgery" that looked more like a study than an examining room; and well-child examinations and immunizations were offered one afternoon a week by health visitors and doctors at a clinic in our neighborhood. When I took my children to pediatricians during summer visits to the United States, I found myself translating cross-cultural information and making unexpected decisions: Should I have my little boys circumcised (usual in the United States, but not in England)? Should I have them immunized against whooping cough (greater concern about side effects in England than in the United States)?

These similarities, differences, and negotiations, which permeated my experience of illness, childbearing, and health care during twelve important years, also informed conceptualization of the research I did during the 1980s and '90s on early modern English suffering and healing.[2] Eager to

1. A short article describing my personal experience of health services in Lancaster appears as "My twelve years in the UK health system," *Health Affairs* 19:3 (2000): 185–90.

2. Publications from this research include *Sufferers and healers: The experience of illness in seventeenth-century England* (Routledge and Kegan Paul, 1987); "Seventeenth-century English

1

explore what Roy Porter most famously was beginning to call the "patient's view," I was prompted by my own experience to broaden my perspective from the doctor-patient relationship to the larger social and cultural arenas where health is maintained and ill-health managed or endured.[3] Using diaries, autobiographies, and casebooks, I searched the past for the contexts within which people gave birth, suffered injury and disease, received or provided treatment and care, and died. I found complex circumstances, where information, authority, decision making, and services straddled the porous boundaries between practitioners, sufferers, and their families, and where gender, class, resources, and community settings influenced people's choices, roles, and experiences. However, my sources were patchy and rarely transparent. Because their creators were long dead, it was not possible to ask for clarification or amplification.

When in 1987 I was given the opportunity to work with Elizabeth Roberts, Administrator and later Director of the Centre for North-West Regional Studies at Lancaster University (United Kingdom), on an oral history project concerning familial and social change in mid-twentieth-century working-class Lancashire communities, I brought my questions about the ways people thought about and dealt with health and ill-health to the project.[4] The opportunity to talk with living informants and to review transcripts of interviews Roberts conducted during the 1970s and early '80s was both liberating and far more informative than I could possibly have predicted. As even the most casual eavesdropping in supermarket queues reveals, people love to talk about their experiences of ill-health and medical care; their talk offers a wealth of information about the cultural contexts for those experiences. This book emerged from hours of listening and identifying patterns, and my growing perception that no scholar has yet told a story that seems, in some respects, too ordinary to be interesting, and in others, too remote and obsolete to be useful. Why should we care that virtually all working-class residents of Barrow, Lancaster, and Preston born before about 1940 as children had goose grease rubbed on their chests to ease congestion?

surgery: The casebook of Joseph Binns," in Christopher Lawrence, ed., *Medical theory, surgical practice: Studies in the history of surgery* (London: Routledge, 1992), 48–84; "Experience and experiment: Robert Hooke, illness and medicine," in Michael Hunter and Simon Schaffer, eds., *Robert Hooke: New studies* (Woodbridge, Suffolk: The Boydell Press, 1989), 235–52; "The good death in seventeenth-century England," in Ralph Houlbrooke, ed., *Death, ritual and bereavement* (London: Routledge, 1989), 43–61; and "In sickness and in health: The Josselins' experience," in Roy Porter, ed., *Patients and practitioners: Lay perceptions of medicine in pre-industrial society* (Cambridge: Cambridge University Press, 1985), 101–28.

3. Porter first called for history from the patient's viewpoint in Roy Porter, "The patient's view. Doing medical history from below," *Theory and Society* 14 (1985): 175–98. F. B. Smith similarly observed the lack of historical scholarship about the patient's experience and agency in *The people's health 1830–1910* (New York: Holmes and Meier Publishers, 1979), 9–12.

4. This project, entitled "Familial and social change and continuity in working-class families, 1940–1970" and conducted between 1987 and 1989, was funded by an Economic and Social Research Council grant.

Why is it important to know about the mutual aid networks that supported working-class families at times of birth, illness, and death until at least the 1950s?

For me, the explanation is that, despite widespread interest in history from the bottom up and scholarly rejection of old-fashioned hagiographical history of medicine, both increasing since the 1960s, the histories of public health and medicine have continued to be physician-centered and dominated by use of professional and institutional records. These sources inevitably skew scholarly perspectives, highlighting the importance of shifting medical theories, formal health care provision, and related governmental policies, and rendering the sufferer a shadowy, passive presence. This process has arguably ghettoized research on prevention, intervention, and care, limiting foci to areas of professional interest and agency. Yet, most experience of health management and ill-health happens far from hospitals, public health clinics, doctors' offices, and medical practitioners; it occurs in homes and workplaces, is discussed among family members and friends, and is often first approached using knowledge and tools related to a shared culture that sometimes, but not necessarily, includes consultation of formal authorities who both help to shape and are shaped by that culture. When I ask undergraduate students at our large public university what they do when they get sick, the knee-jerk response, given because it seems conventionally correct, is "I go to the doctor." When I probe, saying, "Really? As soon as you think you might be sick?" they say, "I call my mother." Their responses reveal historical continuity and change, as well as linkages in health cultures that are both diverse, according to students' ethnic and social backgrounds, and common among people living in the early-twenty-first-century United States. They also suggest a reality with global implications in an era of huge public health challenges and tensions between traditional cultures, on the one hand, and "modern" Western biomedicine, on the other.

Thus, although this book is about a particular group of people—239 working-class residents of three north Lancashire cities—during the years between about 1880 and 1970, it also calls for expansion of scholarly approaches to the histories of public health and medicine to include "lay" as well as "professional" sources and perspectives. It observes a shift in responsibility for illness, birth, and death from the informal domestic and neighborhood sphere to the purview of professional, institutionally based authorities—a shift that involved a dramatic transformation of people's beliefs, expectations, and actions.[5] This cultural change has occurred at different times in different places; timing and reasons for the change vary by

5. See Peregrine Horden and Richard Smith, eds., *The locus of care: Families, communities, institutions, and the provision of welfare since antiquity* (London and New York: Routledge, 1998), for a variety of perspectives on the international history of this transition.

motivation and process, as well as "client" (e.g., the mad, the infirm elderly, etc.) and social group (e.g., class, income, sex, age). In working-class Lancashire, with rare exceptions that reinforced rather than altered traditional health culture, it happened during the mid-twentieth century.[6]

Beginning with the oral history evidence affects the way one reads institutional sources. The annual reports of the Medical Officers of Health (MOsH) are available for most English municipalities and counties during the study period and offer rich evidence to historians of public health, providing information about demography, morbidity, causes of death, health care services, school and work environments, and living conditions.[7] Owing their profession and responsibilities to nineteenth-century policymakers' observation of a relationship between poverty, dirt, ignorance, vice, and disease, MOsH focused their attention and services on working-class residents of their communities.[8] During the early and mid-twentieth century, their responsibilities expanded enormously, by 1948 including, in addition to other inspection and regulatory duties, local hospital, infant and maternal welfare, tuberculosis and venereal disease, and school health services.[9] Their reports show that they had a good deal of discretion about the ways national policies were implemented at the local level. Written from their own gender (predominantly male) and class (predominantly middle-) perspectives, their narrative comments project attitudes regarding working-class people that influenced their decisions. I consulted the annual reports of the MOsH for Barrow (1883–1968), Lancaster (1907–60), and Preston (1878–1970) to balance and enhance information obtained from oral history informants.

These two major sources, which will be discussed in greater depth below, reveal some important areas of agreement between MOsH and working-class residents of the study cities. For example, both viewed housing as

---

6. In the late nineteenth century, members of some special groups, including the indigent without family support, the mentally subnormal, and the emotionally ill, were admitted to local institutions, including workhouses and asylums. However, these people comprised a small minority of the population, and oral history informants considered these types of institutionalization highly undesirable and departures from the accepted norm of home and neighborhood care.

7. See Anne Hardy, *The epidemic streets: Infectious disease and the rise of preventive medicine, 1856–1900* (Oxford: Clarendon Press, 1993); and John Welshman, *Municipal medicine: Public health in twentieth-century Britain* (Oxford: Peter Lang, 2000), for excellent recent studies that depend heavily on annual reports of the Medical Officers of Health for London and Leicester respectively.

8. See, for example, Anthony S. Wohl, *Endangered lives: Public health in Victorian Britain* (Cambridge, MA: Harvard University Press, 1983); Gerry Kearns and Charles W. J. Withers, "Introduction: Class, community, and the processes of urbanisation," in Gerry Kearns and Charles W. J. Withers, eds., *Urbanising Britain: Essays on class and community in the nineteenth century* (Cambridge: Cambridge University Press, 1991), 1–11.

9. See Jane Lewis, *What price community medicine: The philosophy, practice and politics of public health since 1919* (Brighton, Sussex: Wheatsheaf Books, 1986).

important to health and quality of life; both were concerned about general issues, such as infant mortality and specific contagious diseases, which shifted in the course of the period under consideration. These sources also, however, illuminate differences in perspective that not only affected people's behavior at the time but also suggest some blind spots in the historical scholarship. For example, introduction of the germ theory stimulated public health officials' determination to isolate sufferers from contagious diseases, either in home quarantine or, increasingly, in isolation hospitals. From a public health perspective, isolation was scientifically based and also made obvious practical sense. However, oral history accounts indicate that isolation threatened traditional working-class mutual aid, which had long provided the most accessible, affordable, and reliable therapeutic advice, nursing, household help, and emotional support in times of sickness.[10] This book, then, aims to fill a need identified by John Welshman in his recent study of public health in twentieth-century Leicester: "Obvious gaps exist in our understanding on such questions as the ways that services were perceived by different classes and social groups, and on the experience of the patient."[11] The oral evidence will help to answer some of these questions.

This evidence will also enable us to range beyond public health issues to explore home and neighborhood management of health, ill-health, birth, and death; relationships between working-class people and practitioners, including chemists (pharmacists), dentists, midwives, nurses, general practitioners (GPs), and consultants; and working-class attitudes toward and use of hospitals. Interview informants talked about how their families tried to prevent, identified, and explained illnesses. Their accounts are threaded by the care of aging or disabled relatives; punctuated by home births, "childhood" diseases, and injuries; and demarcated by deaths, more frequent and familiar than those experienced by later generations. Ever-present in these accounts are the women—mothers, grandmothers, and neighborhood health authorities—who made most health care decisions and provided all of the home-based care. These activities have received little scholarly attention, although Ellen Ross's study of poor London mothers between 1870 and 1918, and Emily Abel's book on family caregiving in the late-nineteenth- and early-twentieth-century United States go some distance toward improving this situation.[12] Yet an important outcome of the growth of the doctor's cultural authority in working-class communities, which was built, in part, on biomedicine's victory over "old wives' tales," was

10. Similarly, Jane Lewis (*The politics of motherhood: Child and maternal welfare in England, 1900–1930* [London: Croom Helm, 1980], 20–21) argues that infant welfare services undermined traditional mutual aid regarding infant care.

11. Welshman, *Municipal medicine*, 299.

12. Ellen Ross, *Love and toil: Motherhood in outcast London, 1870–1918* (New York and Oxford: Oxford University Press, 1993); and Emily K. Abel, *Hearts of wisdom: American women caring for kin* (Cambridge, MA: Harvard University Press, 2000).

a change in women's roles and a reduction in their authority and confidence regarding health matters; in a sense, biomedicine invalidated both the tales and the women who told them.[13] Thus, the transformation of working-class health culture was highly gendered. While I certainly will not argue that this transformation took the form of a crude power struggle between (evil) middle-class male doctors and (good) working-class women, or that it represented a shift from a golden age of family and community care to the impersonal, non–tender mercies of professional and institutional attention, the evidence does suggest a hegemonic process through which working-class people—men and children, as well as women—embraced the health beliefs and practices espoused and prescribed by dominant social and professional groups.[14] This book both documents and interprets this transformation.

DEFINITIONS

Before moving forward, I want to discuss two phrases that are central to this study and, indeed, that have already been frequently used in this introduction: "working class" and "health culture." To begin with the most hotly contested issue, despite recent critiques that question both the existence of identifiable social classes and the ways scholars have written about those groups, I will make the potentially controversial statement that I believe there was—and perhaps still is—an English working class.[15] I also accept

13. I owe the phrase "cultural authority" to Paul Starr (*The social transformation of American medicine* [New York: Basic Books, 1982]).

14. I extrapolate my concept of hegemony from Gramsci's theory, which was rooted in his observations regarding political and historical change. As other scholars have noted, the concept helps to interpret cultural processes through which dominant groups negotiate both leadership and willing acceptance of their ideologies by members of nondominant groups. See Antonio Gramsci, *Selections from the prison notebooks*, Quentin Hoare and Geoffrey Nowell Smith, eds. (New York: International Publishers, 2003 ed.), 12–13, 106–7, 125, 161, 182, 207; Graeme Turner, *British cultural studies: An introduction*, 2nd ed. (London and New York: Routledge, 1996), 182–213.

15. For some recent discussions of these issues, see William M. Reddy, "The concept of class," in M. L. Bush, ed., *Social orders and social classes in Europe since 1500: Studies in social stratification* (London and New York: Longman, 1992), 13–25; Stuart Woolf, "Order, class and the urban poor," in M. L. Bush, ed., *Social orders and social classes in Europe since 1500*, 185–98; Gareth Stedman Jones, *Languages of class: Studies in English working class history 1832–1982* (Cambridge: Cambridge University Press, 1983), especially 1–24; Patrick Joyce, *Visions of the people: Industrial England and the question of class, 1848–1914* (Cambridge University Press, 1991, pb. ed. 1994), especially 1–26. The qualification of my statement that there is still an English working class emerges from post–World War II changes in working-class life that relate both to deindustrialization, on the one hand, and to development of a national mass culture, on the other. Both developments altered key elements in working-class culture—not least of which (and most germane to my study), the importance of local mutual aid networks to resource sharing, social interaction, and reputation.

E. P. Thompson's contention that social class is a relationship, not a thing.[16] While Thompson focused on consciousness of this relationship as it affected workers and employers, as well as dominant and subordinate political groups, I observed what Joanna Bourke referred to as "class awareness" at the local level of an "us," subsuming relatives, neighbors, coworkers, and members of other "communities," such as co-religionists or labor union comrades, and a "them," that mainly included middle-class people and sometimes health care providers.[17] That these relationships shifted over time—and that it became possible, for example, for people to continue to identify themselves as working-class, or of working-class origins, even after taking up stereotypically middle-class occupations such as clerical work or teaching—if anything strengthens the argument that working-class identity involves perception of difference from members of other classes. This argument is also supported by the consciousness expressed by Medical Officers of Health that their primary responsibilities concerned preventing and containing mortality and morbidity among working-class residents of the cities they served. Thus, the MOsH studied working-class physical, occupational, and housing conditions; visited schools where working-class pupils' health status received special attention; and, in the course of the twentieth century, manifested at the local level national changes in public health foci, which shifted from ignorant factory girls and working mothers in the first half of the century to "problem families" after World War II.[18]

The notion of class identity as relationship also applies to the diversity within the working class. In her useful social history of council housing, Alison Ravetz points out that "In practice, council housing had to deal with a divided tenant population that corresponded better to the Victorian notion of layered and plural working classes than to the twentieth-century concept of a single, unified 'working class.'"[19] This insight helps to explain and justify the inclusion of comparatively prosperous artisan families and those of casually employed laborers, self-consciously "respectable" and carelessly "rough" people, within the umbrella category, "working-class." Oral history informants to this study recognized the complexity and reality of this class identity and culture.

16. E. P. Thompson, *The making of the English working class* (New York: Vintage Books, 1966).

17. Joanna Bourke, *Working-class cultures in Britain 1890–1960: Gender, class and ethnicity* (London and New York: Routledge, 1994), 4.

18. See, for example, Lewis, *Politics of motherhood;* David Armstrong, *Political anatomy of the body: Medical knowledge in Britain in the twentieth century* (Cambridge: Cambridge University Press, 1983); Bernard Harris, *The health of the schoolchild: A history of the school medical service in England and Wales* (Buckingham and Philadelphia: Open University Press, 1995); and John Welshman, "In search of the 'problem family': Public health and social work in England and Wales, 1940–70," *Social History of Medicine* 9:3 (1996): 447–65.

19. Alison Ravetz, *Council housing and culture: The history of a social experiment* (London: Routledge, 2001), 6.

In addition to perception of social class as relationship, I also find useful Patrick Joyce's observation that

> a common socio-economic condition as proletarians, or dependent, manual, waged workers, would in fact seem central to any definition of what "working class" might mean, as would a shared perception of this common condition. Now, the actual nature of proletarianisation in practice varied considerably, but nonetheless a certain level of common condition and outlook would have to prevail. Therefore, broadly speaking, "economic" criteria would seem to be uppermost.[20]

While, as Joyce also observed, nonmanual workers such as small neighborhood shopkeepers and hospital porters, as well as nonindustrial workers such as domestic servants, may justifiably be considered working-class, manual work, both skilled and unskilled, usually in a factory setting, was, together with comparatively low waged earnings, a constant element of individual and group identity that will, in the discussion that follows, be called working-class. However, Bourke and other gender historians point out the limitations of occupational and economic factors in the class identification of women, by contrast with that of men. I believe that shared meanings, outlooks, and experience of everyday life, linked as they were to limited resources, are actually the central components of class awareness among working-class women, children, and men.[21]

Joyce and other scholars, most notably Gareth Stedman Jones, have focused on language as the signifier and vehicle for working-class identity. In this study, rather than exploring genres such as popular ballads or political speeches and publications for key elements of working-class culture, I depend instead on the language of self-identified working-class oral history informants, which is composed of words, usage, and (inevitably) accents that to themselves and others expressed both their working-class identities and their health culture. Thus, for example, the "doctor's man" (bill collector), "working medicine" (laxatives) and "Nitty Nora" (school nurse or health visitor) belong to a discourse that reveals a class culture regarding health care personnel, economics, and theories about prevention and cure of disease. Informants' memories, expressed through the language and other signifiers of daily life, including dress (e.g., shawls and clogs before the interwar years), housing (e.g., terraced cottages), food (e.g., bread and milk "pobs" for babies), leisure activities (e.g., public houses, day trips to the seaside), hygiene (e.g., rags used as sanitary towels, cleaning of shared

---

20. Joyce, *Visions*, 10. See also Elizabeth Roberts, *Women and families: An oral history, 1940–1970* (Oxford: Basil Blackwell, 1995), 237.

21. Bourke, *Working class cultures*, 2–5; Laura Oren, "The welfare of women in laboring families: England, 1860–1950," in *Clio's consciousness raised: New perspectives on the history of women*, Mary Hartman and Lois W. Banner, eds. (New York: Harper Torchbooks, 1974), 226–44.

lavatories), and remedies (e.g., "knitbone" [comfrey] and goose grease) embody a shared set of meanings and behaviors that, for this study, will be explored for health-related content.

This concept of a shared set of meanings and behaviors associated with health-related events and activities will also do as a broad definition for health culture.[22] While it is sometimes easier to express what working-class health culture was *not* (e.g., it did not, before the interwar period, include routine dependence on professional institutional medicine for most minor or even major health problems), it is possible to identify some important characteristics that differentiate the working-class health culture of the late nineteenth and early twentieth centuries from either middle-class health culture of the same period, or the health beliefs and practices of working-class people after about World War II.

What may be called traditional working-class health culture had its roots in preindustrial times and places, sometimes transported within informants' remembered experience from rural communities.[23] It was a dominantly self-help culture, where adults (mainly women) took charge of disease prevention, diagnosis, and treatment for themselves, their families, and sometimes their neighbors. Closely related to this issue was traditional dependence on informal knowledge and expertise of mothers, grandmothers, more rarely interested fathers or grandfathers, and informal neighborhood authorities (sometimes referred to as "handywomen" by Medical Officers of Health, although never by working-class oral history informants, who were more likely to call them "Aunty," "Nurse," or simply "Mrs.") who delivered babies, laid out the dead, and offered health advice and nursing care to neighbors. Working-class health-related knowledge and expertise were pluralistic, drawing from diverse traditions ranging from humoral theory and magical beliefs to empirical and biomedical approaches. Working-class neighborhoods were face-to-face societies where identity was personal rather than functional and where trust was based on day-to-day contact, relationship histories, and reputations; while this characteristic affected most aspects of life, it was exceptionally important in times of illness when family comfort, livelihood, and even survival were threatened.

22. See Elizabeth D. Whitaker, "The idea of health: History, medical pluralism, and the management of the body in Emilia-Romagna, Italy," *Medical Anthropology Quarterly* 17:3 (2003): 348–75, for an anthropological study of a regional Italian health culture that bears some similarity to my approach.

23. I observed elements that would later characterize Lancashire working-class health culture in health-related practices of seventeenth-century England, including self-help; mutual aid; female-dominated, home-based treatment and care; and dependence on informal knowledge and expertise. See Beier, *Sufferers and Healers,* particularly 154–241. Social childbearing in that period was ably discussed by Adrian Wilson in "Participant or patient? Seventeenth-century childbirth from the mother's point of view," in Roy Porter, ed., *Patients and practitioners: Lay perceptions of medicine in pre-industrial society* (Cambridge: Cambridge University Press, 1985), 129–44.

In these communities, health culture was home- and neighborhood-based; before the interwar period, almost all births, suffering, and deaths occurred at home. (It is noteworthy that physicians, midwives, and nurses generally did their work in patients' homes; thus, theirs was also a home-based health culture.) Finally, in times of childbearing, ill-health, and death, working-class people depended on mutual aid exchanged within family and neighborhood networks. Indeed, the question of what an informant's childhood neighborhood had been like almost always elicited a response about the help neighbors gave each other during health crises.

Working-class health culture was not static, even during the comparatively short time from approximately 1880 to 1948, when the introduction of the National Health Service definitively tipped the balance toward a national health culture. Instead, it was fluid, responding to new conditions and resources, and incorporating some while rejecting others. For example, in most households the homemade home remedies of the late nineteenth century were replaced by over-the-counter patent medicines by the 1920s; during the same period, the more expensive "doctor's medicine" continued often to be rejected in favor of the cheaper "chemist's medicine." In 1880 working-class self-help and mutual aid had already expanded to include membership in friendly societies that created bridges to official health care for some individuals and families.[24] Similarly, the model of the clothing or Christmas club and hire purchase (buying things "on the installment plan"), increasingly popular among working-class families, made culturally acceptable weekly contributions to hospital schemes and payments to collectors for GPs' services. Nonetheless, working-class patients continued to avoid hospitalization whenever possible until the mid-twentieth century. Beginning in 1902, successive Midwives Acts undermined the roles of neighborhood health authorities and made more common recourse to licensed midwives and general practitioners. However, until the activities of handywomen were outlawed in 1936, many working-class women preferred the services of old-fashioned "bona fide" midwives. Furthermore, increasing consultation of officially sanctioned health care providers, including chemists, licensed midwives, and "family doctors," was similarly fostered by long-term face-to-face relationships where familiarity and personal knowledge was at least as important as perceived expertise or even quality of service. And, finally, the pluralism of working-class health culture, together with traditional deference to authority, enabled it gradually to absorb new messages about illness, treatment, and appropriate care providers as these were transmitted by a range of sources including public health workers, school-based health education, and popular media (principally periodical literature, radio programs, and films).

24. See James C. Riley, *Sick, not dead: The health of British workingmen during the mortality decline* (Baltimore and London: Johns Hopkins University Press, 1997), for an account of working-class health conditions based on friendly society records.

The working-class health culture discussed in this book was unique nei-ther to industrial, urban Lancashire nor to exclusively working-class peo-ple. As I have said, informants with rural connections remembered similar health cultures in mainly northern rural villages. Furthermore, the poor mothers managing family health between 1870 and 1918 in Ellen Ross's "Outcast London," and Margery Spring Rice's Depression-era working-class wives, who lived in both urban and rural settings distributed around the country, operated within a health culture that was quite similar to that remembered by this study's informants—and would also have been recog-nizable to Robert Roberts from his early-twentieth-century Salford neigh-borhood.[25] Thus, it is possible that what I have perceived as Lancashire working-class health culture might more accurately be designated the tradi-tional health culture of the English poor.[26] However, my evidence expresses with certainty only the experience of working-class residents of Lancaster, Barrow, and Preston.

I do not intend to argue that working-class health culture was com-pletely different from the health cultures of, say, middle-class people or officially trained and licensed health care professionals. Indeed, to some degree, all members of English society shared some elements of the same health culture. It may be useful to visualize health cultures as overlapping, rather than as mutually exclusive, with social class and status, together with the shared meanings engendered by similar education and socialization, helping to determine the extent of the overlap. Physicians, the leading representatives of both biomedicine and public health, tended to come from middle-class backgrounds. Thus, it should not be surprising that middle-class people embraced biomedicine and official health care earlier than working-class people and, indeed, became advocates for change of working-class beliefs and behaviors as they related to hygiene and medi-cal care. Nonetheless, most people were essentially multilingual in their health cultures, retaining elements of older beliefs and practices (e.g., the humoral concept of a "cold" caused by a "chill," which a "hot" remedy such as whiskey helped, and keeping the feet, chest, and head warm prevented) combined with a newer health culture (e.g., the conviction that germs cause upper respiratory infections). While the learned health culture and terminology of health care professionals to some extent separated them from all laypeople, medical practitioners were also multilingual, retaining and using both biomedical and traditional concepts and terminology. So, for example, Mrs. Melling, born in 1917, remembered:

25. Ellen Ross, *Love and toil,* 169–94; Margery Spring Rice, *Working-class wives,* 2nd ed. (London: Virago, 1981. First published 1939); Robert Roberts, *The classic slum: Salford life in the first quarter of the century* (Harmondsworth, Middlesex: Penguin, 1987. First published 1971), 124–28.

26. This observation is supported by evidence provided by Carl Chinn, *Poverty amidst prosperity: The urban poor in England, 1834–1914* (Manchester and New York: Manchester University Press, 1995), 144.

> There was a lot of diphtheria going around at one time . . . and I
> remember m'dad saying that he had to call the doctor. Old Dr. Aitken,
> who was a very old doctor in Lancaster, and he was Scotch, m'dad said
> that he came in and said what he wanted him for, I don't know what it
> was for particularly. Anyway, m'dad was saying why *his* kids hadn't got
> these sore throats and that, and old Dr. Aitken just looked up and there
> was an old clothes rack as they used to have in those days, and hanging
> from the clothes rack was a big bunch of onions. Aitken said, "How long
> have you had that up there?" You know, you always got a string of onions
> up. He said, "Now, that is where your disease is going. Take them down
> and try one." He took them down and there wasn't a sound onion, all
> rotten. Dr. Aitken said that *they* had got the disease that was going about
> instead of the children.[27]

In this example, the physician, whether seriously or in jest, authoritatively
validated an explanation for something that has never been definitively
explained: why some people catch communicable diseases while other
people do not. He linked that explanation to onions, which were commonly used in a variety of homemade internal remedies and poultices and
were thought to be generally good for people's blood. The explanation
was culturally coherent and remembered by this informant for approximately fifty years. It also indicates this doctor's familiarity with working-class
health culture. Other trained health care providers, especially chemists,
who arguably served as a bridge between working-class families and official
medicine, both understood and facilitated the self-help health culture that
sustained working-class Lancashire communities in the nineteenth and
early twentieth centuries.[28]

At the same time, official health care providers threatened that culture.
Gerry Kearns and Charles Withers remind us that there has been little
scholarly attention

> paid to the construction, from within working-class communities, of
> shared values out of the repetitive routines of daily life. Yet, in certain
> respects, the tenacity of working-class communities, their responses to
> their exclusion from the hegemonic equation of the public sphere with
> that of the middle class and their resistances to direct assaults on their

---

27. Oral history informants were promised confidentiality; thus, pseudonyms are used in
this book. References to interview transcripts (housed by the Elizabeth Roberts Oral History
Archive, Lancaster University) are given by the informant's code number and transcript page
number: Barrow informants are indicated by the suffix "B," Lancaster informants by the suffix
"L," and Preston informants by the suffix "P." For this quotation, the reference is Mrs. M3L,
31. Roberts and I created aliases for informants that, unlike code numbers, are not necessarily
consistent from one publication to another.

28. Whitaker's "The idea of health" observes similar types of communication in northern
Italy.

living standards through changing labor relations were all rooted in a militantly local culture that . . . often successfully rejected and subverted external pressures.[29]

Working-class adherence to traditional health culture, in the face of tremendous pressure to change or jettison that culture, is an important theme of this book.

ORAL HISTORY AND THIS PROJECT

As many scholars argue, oral history techniques provide an exceptionally useful way to explore the experiences and perspectives of "ordinary" working-class people, which would not otherwise inform a historical scholarship that tends to rely on evidence from male, and to a lesser extent female, members of social elites.[30] Widely used by feminist researchers and scholars concerned with other disenfranchised groups (e.g., African Americans, Holocaust survivors, immigrants, gays and lesbians, etc.), oral history methods draw their strength, according to Penny Summerfield, from "the importance of language within social relations. We are dependent upon language for understanding who we are and what we are doing. The meanings within language are cultural constructions collectively generated, historical deposits within the way we think, which constitute the framework within which we act."[31] The challenge to the oral historian is to tease out and contextualize these meanings, which can include contradictions or be deliberately skewed by the informant, potentially be misunderstood by the researcher, and convey as much by silence as by what is said.[32] While this challenge also affects the interpretation of documentary or other (e.g., statistical or visual) evidence, it is particularly important in the use of oral

29. Kearns and Withers, "Introduction," 10.

30. Paul Thompson, *The voice of the past: Oral history,* 2nd ed. (Oxford: Oxford University Press, 1988); Elizabeth Roberts, *A woman's place: An oral history of working-class women 1890–1940* (Oxford: Basil Blackwell, 1984); Elizabeth Roberts, *Women and families;* Steve Humphries, *The handbook of oral history. Recording life stories* (London: Inter-Action Trust, 1984); Luisa Passerini, *Fascism in popular memory: The cultural experience of the Turin working class,* trans. Robert Lumley and Jude Bloomfield (Cambridge: Cambridge University Press, 1988); Alessandro Portelli, *The battle of Valle Giulia: Oral history and the art of dialogue* (Madison: University of Wisconsin Press, 1997).

31. Penny Summerfield, *Reconstructing women's wartime lives: Discourse and subjectivity in oral histories of the Second World War* (Manchester and New York: Manchester University Press, 1998), 11.

32. Summerfield points out that Luisa Passerini "is often credited with being the first to urge on oral historians the need to listen for and interpret women's silences and contradictions as part of the endeavor to gain access to the deeper meanings of what women are saying" (*Reconstructing Women's Wartime Lives,* 40n.88). I believe that this statement can be generalized to men and, thus, all oral history informants.

history, which is both a technique and a source, and is the only form of historical evidence deliberately created by the historian, who devises the questions, selects the informants, initiates the conversations, and makes sure that the resulting information can be accessed by scholars.

I was fortunate to have as my guide and partner in the interviews on which this book is based Elizabeth Roberts, who helped to pioneer oral history studies in England during the 1970s and had published her classic *A Woman's Place: An Oral History of Working-Class Women 1890–1940* (Blackwell, 1984) before we began working together. *A Woman's Place* drew on approximately 160 life history interviews Roberts recorded in 1974–76 (in Preston) and 1978–81 (in Barrow and Lancaster). In the project we worked on together between 1987 and 1989, Roberts's goal was to extend her study of working-class family, work, and social life from 1940 to 1970. The 98 interviews we conducted, with each of us doing approximately half, benefited from Roberts's earlier experiences and choices and resulted in her book *Women and Families: An Oral History, 1940–1970* (Blackwell, 1995).

Based on questionnaires she had used for her earlier projects, Roberts and I composed a lengthy interview instrument. Employed not as a straitjacket but as a guide for our semistructured interviews, it was thirteen pages long and included 236 questions covering multiple aspects of personal, family, and community life, including health maintenance, childbearing, illness and injury, medical and home care, and death. We did not ask every informant every question, nor did we hesitate to depart from the interview instrument if an informant led us in an unexpected direction. However, the instrument served as a springboard to stimulate our guided conversations and an *aide-mémoire* between multiple interviews; its structure also facilitated comparison of information we obtained from numerous informants. Our intent was to elicit the type of life stories that Alessandro Portelli describes as full, coherent narratives that do not exist in nature but are created through the interview situation.[33] Each interview lasted an average of six hours and took place during an average of three visits to the informant's home. Each recording was transcribed; each transcript was subject-indexed. Audiotapes, transcripts, indexes, and biography sheets for each informant are housed by the Elizabeth Roberts Oral History Archive, Lancaster University (United Kingdom).

The identity, appearance, and demeanor of the interviewer affect the quality of the interview and the information it elicits. Both Roberts and I were female, middle-class academics, happily married, with children. Roberts was in early middle age when she conducted her three major sets of interviews; I was 36 in 1987. Roberts was born and raised in Barrow; thus, as a "Lancashire lass," she had a local connection. Although I had lived in England for a decade when I began work on the project, I was very obvi-

---

33. Portelli, *The battle of Valle Giulia*, 4.

ously a foreigner with an American accent. Sometimes our identities created challenges. For example, on one occasion, a single, middle-aged man
paused after about the first hour of his interview and said to me, "Here,
then: who made up these questions?" I told him that Elizabeth Roberts
and I had worked on the interview instrument together. He asked, "Are
you both married ladies?" I admitted the obvious. He pointed out that our
questions about family and neighborhood life bore little relevance to his
own experience, and proceeded to interview himself. From his account I
found out more about both pub life in 1960s Lancaster and Morecambe
(a nearby seaside resort town) and my own unconscious biases as a scholar
than I ever expected to learn.[34] Rather to Roberts's and my surprise, however, my foreignness was only comment-worthy at the beginning of each first
interview and probably elicited fuller explanations of matters that interview
informants might have expected a "local lass" to understand without aid,
thus arguably increasing the quality of the information given. In addition,
since I was a complete outsider with respect to informants' social networks,
talking honestly to me arguably may have posed less risk than revealing
personal and family secrets to someone who was truly *of* the community.

Interviewers and informants develop intense relationships during the
period when interviews are being conducted. While these relationships are
not exactly friendships, they are intimate and confidential. And, although
within any interview situation there are both power dynamics and the
desire of the informant to present him- or herself in the best possible light,
any perceived "power" of the interviewer was mitigated by the power of the
informant to give or withhold information, while the interviewee's concern
about how she or he appeared to the interviewer declined as the relationship between informant and interviewer developed.[35] Multiple interviews
were important, since with each interview trust grew between informant
and interviewer, and the quality of information improved. For instance,
denial of knowledge about illegal abortions in a first interview was sometimes followed by an account of such activities in a later conversation. In
the course of these discussions, people told me things about their lives that
even their partners and children did not know. Many informants appeared
to eagerly await interview appointments, sometimes having made notes
about things they wanted to say during that day's conversation. It is possible that the guarantee of confidentiality, which in this book is protected
by the use of aliases and code numbers for informants, made interviews
especially candid. Conducted in informants' homes, usually one-to-one
but sometimes with the interviewee's spouse, children, other relatives, or

34. See interview with Mr. H7L.
35. The power relationships inherent in the interview situation are well discussed by Penny
Summerfield in *Reconstructing women's wartime lives*, 23–26, and Kate Fisher in "'She was quite
satisfied with the arrangements I made': Gender and birth control in Britain 1920–1950," *Past
and Present* 169 (2000): 161–93.

friends present; lubricated by endless milky tea or instant coffee and sweet biscuits; the interviews were important and special for everyone who took part.

This book draws on both Roberts's earlier interviews and those we conducted during the 1987–89 project. In all, there are 239 usable interview transcripts. The informants' years of birth span the years from 1872 to 1958, with the preponderance of interviewees having been born between 1890 and 1940. Almost all identified themselves as working-class, or of working-class origin.[36] One hundred twenty-five informants were women; 114 were men (see table 1.1).[37]

Informants were recruited mainly through personal networks (of both interviewees and interviewers), interest groups (e.g., local history organizations), and services (e.g., adult literacy programs). The final group can be regarded as a snowball sample. It cannot be argued that information elicited from this group is as generalizable as, say, survey data provided by 400 respondents from a randomly selected population of 1,500. The criticism about interviewees who contributed to *A Woman's Place*, that "Elizabeth Roberts's interview sample is in any case insufficient to form a numerical basis for quantitative statements (such as 'The majority of working-class women in Barrow and Lancaster were enthusiastic bakers')," is probably justified, but perhaps unimportant: what does it mean to be an "enthusiastic baker," after all?[38] Does it matter whether the baker is enthusiastic? Is an enthusiastic baker necessarily a good one? Perhaps, given the opportunity, Roberts would rephrase the statement. My impression from the interviews in the archive is that Barrow, Lancaster, and Preston women who did not work outside the home did a great deal of baking and cooking "from scratch," especially before World War II, partly because they had learned this type of cooking as young girls and partly because it helped to stretch family budgets. This statement is not particularly controversial except as it counters some contemporary views including those of the Medical Officer of Health

36. By accepting informants' self-identification as working-class, Roberts and I took an approach similar to that adopted by Joanna Bourke in *Working-class cultures in Britain 1890–1960*. Two of the informants who contributed to this study were physicians, who did not identify themselves as working-class; two were chemists who lived and worked in working-class neighborhoods and served a predominantly working-class clientele. Several other informants were of working-class origin but arguably moved into the middle class due to combinations of education, occupation, marriage, and income.

37. This figure differs slightly from those used in my other publications based on the complete oral history collection: Beier, "Expertise and control: Childbearing in three twentieth-century working-class Lancashire communities," *Bulletin of the History of Medicine* 78:2 (2004): 379–409; and "'We were green as grass: Learning about sex and reproduction in three working-class Lancashire communities, 1900–1970," *Social History of Medicine* 16:3 (2003): 461–80. In reviewing evidence used for this study, I decided not to include in the final interview group informants I did not quote.

38. John K. Walton, *Lancashire social history, 1558–1939* (Manchester: Manchester University Press, 1987), 293.

Table 1.1 Oral History Informants by Sex and Decade of Birth

	1870s		1880s		1890s		1900s		1910s		1920s		1930s		1940s		1950s		Total
	F	M	F	M	F	M	F	M	F	M	F	M	F	M	F	M	F	M	
TOWN																			
Barrow	2	0	9	2	7	10	6	8	3	1	4	6	6	5	3	2	2	2	78
Lancaster	0	1	4	2	7	7	6	12	4	6	4	4	5	5	7	4	0	0	78
Preston	1	0	0	3	11	8	13	8	9	4	2	5	5	3	4	6	1	0	83
Total	3	1	13	7	25	25	25	28	16	11	10	15	16	13	14	12	3	2	239

for Preston for over forty years, Dr. H. O. Pilkington, who regularly disparaged the housekeeping skills of working-class women—a critique regarding
which one must carefully consider the source.[39] Roberts's critic also con-
tends that "some of the comments made by Elizabeth Roberts's interviewees
were prompted by leading questions," although since no examples of this
practice are given, I cannot offer a specific defense. Nonetheless, the main
question about diet appearing in the interview guide (e.g., 42. "Can you
describe your meals? What did you normally have for breakfast, at midday,
evening meal, snacks? Did your eating habits change as you grew older?")
did *not* suggest a desired response, but *did* elicit information that would
enable me to make the generalization, say, that it was quite usual between
1880 and at least the 1950s for people to eat porridge for breakfast.

The issue at hand, however, is representativeness: do the 239 life history
interviews on which this study depends offer a reliable basis for making gen-
eralizations about working-class lifestyles and cultures in Barrow, Lancaster,
and Preston between 1880 and 1970? According to Roberts, regarding the
interviews for *A Woman's Place,* "About 160 people, both men and women,
were interviewed . . . in these towns, and I am confident that they are a representative sample of the working class in all three areas. They come from
a wide variety of family sizes and occupations, and represent a good spread
of wage levels and religious and political beliefs."[40] The same could be said
for the group of 98 informants that Roberts and I interviewed in 1987–89.
I would argue that oral history provides a depth of qualitative information that the blunt instrument of a forced-choice social survey—however
random or large the survey sample—cannot hope to obtain, and at the
same time offers a much more balanced view than does a memoir such
as Robert Roberts's often-quoted *The Classic Slum: Salford Life in the First
Quarter of the Century,* which, after all, represents only one set of memories
and perceptions. Furthermore, the unusually large number of informants
who contributed to this study allows comparison of many accounts and
the opportunity to intuit representative or contrasting stories, as well as to
identify common myths (e.g., "We were happier then"), which, as much as
common experiences (e.g., of home remedies and care), can flesh out our
understanding of culture.

Most oral history studies depend on the memories of far fewer informants representing a broader range of geographical location and class origins. For example, Penny Summerfield's respected *Reconstructing Women's
Wartime Lives* (Manchester University Press, 1998) is based on 42 oral histories of women from various social backgrounds and locations scattered

---

39. *Borough of Preston: Annual report of the Medical Officer of Health for 1896,* 10. Since the
titles of the annual reports of Medical Officers of Health vary from year to year and place to
place, these documents will henceforth be referred to as "[Place] MOH Report, [Year], [Page
Number].

40. Roberts, *A woman's place,* 6.

around Britain and its former empire. For her excellent *Women, Identity and Private Life in Britain, 1900–50* (St. Martin's Press, 1995), Judy Giles interviewed 21 working-class women from several urban and suburban areas. I believe that because of its many informants, my study enables an exceptionally nuanced view of working-class health culture, as well as supporting confidence in interpretation of both the oral and other evidence. However, as with any other type of historical source, reconstruction of a past reality produces as many doubts and questions as it satisfies. With Giles, I observe,

> There are no primary sources by which I can verify the "truth" of the many things I was told, nor can I provide quantitative or empirical data to reinforce some of my interpretations. I can, however, identify common patterns and tropes in the narratives, and I can use these judiciously to ask questions about how myth and chronology, fact and story, memory and history are used to reinvent subjectivities that both expose and hide selfhood, and that tell us not only about the individuals who created these definitions, but also about the historical circumstances from which they produced and in which they intervened.[41]

Together with other evidence, the oral history accounts are used in this book "as textual verifications of a historical interpretation."[42] The book is intended as a contribution to the growing body of interview-based research on health-related issues.[43]

41. Judy Giles, *Women, identity and private life in Britain, 1900–50* (New York: St. Martin's Press, 1995), 26.

42. Portelli, *Battle of Valle Giulia,* 17n14.

43. See, for example, Joanna Bornat, Robert Perks, Paul Thompson, and Jan Walmsley, eds., *Oral history, health and welfare* (London and New York: Routledge, 2000); Jocelyn Cornwell, *Hard-earned lives: Accounts of health and illness from East London* (London: Tavistock, 1984); Sophie Laws, *Issues of blood: The politics of menstruation* (Basingstoke: Macmillan, 1990); Ann Cartwright, *Parents and family planning services* (New York: Atherton Press, 1970); Steve Humphries, *A secret world of sex: Forbidden fruit: The British experience 1900–1950* (London: Sidgwick and Jackson, 1988); Maureen Sutton, *"We didn't know aught": A study of sexuality, superstition and death in women's lives in Lincolnshire during the 1930s, '40s, and '50s* (Stamford: Watkinds, 1992); Ann Oakley, *The captured womb: A history of the medical care of pregnant women* (Oxford: Blackwell, 1984); Nicky Leap and Billie Hunter, eds., *The midwife's tale: An oral history from handywoman to professional midwife* (London: Scarlet Press, 1993); Fisher, "'She was quite satisfied'"; Elizabeth Roberts, "Oral history investigations of disease and its management by the Lancashire working class 1890–1939," in *Health, disease and medicine in Lancashire 1750–1950,* Occasional Publications, 2, Department of History, Science, and Technology, UMIST (1980), 33–51; Lucinda McCray Beier, "Contagion, policy, class, gender, and mid-twentieth-century Lancashire working-class health culture," *Hygiea International* 2:1 (2001): 7–24; Beier, "'I used to take her to the doctor's and get the *proper* thing': Twentieth-century health care choices in Lancashire working-class communities," in *Splendidly Victorian: Essays in nineteenth- and twentieth-century British history in honor of Walter L. Arnstein,* Michael H. Shirley and Todd E. A. Larson, eds. (Aldershot: Ashgate Press, 2001), 331–41; Beier, "Expertise and control: Childbearing in three twentieth-century working-class Lancashire communities," *Bulletin of the History of Medicine* 78:2 (2004): 379–409; and "'We were green as grass: Learning about sex and reproduction in three working-class Lancashire communities,

Every oral historian must decide how to refer to the people who contribute their memories to a research project. The usual choices are "interviewees," "respondents," "narrators," or "informants." The terms "interviewees" and "respondents" reflect one truth—that interviewers ask questions. However, these terms also imply lack of recognition of a more important truth—that people who are interviewed have a great deal of control over what they say. A "narrator" is a person who tells a story about a situation or event in which he or she may or may not have participated; oral history includes more than stories, but always involves personal experience and point of view. Thus, the term "informant," which I mainly use in this book, implies both the speaker's discretion about the content and credit for the quality of the information provided.

ANNUAL REPORTS OF THE
MEDICAL OFFICERS OF HEALTH

As Anthony Wohl points out, "Public health codes might be devised and laws passed, local authorities might form boards of health or sanitary committees, but for much of the second half of the [nineteenth] century the effectiveness of public health at the local level rested in the hands of the M[edical] O[fficer of] H[ealth]."[44] This could certainly also be said for the first three quarters of the twentieth century. While some cities employed medical officers beginning in the 1840s, most did not take this step until it was required by the 1872 Public Health Act, although Barrow anticipated the requirement, appointing an MOH in 1871.[45] Preston hired its first MOH in 1874—Dr. H. O. Pilkington, who served until his death in 1920— and Lancaster made a similar appointment in 1878.[46] With the exception of a year or two here and there, I obtained annual reports of the Medical Officers of Health for Barrow from 1883, Preston from 1889, and Lancaster from 1907. These reports document the expansion of the MOH's responsibilities up to the introduction of the National Health Service in 1948, and the alteration and contraction of those duties up to the abolition of the position in 1974.

1900–1970," *Social History of Medicine* 16:3 (2003): 461–80.

44. Wohl, *Endangered lives,* 179.

45. Wohl, *Endangered lives,* 181–82; Hardy, *Epidemic streets,* 4; J. D. Marshall, *Furness and the Industrial Revolution: An economic history of Furness (1711–1900) and the Town of Barrow (1757–1897) with an epilogue* (Barrow-in-Furness: Barrow-in-Furness Library and Museum Committee, 1958), 377.

46. Preston MOH Report, 1919, introductory letter "To the Chairman and Members of the Health Committee" written as a tribute to Dr. Pilkington by Acting Medical Officer of Health, Mary Lowry; Michael Winstanley, "The town transformed 1815–1914," in *A history of Lancaster 1193–1993,* Andrew White, ed. (Keele, Staffordshire: Ryburn Publishing, Keele University Press, 1993), 181.

Local reports vary dramatically in length and quality. Barrow's reports are brief, often (particularly in the early years) comprising fewer than ten pages and offering little narrative contextualizing the vital statistics, morbidity, and mortality data provided. By contrast, reports for Preston and Lancaster are lengthy, with text and tables generally running to over one hundred pages—particularly after 1907 when the Medical Officer assumed administration of the school medical service. Indeed, Lancaster's reports are more detailed than Preston's, despite disparities in city size and mortality from contagious diseases. Report lengths inevitably affected use of the documents and representation of each study city's experience in this book.

While much of the information offered by the MOH reports is not of particular interest for this study (e.g., climate data and accounts of canal boat inspections), total report contents aid understanding and comparison of the changing perspectives of each city's Medical Officers. Report contents, to some extent mandated by the central government, also illustrate the degree to which localities contested or supported national public health policies and priorities. For example, Dr. Pilkington strongly favored notification of births in Preston (mandated in 1908) as a means for increasing health visitors' access to working-class homes, reducing infant mortality, and preventing abortion, but objected to making measles a notifiable disease (1916), because this created a lot of work for his office and was, he thought, unlikely to prevent the spread of this highly contagious ailment.[47]

In addition, the reports illustrate contrasts in public health conditions, preoccupations, and interpretations between the three study cities. For instance, while all late-nineteenth- and early-twentieth-century MOsH were concerned about infant mortality, Barrow's MOH focused on especially high rates among illegitimate infants, Preston's MOH was most worried by diarrhea and efforts to limit family size, and Lancaster's MOH emphasized prematurity and its relationship to the health of the mother during pregnancy.[48] By contrast, only Preston had to deal with significant smallpox outbreaks during the twentieth century, while Lancaster and Barrow maintained smallpox hospitals that were almost never used. Responsible for sanitation in older cities, Lancaster and Preston MOsH mounted campaigns for installation of water closets and improvement or demolition of unhygienic housing, while Barrow's MOsH focused on planning and installing sanitation in a new town, as well as addressing the problems generated by rapid growth.

Reports of Medical Officers of Health were, of course, the voice of official public health policy, informed by contemporary medical and social

47. Preston MOH Report, 1907, 10; 1908, 12; and 1915, 6.
48. Barrow MOH Reports, 1894, 191; 1895, 186–87; 1901, 187; 1906, 197; 1907, 193; 1908, 245; 1910, 213. Lancaster MOH Reports, 1913, 88; 1919, 27; 1930, 39. Preston MOH Reports, see especially 1902, 11; 1903, 15; 1917, 10.

theories as well as middle-class outlooks. Thus, they offer a top-down alternative to the bottom-up viewpoints provided by the oral history accounts. However, like each oral history, each MOH's report is an account produced by an individual with perspectives and opinions of his, or more rarely her, own. Despite central government requirement of specific (and expanding) types of data (e.g., incidence of notifiable diseases, causes of death, heights of schoolchildren), early MOsH for each city developed a format that tended to be followed by later MOsH. However, it is clear that each MOH set out to both update his or her predecessor's approach to public health administration and put his or her own personal stamp on the annual reports s/he wrote. For example, Dr. Mary Lowry's 1920 tribute to Preston's long-standing MOH suggests impatience with his old-fashioned ways. She wrote of "Dr. Pilkington, who, for so many years furnished reports which were the envy and wonder of many of us less gifted with literary ability than he was. . . . Dr. Pilkington was an able administrator with a wonderful grasp of detail and a marvelous memory, and the fact that he accepted new schemes reluctantly was the result of long experience and sound judgment."[49]

The MOsH also inevitably set the tone for the people they supervised—Inspectors of Nuisances, Health Visitors, qualified Midwives, School Medical Officers, School Nurses, School Dentists, isolation hospital staff, ambulance attendants, and clerical workers. Medical Officers' comments reveal their belief in science as the way to conceptualize health challenges and solutions, their faith in educated expertise, and their value for temperate, fastidious, and restrained behavior. They viewed the working class as the location and cause of community health problems and targeted working-class individuals and families for the inspection, education, re-housing, and enforcement of measures that included isolation, disinfection, and medical treatment that were the health officials' main tools for disease prevention and control.[50] While they recognized the responsibility of landlords and employers for poor living and working conditions and negotiated public works and other reforms with local governmental agencies, their comments show both lack of a systemic view of poverty as a solvable root cause of many working-class health problems and impatience with a working-class culture that to them seemed passive, ignorant, and often destructive. Furthermore, it should not be forgotten that public health professionals *needed* the poor

49. Preston MOH Report, 1919, introductory letter "To the Chairman and Members of the Health Committee" written as a tribute to Dr. Pilkington by Acting Medical Officer of Health, Mary Lowry. This report on health conditions for 1919 was written and published after Pilkington's death in 1920.

50. In their *A social history of nursing* (London: Routledge, 1988), Robert Dingwall, Anne Marie Rafferty, and Charles Webster point out, "Middle-class women remained largely unexposed to health visiting until the 1920s. Health visiting was thus a more class-bound service than many subsequent accounts have suggested" (188). The same could be said for most public health services.

and their problems, which provided both a raison d'être and opportunities for expansion for this growing area of occupational endeavor. These perspectives make the MOH reports both a limited and a valuable source for this book.

TIME FRAME: 1880–1970

In 1880 Barrow-in-Furness (hereafter referred to as "Barrow"), Lancaster, and Preston were poised on the brink of a major change in official health care provision—the introduction of local public health services, which especially focused on dealing with dirt and disease among working-class residents.[51] Although each city had a health care delivery system that included private physicians, dentists, and chemists; voluntary hospitals; and Poor Law provision for health care of the indigent, most working-class people made little use of those services. Instead, the dominant childhood experience of the oldest informants in this study was of the traditional health culture described above—home- and neighborhood-based, characterized by self-help and mutual aid, avoiding charitable or institutional care when possible, and having only rare recourse to formally trained and licensed health care providers. Because the earliest memories of the oral history informants date from the 1880s and local Medical Officer of Health reports were also available from that decade, 1880 is an appropriate starting point for this book.[52]

The study spans policy-driven changes in public health activities that, with popularization of the germ theory, picked up steam after 1880—surveillance, notification, isolation, disinfection, education, immunization, and mandated treatment for specified conditions—that had an enormous impact on working-class residents of the study communities.[53] This impact was highly personal, taking the form of enforced interference with and confinement of bodies, substitution of official for traditional authorities, and intrusion into homes. There is no doubt that public health authorities at the national and local levels were altruistically motivated and sometimes effective in their efforts to reduce, in particular, the infant mortality and infectious diseases that especially devastated working-class families in northern industrial cities.[54] However, it is also true that official efforts to

51. See Wohl, *Endangered lives,* and Robert Woods and John Woodward, eds., *Urban disease and mortality in nineteenth-century England* (New York: St. Martins Press, 1984).

52. The earliest MOH report for Lancaster I could obtain was for 1907.

53. Helen Jones, *Health and society in twentieth-century Britain* (London and New York: Longman, 1994), provides an excellent survey of these developments.

54. See, in particular, Anne Hardy, *The epidemic streets,* for detailed discussion of late-nineteenth-century public health attacks on, and efficacy regarding, specific contagious diseases, including whooping cough, measles, scarlet fever, diphtheria, smallpox, typhoid, typhus, and tuberculosis. Depending mainly on London MOH reports, Hardy's conclusions pinpoint

help the community were sometimes experienced as attacks on working-class individuals and families, and that class and power differences and relationships influenced perceptions of both public health personnel and working-class people. As Kearns and Withers argue, "Ideas of contagion and environment were basic to the ways people wrote about class as well as disease. When a medical view of society was offered, there was an implicit conflation of social and biological relations. Class infused social epidemiology. Ideas of biological separateness reinforced a more primitive sense of the alienation of classes from one another."[55] And, extrapolating from Michel Foucault's arguments regarding shifting medical views of the body and uses of elite power to discipline bodies, David Armstrong observes that British social medicine, emerging in the late nineteenth century,

> constructed the outlines of a social map in which particular social relationships came into increasing focus through their constant and meticulous scrutiny. At the same time both justification and explanation were provided for this surveillance by the "invention" of new medical problems—venereal diseases, tuberculosis, the nervous child, infant mortality, the feckless mother—which, if left unsupervised, might have threatened the very fabric of society, but which, when adequately monitored, could serve instead to throw into relief the essential bonds that linked one person with another.[56]

These developments were experienced by the vast majority of working-class people after 1880. Thus, while many informants' parents grew up before the introduction of compulsory free elementary education in 1870, all but the oldest interviewees remembered medical inspections mandated by the School Medical Service established in 1907, while younger informants remembered treatment by the school dentist, interwar school-based administration of "emulsion" to prevent illness, and special interventions including ultraviolet light treatment and open-air schools for frail children.[57] The 1889 Notification Act that required reporting of diseases such as smallpox, diphtheria, scarlet fever, and typhoid also stimulated official examination of the sick, construction of isolation hospitals to which the sufferers from a growing list of diseases were involuntarily admitted, and enforcement

---

comparative successes and failures of these activities. Simon Szreter, "The importance of social intervention in Britain's mortality decline *c.* 1850–1914: A re-interpretation of the role of public health," *Social History of Medicine* 1:1 (1988): 1–37, argues that public health services reduced morbidity and mortality from contagious diseases.

55. Kearns and Withers, "Introduction," 9.

56. Armstrong, *Political anatomy*, 18.

57. See Harris, *The health of the schoolchild*. It is worthy of remark that public health authorities were increasingly dubious about the value of universal, compulsory, school-based medical examinations and the value of the resulting data collected. See 104–7 in particular.

of home quarantine and fumigation. The 1902 Midwives Act, intended to improve standards of midwifery services for working-class mothers, began the process of limiting working-class access to traditional neighborhood midwives, few of whom had formal training but many of whom were very popular.[58] Health visitors, employed by all of the study communities in the early years of the twentieth century to provide health information to working-class mothers and to inspect the condition of babies and homes, were occasionally welcomed but also often resented as "interfering busybodies."[59]

This is not to say that public policies regarding health matters were uniformly unpopular among working-class people. The National Insurance Act of 1911, which in return for minimal contributions provided medical services and sick- and disability pay to manual workers earning less than £160 per year, was viewed as a good thing by those oral history informants whose families benefited.[60] Some informants even commented on the Act's maternity provision, which offered covered wage earners 30s. per delivery for the services of a registered midwife.[61] However, with this exception, the "Lloyd George Act" did not cover wives and children so had a minimal impact on working-class health culture, particularly by comparison to the introduction of the National Health Service in 1948. Similarly, care provided by general practitioners and infirmaries via application to the Poor Law Guardians was avoided by members of the respectable working class and thus did little to change, but instead reinforced, its health culture.[62]

Friendly society coverage, sturdy and increasing in the early twentieth century, particularly in Barrow and Lancaster, may have had a larger effect on families with memberships. Mainly involving men, but also sometimes including children—particularly in temperance organizations such as the Rechabites, which was especially strong in Barrow—friendly society membership made consultation of general practitioners affordable. While this development probably hastened inclusion of biomedicine in working-class culture, that process was arguably slowed by the exclusion of most women, who made family budgetary and health decisions and provided home-based

---

58. See Oakley, *The captured womb;* Leap and Hunter, eds., *The midwife's tale;* and Jan Williams, "The controlling power of childbirth in Britain," in *Midwives, society and childbirth: Debates and controversies in the modern period,* Hilary Marland and Anne Marie Rafferty, eds. (London: Routledge, 1997), 232–47.

59. Mrs. J1B, 64. See also Mr. G1P, 60; Mrs. H4P, 16; Mrs. M1P, 50; Mrs. A3B, 51; Mrs. B5P, 48; Preston MOH Report, 1901, 17; and Celia Davies, "The health visitor as mother's friend: A woman's place in public health, 1900–14," *Social History of Medicine* 1:1 (1988): 39–59.

60. Jones, *Health and society,* 26–28.

61. See, for example, Mr. G1P, 7.

62. The classic study of medical care provided under the New Poor Law of 1834 is Ruth G. Hodgkinson. *The origins of the National Health Service: The medical services of the New Poor Law, 1834–1871* (Berkeley and Los Angeles: University of California Press, 1967).

care. The doctor's bill was a consideration before he was consulted and a dreaded obligation after his visit. This, in addition to the social class gap between physicians and working-class patients, made calling the doctor the last resort for most working families until the mid-twentieth century.

Before the interwar period, working-class residents of the study cities had little experience of hospitalization, except for injuries (particularly those experienced at work) and communicable diseases. Voluntary hospitals were small and were not considered desirable substitutes for home treatment and care. By the turn of the twentieth century, each city had a hospital prepayment "scheme" to which working-class people contributed—sometimes voluntarily, but more often involuntarily, through deductions made from pay packets by major industrial employers.[63] As a result, most people who were hospitalized paid little or nothing for their bed and nursing care, although they might be charged for the doctor's attendance and medication. Nonetheless, isolation hospitals and (after their introduction in the 1910s) tuberculosis sanatoria were feared, and any hospitalization avoided—in part, because it took sufferers out of their homes and removed both contact and control from the women whose normative roles included health care decision-making and provision. However, after 1929 local health authorities assumed management of many Poor Law hospital facilities, whose negative images they deliberately tried to transform, and both professional medicine and policymakers agreed that hospitalization was desirable for an expanding range of conditions—especially childbirth and anything requiring surgery.[64] The number of working-class people with experience of hospitalization increased, and by the 1940s hospitalization had become a routine part of everyday life.

The most important catalyst in the transformation of working-class health culture was the introduction of the National Health Service (NHS) in 1948.[65] By eliminating both the financial burden of calling the doctor and the shame of accepting charity, the NHS made it possible for working families to take the advice they had been given by official health authorities for more than half a century to jettison informal home and neighborhood health care in favor of professional institutional medicine. Arriving at about the same time that antibacterials made the "doctor's medicine" demonstrably more effective than home or patent remedies, the NHS was

63. See John G. Blacktop, *In times of need: The history and origin of the Royal Lancaster Infirmary* (no publisher, no date), available at the Lancaster Public Library; John Wilkinson, *Preston's Royal Infirmary: A history of health care in Preston 1809–1986* (Preston: Carnegie Press, 1987); and J. D. Marshall, *Furness and the Industrial Revolution*, 373–78, for information about hospitals and hospital schemes in the three study cities.

64. Lewis, *What price community medicine*, 15.

65. See, for example, Charles Webster, *The National Health Service: A political history*, 2nd ed. (Oxford: Oxford University Press, 2002); Brian Watkin, *The National Health Service: The first phase, 1948–1974 and after* (London: George Allen and Unwin, 1978).

welcomed by all but the most conservative families. Surprisingly quickly, visits to the general practitioner, use of antenatal and child health clinics, and hospitalization for a proliferating range of health events became usual for the Lancashire working class, which after World War II fully embraced the dominant national health culture.

It should here be observed that other important developments facilitated this change. During the interwar years, radio and cinema transformed popular entertainment for working families in Barrow, Lancaster, and Preston, as in other parts of the country. These media, together with magazines and popular fiction and, after World War II, television, glamorized official medicine. Crusty old general practitioners, beautiful self-sacrificing hospital nurses, and idealistic (handsome) young surgeons with poor social skills rode the airwaves and the silver screen, rendering biomedicine attractive and modern, and traditional working-class health culture dangerous and old-fashioned.[66] As working-class participation in secondary school increased and lengthened, school-based health education reinforced these messages.

However, more important than the marketing of biomedicine through entertainment and education was the decline of working-class dependence on mutual aid. After World War II, working-class incomes rose and employment opportunities increased.[67] The trend, observable before the war, in favor of "keeping myself to myself," which has been interpreted by Judy Giles as a manifestation of "a need and a desire for certain forms of privacy in the face of constant attempts to regulate the lives of working-class women by innumerable 'theys,'" including health care professionals, became much more possible and viable for the majority in the flush years of the 1950s and '60s, while the post-1948 welfare state addressed the needs of the less prosperous.[68] At the same time, increasing mobility undermined the stability of working-class neighborhoods and the long acquaintance and interdependence that had supported normative mutual aid.[69] Thus, reliance on professional medicine and public health became both conve-

66. See especially Susan E. Lederer and Naomi Rogers, "Media," in *Medicine in the twentieth century,* Roger Cooter and John Pickstone, eds. (Amsterdam: Harwood Academic Publishers, 2000), 487–502; Ann Karpf, *Doctoring the media: The reporting of health and medicine* (London: Routledge, 1988); Michael Shortland, *Medicine and film: A checklist, survey, and research resource* (Oxford: Wellcome Unit for the History of Medicine, 1989); and Joseph Turow, *Playing doctor: Television, storytelling, and medical power* (Oxford and New York: Oxford University Press, 1989).

67. See, for example, Andrew Rosen, *The transformation of British life 1950–2000: A social history* (Manchester and New York: Manchester University Press, 2003); Edward Royle, "Trends in post-war British social history," in *Understanding post-war British society,* James Obekevich and Peter Catterall, eds. (London and New York: Routledge, 1994), 9–18.

68. Giles, *Women, identity, and private life,* 101; Ann Digby, *British welfare policy: Workhouse to workfare* (London and Boston: Faber and Faber, 1989).

69. See Roberts, *Women and families,* 199–231.

nient and appropriate. By 1970 that dependence, both in terms of policy support and in terms of the dominant national culture, had reached its zenith.

PLACE

Because the oral history evidence used for this book was collected in Barrow, Lancaster, and Preston, to some extent its geography was a foregone conclusion since the interviews are a hugely valuable source of information about working-class health culture, which because of their age and number could never be replicated. However, selection of these cities for this case study can also be justified by factors other than serendipity or opportunism. All are located within the boundaries of the old County of Lancashire, selected by Michael Anderson for his authoritative research because it "typified or led industrializing Britain" in terms of the proportion of its population employed in manufacturing industry.[70] Similarly, Patrick Joyce focused his research on working-class culture on Lancashire, which he calls "as good an example of 'industrial England' as anywhere. Indeed, to contemporaries for much of this period [1848–1914] Lancashire *was* industrial England, its factories and mines the *locus classicus* of a new urban, industrial civilization."[71]

It is clear, of course, that Lancashire is quite diverse and, according to John Walton, "more a geographical expression than a cultural unity."[72] Its textile manufacturing, mining, engineering, and port cities both cradled British industrialization, and contrasted not only with each other but also with the county's rural areas, the Fylde and Furness, west Lancashire and the Pennine uplands. For this reason, many researchers focus on one region or community. Anderson's study was based on Preston data, Trevor Griffith's *The Lancashire Working Classes, c. 1880–1930* focused on south-central Wigan (mining) and Bolton (cotton textile manufacturing), and even Walton's county history emphasized developments in Liverpool and the cotton towns south of the Ribble River.[73] My own study is therefore in good company, and following Elizabeth Roberts's lead, I intend to enhance understanding of working-class Lancashire experience through evidence from Barrow, Lancaster, and Preston. In *A Woman's Place* and *Women and Families*, Roberts provides excellent introductions to the industrial and occupational profiles of these cities in the early and mid-twentieth century,

70. Michael Anderson, *Family structure in nineteenth century Lancashire* (Cambridge: Cambridge University Press, 1971), 18.

71. Joyce, *Visions*, 19.

72. Walton, *Lancashire social history*, 1.

73. Anderson, *Family structure;* Trevor Griffiths, *The Lancashire working classes c. 1880–1930* (Oxford: Clarendon Press, 2001); Walton, *Social history*.

while Walton offers useful information about their economic and social development compared to other Lancashire industrial communities.[74] Because of the valuable work of these scholars, I hope that a brief description will suffice here to set the scene for what follows in later chapters.

In the nineteenth and twentieth centuries, Preston was the largest of the study cities.[75] Like Lancaster, dating back to Roman times, Preston was an administrative and market center, and from the late seventeenth century it fostered a provincial social elite that left its mark on domestic and civic architecture.[76] From the early nineteenth century, Preston was also a cotton town, specializing in spinning and weaving "high-class cloths for the home, European and United States markets."[77] In 1891, 28 percent of the city's male workers and 42 percent of its female workers were employed in textile manufacturing; in 1911, 45 percent of its working population were textile workers.[78] Attracting migrants, particularly from rural areas within a 30-mile radius, Preston more than doubled its population between 1831 and 1851, when it stood at 69,542; the population increased by another 40 percent to 96,532 by 1881.[79] While Preston had a large English Roman Catholic population, it also had a large proportion of Irish-born residents (approximately 10% in 1851), most of whom were also Catholic.[80]

Despite Preston's booming textile factories, engineering works, and growing port, wages there were comparatively low—perhaps reflecting the large number of women who worked after marriage, mainly in the cotton mills.[81] The city's dependence on cotton manufacturing made it vulnerable to market fluctuations and ultimately (after World War I) decline in that trade, with resulting hardship for textile workers. In addition, working-class Preston suffered especially from poor housing and overcrowding.[82] Michael Anderson's description of working-class Preston neighborhoods in 1851 would still have been depressingly familiar in 1880:

74. Roberts, *A woman's place*, 6–8, 204–6; Roberts, *Women and families*, 3–6; Walton, *Social history*, for example, 25, 219, 225, 253, 283–360.

75. This was not always the case. Walton points out (*Social history*, 77) that in the 1780s, Lancaster, then in its heyday as a port, had 8,584 residents compared to Preston's five or six thousand.

76. Walton, *Social history*, 80–81. According to David Hunt, *A history of Preston* (Preston: Carnegie Publishing, 1992), "Preston has produced little archaeological evidence of the Roman occupation" (6–7), but the area was inhabited at the same time as the Romans were present in nearby Ribchester, Walton, and Kirkham.

77. Walton, *Social history*, 200.

78. Michael Savage, *The dynamics of working-class politics: The labor movement in Preston, 1880–1940* (Cambridge: Cambridge University Press, 1987), 202–3; Roberts, *A woman's place*, 7.

79. Anderson, *Family structure*, 24, 33–37.

80. Compared, for example, to 17% in Manchester. Walton, *Social history*, 252.

81. Walton, *Social history*, 169, 288.

82. Nigel Morgan, *Deadly dwellings: Housing and health in a Lancashire cotton town. Preston from 1840 to 1914* (Preston: Mullion Books, 1993).

Many of the main streets were respectable enough. Behind them, however, lay a different world. There were long rows of blackened two-story
terraced cottages, some built back-to-back. There were also narrow twisting lanes and enclosed courts of a dozen or fewer houses. Overshadow-
ing all were the factory chimneys. Here and there were shops and
chapels and public houses. . . . Some of the houses were so badly built
that they were damp and in need of repair almost immediately. . . . Preston was one of the worst towns. Inside, the houses were very cramped.
Two bedrooms was the rule.[83]

Perhaps not surprisingly, Preston experienced persistently high infant mortality rates, even by comparison with other industrial cities in the county.[84]
However, it also developed strong and stable working-class neighborhoods.
In his analysis of the 1851 census for Preston, Anderson found that almost
40 percent of men "were found in the same house or within 200 yards
of the house that they had occupied ten years earlier."[85] Walton observes,
"This was enough to form a substantial and influential core of shared experiences and norms, especially where neighbors shared the same workplace.
Such neighborhoods could be hostile to outsiders, but they looked after
their own, sometimes against police or bailiffs as well as sickness or unemployment."[86]

Having been a successful port city in the eighteenth century, Lancaster
lost its maritime trade to the silt filling the estuarial River Lune and to competition from other northwestern ports—notably Liverpool—leaving only
some striking Georgian buildings on the quayside and in the city center to
mark its heyday. A comparative economic backwater during the early and
mid-nineteenth century, the city was transformed after 1870 by the advent of
"a new manufacturing empire providing work for thousands which specialized in the production of table baize, oilcloth, and linoleum."[87] The success
of this industry, dominated by Williamson's and Storey's mills, stimulated
growth of Lancaster's population, which almost tripled between 1861 and
1901, and stood at 20,724 in 1881.[88] Home to other industries, notably an
internationally known furniture maker (Waring and Gillow) and a successful wagon works, the city was also a market town employing many retail
workers, and a service center with institutions drawing from a large area
beyond its boundaries.[89] Its court facilities and prison, housed in a castle

83. Anderson, *Family structure*, 33.
84. Walton, *Social history*, 310.
85. Anderson, *Family structure*, 42.
86. Walton, *Social history*, 181.
87. Michael Winstanley, "The town transformed," 145; Walton, *Social history*, 216; Philip
J. Gooderson, *Lord Linoleum: Lord Ashton, Lancaster and the rise of the British oilcloth and linoleum
industry* (Keele: Keele Univerity Press, 1996).
88. Winstanley, "The town transformed," 162.
89. Roberts, *A woman's place*, 7.

with medieval foundations, had originally served the entire county and, after 1835, continued to serve north Lancashire. The Lancaster County Asylum (locally called the Moor Hospital) was established to accommodate "lunatics" in 1811 and by 1911 housed 2,327 inmates and 268 resident staff members and their families. The "Royal Albert Asylum for Idiots and Imbeciles in the Northern Counties" was opened in 1870 and by 1911 housed 678 inmates and 110 staff and their families.[90] These facilities were still operating at full capacity in 1970.

Less dominantly working-class than the other study cities, Lancaster possessed a mixed economy and expanding service sector that arguably protected it from the economic fluctuations affecting Preston, which relied on the cotton trade, and Barrow, which depended on shipbuilding and heavy engineering.[91] According to Elizabeth Roberts, "Lancaster was one of the Lancashire towns least affected by the Depression" of the interwar years.[92] Its working-class housing, which before 1870 had generally been confined to cramped inner-city courts and terraces, improved greatly after that date with construction by private speculative builders of a number of new housing estates, most of them composed of dressed-stone terraced housing of a much higher quality than the accommodation previously available to workers.[93]

Located at the northern edge of the county and separated from it by the mountains of the Lake District to the northeast and the waters of Morecambe Bay to the southeast, Barrow was a tiny hamlet on the shore of the Irish Sea before its natural harbor attracted the attention of iron, railway, and shipping entrepreneurs in the mid-nineteenth century. Its 1851 population of 600 had swelled to 16,000 by 1866 and to 47,111 by 1881.[94] Unlike Lancaster and Preston, Barrow was a planned city, built by industrialists on land provided by aristocratic investors. Its wide main thoroughfares and grid-patterned housing areas surrounded the docks and, eventually, the great shipyards that still straddle the harbor to Walney Island, where many Barrovians live. Early industrial development focused on steel-making (based on local hematite iron ore), jute manufacturing, and railway and shipping links. However, from 1869, shipbuilding determined Barrow's character and primary industrial focus. In 1911, 37.5 percent of the city's workforce was employed by Vickers, the firm that still justifies characterization of Barrow as a company town.[95] In the late nineteenth century, Barrow was a boomtown with a primarily male population, rudimentary sanitation

90. Winstanley, "The town transformed," 155–61.

91. Steven Constantine and Alan Warde, "Challenge and change in the twentieth century," in *A history of Lancaster 1193–1993*, Andrew White, ed. (Keele, Staffordshire: Ryburn Publishing, Keele University Press, 1993), 207. Walton, *Social history*, 216.

92. Roberts, *A woman's place*, 7.

93. Winstanley, "The town transformed," 166–67.

94. J. D. Marshall, *Furness and the Industrial Revolution*, 288–306, 407.

95. Roberts, *A woman's place*, 6.

TABLE 1.2 Populations of Barrow, Lancaster, and Preston, 1881–1971

Year	Barrow	Lancaster	Preston
1881	47,111	20,724	96,532
1891	51,712	31,038	107,573
1901	57,586	40,329	112,989
1911	63,770	41,410	117,088
1921	74,244	40,212	117,406
1931	66,202	43,383	119,001
1939	69,235	51,261	111,385
1951	67,476	51,661	119,250
1961	64,927	48,253	113,341
1971	64,034	49,584	98,088

Sources: 1881–1931, Censuses for England and Wales, Summary Tables; 1951–1971, A Vision of Britain, "Place Information," http://www.visionofbritain.org.uk/; 1939, "The 1939 National Registration." No census was taken in 1941 owing to World War II.

and services, and an ongoing housing shortage. Blocks of sandstone flats, modeled on Glasgow's working-class housing (locally called the "Scotch Buildings"), and streets of small terraced cottages housed the workers and their families who thronged to new, well-paid job opportunities. However, as Barrow stabilized by the turn of the twentieth century, neither living up to the hopes of its founders that it would become the Liverpool of the north, nor returning to its previous insignificance, it became a prosperous small city that was nonetheless especially vulnerable to periodic economic crises that created mass unemployment and caused workers to leave for job opportunities elsewhere. (See table 1.2 for population data for Barrow, Lancaster, and Preston.)

STRUCTURE

The chapters that follow will consider diverse aspects of working-class health culture from a variety of perspectives. Chapter 2 discusses traditional management of health and health events (birth, illness, injury, disability, and death) in working-class Barrow, Lancaster, and Preston. It begins by describing houses and neighborhoods, then goes on to document the home-based environment for care, consultation of informal female health authorities, dependence on neighborhood mutual aid networks, and use of home and patent remedies. The chapter concludes with public health officials' contribution to construction of a negative image of the working-class woman, which supported the professionalization of public health occupations.

Located in the context of both national policies and local resources (such as friendly societies, hospital schemes, and installment payments for medical services), chapter 3 addresses formal health care provision in Barrow, Lancaster, and Preston. It considers the increasing scope of clinical medical provision and hospitals during the first half of the twentieth century. It discusses working-class perspectives regarding official health care providers and institutions as well as financial, cultural, gender, and social class issues affecting working-class health care choices. Finally, it explores the attitudes of some health care providers toward working-class people.

Chapter 4 focuses on the incidence, experience, and management of contagious diseases in the study cities. It discusses public health attempts to prevent or contain these ailments, and explores working-class people's experiences of and responses to these efforts. It also considers working-class perceptions of contagion within their social and physical environments, and links between hygiene, on the one hand, and respectability, on the other.

Chapter 5 explores the related issues of working-class respectability, sex, family planning, and birth control. Locating discussion within the context of national concerns about the fertility decline, on the one hand, and population fitness, on the other, it observes growing interest in working-class sexuality among policymakers, educators, medical authorities, and social advocates that resulted in pressure on working-class families to change the ways they dealt with sex. It considers changing working-class attitudes toward and use of various approaches to family planning (including abortion, abstinence, and contraception) and associates these changes with shifting norms regarding extramarital pregnancy as well as marital and parent-child relationships during the course of the study period.

Chapter 6 observes sweeping changes in authority regarding and management of working-class pregnancy, childbirth, and child care in the study cities. It contrasts traditional ways of dealing with these matters in the late nineteenth and early twentieth centuries with the medicalization and institutionalization of childbearing and child care that gathered steam during the interwar period. It explores motivation and policy support for these changes, together with working-class responses to them. Finally, it identifies some results of these changes, including waning confidence of working-class women in their own capacity to deal with childbearing and child care and their increasing dependence on professional experts for advice and support.

Chapter 7 considers the contribution of health messages delivered by the popular media (e.g., films, radio programs, and magazines) to the transformation of working-class health culture in the study cities. It argues that these messages promoted official health care as modern, safe, and respectable, while invalidating traditional health information and practices. These messages also glamorized health experts—doctors and nurses,

in particular—while ascribing to them altruistic motives and blaming ignorant noncompliant "patients" (and their families) for their own problems.
Increasing acceptance of biomedical theories and therapies, together with
growing familiarity with formal health services, developed a working-class
market that enthusiastically welcomed the introduction of the National
Health Service (NHS) in 1948.

Chapter 8 opens with local working-class perspectives on the establishment of the NHS. Dovetailing with an explosion in effective therapeutic
interventions, as well as elimination of the Poor Law and the hated means
test, the NHS removed financial and social barriers to working-class use
of official health care. For the first time, after World War II the general
practitioner (GP), school doctor and dentist, health visitor, and licensed
midwife took the place of the neighborhood health authority and mutual
aid network in working-class health culture. At the same time, it is arguable that after World War II the distinctive working-class Lancashire culture
that endured until mid-century began to fade. Factors including deindustrialization, growing prosperity and mobility, expanding consumerism,
lengthening participation in formal education, and proliferating media
influence diluted neighborhood influence on working-class values, interests, and behavior. In addition, the postwar social safety net (including the
NHS) both eliminated the stigma of the means test and reduced working-class dependence on neighborhood and family mutual aid networks
that had been central to management of ill-health and other challenges
before the war. Official health care, free at the point of use and accorded
unquestioned reverence by virtually all authorities, gained hegemonic
sway among members of the Lancashire working class. Although "old
wives' tales" echoed in living memory, new wives and mothers consulted
GPs rather than grannies, went to hospitals and clinics rather than calling in the neighbors during childbearing and illness, and converted to
the gospel of biomedicine that also pervaded the radio and television programs, films, newspaper reports, and magazine stories they consumed. This
chapter considers both "progress" and losses in working-class experience
of health and health incidents. While infant and maternal mortality and
deaths from contagious diseases declined dramatically between 1880 and
1970, experts disagree about the extent to which these improvements can
be viewed as the result of increased provision and use of professional medical and health services. Furthermore, despite extension of official health
care to the entire British population, health disparities by socioeconomic
class continue. Indeed, that extension was accompanied by an attack on
traditional working-class management of health incidents that may have
done as much harm as good, undermining individual and collective competence to deal with these matters and increasing the need for and cost of
professional health care.

Chapter Two

≈

"Every street had its lady"

Working-Class Health Culture
before World War II

INTRODUCTION

Before we can understand transformation, we must know the characteristics of what was transformed. This chapter explores the premise of my
argument, that traditional Lancashire working-class health culture was
home-based and controlled by laywomen. While it implies the lack of centrality to that culture of the usual primary actor in medical and public
health history—the physician—this issue is not its focus. Indeed, as we
will see in chapter 3, many working-class families consulted general practitioners. However, the physician was peripheral to routine household
health management and, in any case, also worked within the home environment to which he (or, more rarely, she) had been invited and where
he depended on adult women in the household to carry out his orders.
In working-class homes, his authority was negotiated within a culture that
employed and often preferred many alternatives to "the doctor's medicine."[1] Furthermore, for most working-class people, his presence was rare
and anything but routine.

By contrast, the expertise and authority of working-class women pervaded matters of health, governing dress, personal and home hygiene,
diet, elimination, reproduction, disease prevention, diagnosis, therapeutics, first aid, nursing, and care of the dead. Female influence and agency
regarding such issues were considered "natural," associated with women's
essential roles as nurturers of children and supporters of men. Indeed,
health authorities and social reformers, whose concern about national

---

1. Phrase used, for example, by Mrs. A3P, 4; Mrs. C2B, 5; Mrs. H2B, 118. In *The evolution
of British general practice 1850–1948* (Oxford: Oxford University Press, 1999), 35–37, Anne
Digby observes the prevalence of self-treatment and consultation of alternative and informal
practitioners, particularly before 1911, despite the oversupply of general practitioners.

(particularly working-class) fitness continued throughout the period under consideration, did not seriously contest the appropriateness of the working-class mother's role as primary health care provider but rather criticized her competence in that role. Much historical evidence about the working-class woman's health-related activities comes from middle-class experts (both female and male), who tended to be highly critical of her housekeeping skills, knowledge of basic hygiene, and, perhaps most damning, judgment regarding childrearing.[2]

Working-class women themselves indicated that their identities and status were based precisely on these contested issues—management of household resources; neatness and cleanliness of the family's home and dress; and childrearing expertise manifested in children's appearance, behavior, and health.[3] However, their most important "judges" were not formal authorities but other working-class women who governed the neighborhood mutual aid networks that provided their most important support. Thus, their need for family respectability, earned through adherence to generally understood "rules," governed women's behavior and much of their influence over their children and husbands. Many of those "rules" concerned health issues, broadly construed: for example, sexual knowledge, behavior, and talk; infant care; and the often-shared responsibility for cleaning outdoor toilets and drains. Such matters were both intensely private, relating to self-image, personality, training, and family relationships, and public, since demeanor and behavior were intended and expected to be observed.

The goals of working-class women often differed from those of health authorities and social reformers; for instance, the Medical Officer's desire to send a child with scarlet fever to an isolation hospital to protect the community from contagion contrasted greatly with the mother's focus on providing the best possible care (as she defined it) for her child in order to either keep the child alive or enable him or her to die (as many children did) surrounded by family and friends. Furthermore, the woman's role as a health authority and care provider was a significant component of her responsibilities and self-image.

2. There is, for example, scholarly disagreement about whether or not working-class women were good housekeepers. See Margaret Hewitt, *Wives and mothers in Victorian industry* (London: Rockliff, 1958); John K. Walton, *Lancashire: A social history, 1558–1939* (Manchester and New York: Manchester University Press, 1987), 293; Peter N. Stearns, "Working-class women in Britain, 1890–1914," in Marsha Vicinus, ed., *Suffer and be still: Women in the Victorian age* (Bloomington and London: Indiana University Press, 1972), 100–120; Carole Dyhouse, "Working-class mothers and infant mortality in England, 1895–1914," *Journal of Social History* 12:2 (1978): 248–67.

3. See, for example, Standish Meacham, *A life apart: The English working class 1890–1914* (London: Thames and Hudson, 1977), 60–94; Joanna Bourke, *Working-class cultures in Britain 1890–1960: Gender, class and ethnicity* (London and New York: Routledge, 1994), 62–67; Melanie Tebbutt, *A social history of 'gossip' in working-class neighborhoods, 1880–1960* (Aldershot, Hants., Scolar Press: Brookfield, VT: Ashgate Publishing Co., 1995).

In addition to the mothers, grandmothers, aunts, and sisters who cared for family health within the home, there were other women who served as health authorities in working-class neighborhoods. These women tended to be middle-aged or elderly and to be married or widowed. Sometimes paid, often unpaid, they included in their ranks unqualified midwives (called "handywomen" by Medical Officers of Health) and monthly nurses (who cared for mothers during the lying-in period); layers-out of the dead; and primary care experts who diagnosed and treated minor ills but also advised on whether the sufferer needed to see a doctor. Scholars tend to consider these caregivers within the history of nursing, categorizing their work as an occupation that was phased out through professionalization processes.[4] However, I think it is more productive to think of neighborhood health authorities as somewhat specialized participants in the mutual aid networks that were essential to working-class family survival. Neighbors and friends as well as functionaries, these women were remembered by oral history informants, with fondness and respect, as "Nana Riley," "Auntie Viv," "Mrs. Mount," "Nurse Garth," or "Nurse Moss." Many recalled that every neighborhood depended on one or two of these women—hence the chapter title, which was drawn from an interview with Mr. Monkham of Lancaster.[5] More than mothers and grannies, they attracted the ire of health authorities who viewed them both as competitors and as destructive, ignorant old women whose influence was to be deplored and eliminated. Hamstrung by Midwives Acts passed between 1902 and 1936 and marginalized by the same processes that undermined working-class health culture in general, neighborhood health authorities literally died out by the 1950s. It is ironic that health visitors and neighborhood clinics were designed to replicate some of the services and techniques of informal health authorities by providing advice to working-class mothers in their own homes and streets, but substituting "correct" for "incorrect" information.

This chapter will focus on home- and neighborhood-based health care provided by working-class women in Barrow, Lancaster, and Preston during the years between about 1880 and 1950. It will deal with general issues and relationships, leaving to later chapters discussion of approaches to specific health challenges, such as family limitation, childbirth, infant care, and management of contagious diseases. Much of the evidence on which the chapter is based was provided by people recounting childhood memories,

4. See, for example, Robert Dingwall, Anne Marie Rafferty, Charles Webster, *A social history of nursing* (London: Routledge, 1988), 1–13.

5. Mr. M10L, 19. See also Mrs. A1P, 39; Mrs. A4L, 37; Mr. A4L, 49–50; Mrs. B2P, 25; Mr. B4B, 31; rs. C2P, 11; Mrs. D1B, 10; Mr. D2P, 27; Mrs. F1L, 52; Mr. F1P, 73; Mr. F2l, 39; Mrs. H5L, 56; Mr. K2P, 81; Mr. L1l, 14; Mrs. L3P, 118; Mrs. M2B, 13; Mr. M3L, 10–11; Mrs. M3P, 2, 5; Mrs. M10B, 12; Mrs. M1L, 32; Mrs. N2L, 50–1, 55; Mr. N3L, 135; Mrs. O1B, 56; Mr. P1B, 42; Mrs. P2B, 10; Mr. P6B; Mr. R1L, 35–6; Mr. R3B, 56; Mrs. S1L, 7, 15; Mrs. T2L, 34; Mr. V1L, 8; Mr. W7B, 42; Mr. W7B, 44; Mrs. Y1L, 15–16.

although many oral history informants maintained very traditional health care approaches in their adult families—behavior that was mediated by financial circumstances, since poorer families remained more dependent on mutual aid than did their more prosperous neighbors. In any case, health culture is both fluid and porous, often supporting several vintages of theories and techniques at once, and stoutly resisting the straitjacket of beginning and end dates. However, working-class health culture did change in the mid-twentieth century through a hegemonic process resulting in the acceptance and internalization of biomedicine by working-class people. This chapter will conclude with a discussion of the ways local public health officials helped to reconstruct the normative health care roles of working-class women and to create a new reality of professional authority in working-class communities.

SETTING THE SCENE:
HOME, STREET, AND NEIGHBORHOOD

Because in working-class Barrow, Lancaster, and Preston before the interwar period birth, ill-health, treatment, care, and death took place almost exclusively at home, consideration of the health culture of working-class people depends on a clear impression of their home environments, which included both dwellings and neighborhoods.[6] The following discussion focuses mainly on the years between 1880 and 1930, after which time development of publicly built council housing, large-scale demolition of inner-city "slum" properties, and rising levels of home ownership influenced working-class experience and expectations of housing quality and neighborhood relationships.[7]

During the period under consideration, in common with their socio-economic counterparts elsewhere in Britain, almost all informants to this study were renters rather than owner-occupiers. Indeed, according to David Englander, "On the eve of the Great War owner-occupation accounted for approximately ten percent of *all* dwellings" in Britain; needless to say, that 10 percent was not composed mainly of working-class housing.[8] While it became more common in the 1920s and '30s for working-class people

6. Elizabeth Roberts discusses working-class housing in the study communities at some length in *A woman's place: An oral history of working-class women 1890–1940* (Oxford: Basil Blackwell, 1984), 125–34, and *Women and families: An oral history, 1940–1970* (Oxford: Blackwell, 1995), 22–44.

7. See, for example, Alison Ravetz, *Council housing and culture: The history of a social experiment* (London: Routledge, 2001). In his Introduction to *The imagined slum: Newspaper representation in three cities 1870–1914* (Leicester, London, and New York: Leicester University Press, 1993), 1–13, Alan Mayne argues that "slums" are myths and stereotypes that hamper historical research regarding the urban poor and their communities.

8. David Englander, *Landlord and tenant in urban Britain 1838–1918* (Oxford: Clarendon Press, 1983), 4. Italics in original text.

to purchase homes, as late as 1940, 76 percent of this study's informants were still renting—many of them from local authorities as council housing became available.[9] Some families moved house frequently—although usually within the same area of the city—sometimes in search of a lower rent or a better house, sometimes ahead of the bailiff because of failure to pay rent, and sometimes because of factors including dampness, unpleasant neighbors, or vermin infestation (bugs or rats).[10] Many stayed in the same rented accommodation for years. However, the oral evidence shows that neither lack of a long tenure in a particular house nor lack of ownership undermined the family's—and particularly the homemaker's—attachment to and responsibility for home—a concept that clearly transcends physical surroundings.[11]

Like their working-class neighbors, the oral history informants mainly lived in dressed-stone or brick two- or three-story terraced (i.e., row) houses with two or three upstairs bedrooms and two rooms (a parlor and a living room) plus a scullery (the "back kitchen") downstairs.[12] The living room, sometimes also called the kitchen, was the location for cooking (often on an iron range that also was the primary heat source in the house), eating, and indoor socializing or relaxation. The back kitchen was where dishwashing and hand-laundering took place; it also sometimes housed a pantry and the "copper" (wash boiler) for laundry. The parlor was used only on special occasions.[13] Many informants—particularly in Preston—lived in "two-up, two-down" houses, which literally contained two rooms on the ground and upper story, respectively. The better properties had entrances at both front and rear, indoor water supplies (very occasionally including a bathtub), and private (outdoor) flush toilets and garbage receptacles ("middens" or "ashpits") in the backyard—a walled or fenced space beyond the back door that was usually paved and provided access to an alley or "ginnel." The worst accommodation was in either back-to-back (particularly in Preston) or courtyard (particularly in Lancaster) houses, which lacked rear entrances and required occupants to share water supplies and lavatories (either dry closets or flush toilets).[14] Houses were heated by coal

9. Roberts, *Women and families,* 25.

10. Frequent moves were not unusual among working-class tenants. See Englander, *Landlord and tenant,* 7–11, for discussion of the many reasons late-Victorian tenants might "flit" or "shoot the moon."

11. See, in particular, Introduction to Judy Giles, *Women, identity, and private life in Britain, 1900–50* (New York: St. Martin's Press, 1995), for discussion of some meanings of home and privacy to working-class women during the first half of the twentieth century.

12. Some Barrow informants lived in flats in what were called the "Scotch Buildings." However, the vast majority of informants lived in terraced houses.

13. In *A life apart,* 34–37, Meacham describes a spectrum of working-class housing, ranging from the squalid, overcrowded dwellings of the very poor to the self-consciously upwardly mobile homes of artisans, which would have been very familiar to our Barrow, Lancaster, and Preston informants.

14. See Roberts, *A woman's place,* 125–35, for further information about informants' homes before 1940.

fires, which were also used for cooking. Some had gas lighting; most used oil lamps. Electric lighting was very rare until after World War I.

Informants' accounts reveal a wide range in quality of housing, which closely related to family financial circumstances. Mrs. Allen, born in 1908 in Lancaster, lived in a courtyard cottage in St. Mary's Place,

> which is now a car park near the Judges Lodgings, and I was there until I was about four. . . . They were very very tiny. [I remember] not a very great deal, only that they were very small, outside communal toilet, and they had to share. . . . There was no running water in the houses and there was a tap out in the yard and you'd to go and fill your kettles or whatever you wanted. . . . No, there were no backs to them at all. You had no back door and you came out through the front door. The toilets and what they called an ashpit, in them days everybody emptied their ashes into a pit, were all at the front of the house. There was a big tap right in the center of the court.[15]

This informant's father was a laborer at Williamson's mill, which manufactured table baize, oilcloth, window-blinds, and linoleum; he was frequently laid off. Her mother, who had been a weaver before marriage, was a homemaker. Mrs. Allen was one of two children.

Similarly, Mr. Quayle, whose father had died before the informant was born in Dalton, near Barrow, in 1897, remembered about the house he shared with his widowed mother:

> There was a pub at the end behind the Castle, the George and Dragon, and our house was the next, number ten. It had no back door and there was no outlet at all bar from the front door. We had to bring the coal in into the coal place in the yard. It was also a pantry, and everything had to come in the front door. If you wanted to use the toilet or anything, you'd as far as from the end there down to the end of those three houses, and it used to be a stable. The modern one had an arch, and that was the cart house. . . . Down there through this gap, that cart house to the toilet, which was also . . . it was there at the back of the pub, but it wasn't used by anyone out of the pub. When I look at them now, I can't believe that if you were taken ill in any way you'd to go down there.[16]

Mr. Eckley, born in 1895 in Preston, recalled, "Nearly all the streets were terraced houses, and you had a lobby between the houses, you had a back

15. Mrs. A1L, 1–2. Information about informants' families comes from biography cards or sheets maintained with the oral history transcripts by the Elizabeth Roberts Oral History Archive, Centre for North West Regional Studies, Lancaster University (UK).

16. Mr. Q1B, 9.

door and you could go in that way instead of using the front door. There was no water closet. It was a proper board, but there were no toilet rolls. They put newspaper up on a string. . . . At the top of the lobby, your toilet is there and behind is what they called the midden."[17] This informant's father ran a pub, which his mother continued to operate after his father's early death. Mr. Eckley was one of four children.

By contrast, Mr. Carson, born in 1902 in Lancaster, remembered "the Windermere Road house. It had three bedrooms, a living room, a parlor, kitchen, and a cellar. The third bedroom was very small and you got to it going through the second bedroom. The stairs were very narrow. . . . The lavatory was outside and it was a flush lavatory. There was a water supply in the house, but only cold, not hot."[18] Mr. Carson's father was a fireman at the Greenfield Mill, which manufactured backing cloth for the oilcloth made by Williamson's works; his mother had been in domestic service as a cook before marriage. Mr. Carson was one of three children.

Mr. Gordon, born in 1879, also from Lancaster, remembered the nice house his family moved into in 1907:

We were in the one on Wingate Saul Road, where that photograph was taken, for a lot of years. It had three bedrooms, a bathroom, and a very big living kitchen and a sitting room.

Interviewer: It was very unusual to have a bathroom, wasn't it?

Informant: Yes, but they started to build bathrooms, but it was a long while before they'd toilets in the house. People thought they were insanitary. It had a bath, but no toilet. The toilet was out in the yard.[19]

This informant's father was employed as a clerk of works; his mother had been a nursery maid in a private home before marriage. Mr. Gordon was the youngest of six children.

In 1930 Lancaster's Medical Officer of Health, Dr. J. D. Buchanan, who had then been serving in that capacity for 18 years, provided a useful description of the city's working-class housing:

The majority of the houses are of the cottage property type. There are, roughly, 500 houses, including those in yards and courts, about 100 years old with two to four bedrooms. The very old houses are often three-storeyed and many have cellars. There is still a considerable number of back-to-back houses, mostly huddled together in yards and courts, with few conveniences. These old houses are often seriously damp, deficient in light and ventilation, and in a bad state of repair.

17. Mr. E1P, 27.
18. Mr. C1L, 2.
19. Mr. G2L, 9.

Few of them are properly drained; many are without a sink or means
for disposing of slop water which is thrown in the gutter. Those in yards
and courts, and built back-to-back have as a rule no internal water supply, nor adequate accommodation for washing or for the preparation or
storage of food. Common yards, the sharing of closet accommodation,
and the common use of ashpits are other conditions found in connection with this old property which make the practice of cleanliness
difficult and a decent standard of living often impossible. During the
nineteenth century there were 2,000–3,000 houses built in the area.
These are self-contained, built in long rows, mostly with two or three
bedrooms, but rarely provided with a bathroom or proper facilities
for storing food. These houses were also, unfortunately, provided with
ashpits instead of sanitary bins, thus allowing for the retention of refuse
close to the dwelling for longer than was desirable.[20]

While this retrospective description of the city's housing was influenced
both by 1930s health science and by then current housing standards, it
nonetheless offers information less anecdotal than oral history informants'
memories, while also substantiating those accounts. Medical officers recognized the connection between rents and house quality. Buchanan's predecessor, Dr. Cates, wrote in 1912, "House rents vary from about three to
seven shillings per week, the former usually entails living in a house of an
undesirable description situated in a court. For about five shillings a week
may be obtained a dwelling containing two kitchens, a scullery, and three
bedrooms, a wash boiler, water closet, and ashpit being in a partly flagged
yard. There are about 570 houses in Lancaster which are not through ventilated, and approximately 450 situated in courts."[21]

Working-class residents of Barrow, Lancaster, and Preston lived very
close together.[22] Crowding within houses generally resulted from the large
family sizes more common among older than among younger oral history
informants.[23] Large families placed pressure on working-class housing—
particularly since ground-floor rooms were rarely used for sleeping and few
homes had more than three bedrooms.[24] Mrs. Anderson, born in 1872 in
Barrow, described her family's home on Devon Street: "It was three rooms
upstairs and three places downstairs—parlor, kitchen, back kitchen." When
they moved in, "I think there were five of us then, but while we were in
Barrow we had another five children, so that there was ten of us. I was the

---

20. Lancaster MOH Report, 1930, 22.

21. Lancaster MOH Report, 1912, 43.

22. This was true of the English generally. In *Friends of the family: The English home and
its guardians, 1850–1940* (Stanford: Stanford University Press, 1998), George K. Behlmer
comments, "As late as 1911, when the first complete figures become available, 75 per cent of the
English people still lived in one- or two-room dwellings" (25).

23. See chapter 5 for more in-depth discussion of family size.

24. Roberts, *A woman's place*, 129.

oldest of ten." The children shared a bedroom, sleeping in two beds.[25] This was unusual; it was more common for there to be a boys' bedroom, a girls' bedroom, and a parents' bedroom, although a two-bedroom house, an uneven number of boys and girls, or coresident adult family members or lodgers could further complicate arrangements. Mrs. Masterson, born in Preston in 1913, remembered, "It was hard because we were a big family and there were only three bedrooms. It meant that all the boys were in one room and I had to sleep with Mum and Dad and they [an older brother and his wife] were in the other room. . . . You would get three sleeping at that end of the bed and two or three at the front of the bed. Every space was made available for use."[26] Mr. Danner, born in 1910 the youngest of seven surviving children, described the additional pressure a lodger placed on sleeping space.[27] "Mother resented paying the big rent for the house we were in and decided to save and buy one. She would take in a lodger and so John Birkett came to live with us. John took over the room of mine and I had a bed made up in the bath; of course, the bedding was moved each day and the bath used as required." This was shortly after World War I.[28]

In addition to experiencing crowded internal space, informants lived close to their neighbors. At a minimum, they shared the walls between houses and back yards, as well as pavements and streets at the front and alleys at the back. However, many also shared water, privies, and laundry facilities. Mrs. Horton, born in 1903 in Lancaster, was asked, "When you lived near the Matting Mill, where was the water?" She responded:

'Round the back. We went through a lobby [passage between houses] and you had a big white bucket and you filled that bucket. We only went through a lobby, but anybody who lived half-way, they had to go right round. There was a tap at the bottom and tap at the top.
Interviewer: How many houses was that for?
Informant: One, two, three, four, five, six, seven, eight, or nine. There was two to a lobby, and then there was Wainmans, Simpsons, Steels, Dowthwaithes, and then Ada and then Carters and Old Tots. How many was that?
Mr. Horton: About twelve altogether.
Interviewer: Fifteen for two taps?
Informant: Yes.
Interviewer: How many toilets did you have?
Informant: There was four and two at the other side. Six. Just one wash house, but with two boilers in it. You see, them that lived on the

25. Mrs. A1B, 2, 8.
26. Mrs. M1P, 57.
27. Elizabeth Roberts explains that only two informants of the 160 to *A woman's place* had unrelated lodgers living in their households, although many more had relatives living with their nuclear families (141).
28. Mr. D2P, 37.

back shared the back boiler and them that lived on the front shared the front boiler.[29]

Mrs. Horton was the eighth of ten children, although the three eldest did not survive infancy. There were nine people in her household before her father's death in 1919. In Lancaster in 1911, there was an average of 5.40 persons per household.[30] At a conservative estimate, then, approximately 76 neighbors shared facilities with Mrs. Horton's family.

Whether or not facilities were shared, working-class people knew their neighbors well. Because they lived in houses that were often less than 20 feet wide, their domestic relationships, activities, and resources were semipublic and spilled from open doors and windows, percolated through shared walls, and were displayed on washing lines, curtain rods, and front steps. Joanna Bourke argues that working-class culture was shaped by this physical closeness: "Most people could hear noises from neighboring homes. In a working-class street in Coventry it was 'possible to sit in the Cannings's living room and to tell the time by the clock in the house over the way' and one 8-year-old boy whimpered that he was spied wearing pajamas by the girl across the road. Individuals would have had to strive hard to be alone since 'You cannot live in a court without knowing a good deal about your neighbors and their concerns, even without deserving the title of a gossip.'"[31]

People's acquaintance was age-related and gendered. Children attended school and "played out" in streets and alleys together. Teens worked and amused themselves in sex-segregated groups. Men met in public houses and garden allotments as well as workplaces and union meetings. Women who worked in factories after marriage (more common in Preston than in Barrow or Lancaster), labored side by side, as did homemakers who chatted over communal washtubs and backyard washing lines, at front steps, or in local shops. And the elderly, who especially before old age pensions became available after 1908 often lived with adult children, continued gendered patterns of socializing. Of course, at church and events such as Preston's annual Whit Monday processions, families came together in groups transcending the boundaries of sex, age, or neighborhood.

NEIGHBORLINESS AND MUTUAL AID

Discussing ways in which "neighborhood" can be identified or defined, Elizabeth Roberts writes that Barrow and Lancaster informants spoke of coming from specific geographically demarcated areas, such as Skerton or

29. Mrs. H3L, 53.
30. Roberts, *A woman's place*, 227.
31. Joanna Bourke, *Working-class cultures in Britain 1890–1960: Gender, class and ethnicity* (London and New York: Routledge, 1994), 140.

Primrose in Lancaster, Vickerstown or Hindpool in Barrow. Preston interviewees were more likely to mention the main road running through the
area in which they lived—Ribbleton Lane or Newhall Lane, for instance.
However, all of these places were large and densely inhabited, with no
opportunity of residents truly "knowing everybody." According to Roberts,
"What seems to have been of considerably greater importance to working-class people was the street, or possibly the small group of streets, in
which they lived. Respondents often claim to have known everyone in their
neighborhood, but this usually turns out to have been no more than three
streets. Some only knew those in their own street."[32] She agrees, however,
with Standish Meacham, who argues, "Neighborhood meant more than
houses and streets. It meant the mutually beneficial relationships one
formed with others; a sort of social symbiosis."[33]

These relationships could not—and should not—be presumed. Streets
and neighborhoods varied in terms of social composition, reputation, and
cohesiveness. Thus, oral history informants' experiences of neighborhood
differed. The age and stability of the neighborhood were influential. For
example, Mr. Eckley, whose daughter was born after he and his wife had
moved to a new Preston housing area in the 1920s, responded to the question, "Did the other neighbors come in and help, did they bring in food
or anything?" by saying, "They were all new people, they were new houses."
By contrast, when he was a little boy, the neighbors "were more sociable"—something he obviously considered normative and desirable.[34] Some
streets, considered "rough," did not nurture close relationships between
neighbors. The brother of an informant, Mrs. Hancock (born in 1893),
who was present during her interview, commented on the reputation of a
Barrow neighborhood during their pre–World War I childhood: "Arthur
Street was one of those streets where careless people lived. You've only to
get one in there in a decent street until it starts to deteriorate and so Arthur
Street became the home of down-and-outs, drunkards, and even prostitutes
lived there. It did get a name in the music halls, comedians coming along
and pick out Arthur Street and Hartington Street. Of course, one was supposed to be good respectable ruffians in Hartington Street and Arthur
Street was more or less the incorrigible types."[35] Mrs. Parton, born in Barrow in 1873, agreed, saying, "You wouldn't go past Arthur Street, because
we didn't want to get mixed up with them. Perhaps a bit snobbish, but
they were really what they called the scum of Barrow. They'd no ambitions
to be any better. Many a time they could have been better."[36] Such areas
were thought to be aberrations—departures from the norm where people

32. Roberts, *A woman's place,* 184.
33. Meacham, *A life apart,* 45.
34. Mr. E1P, 42–43.
35. Mrs. H1B, 8.
36. Mrs. P3B, 33–34.

were not "careless," but cared about and looked after their homes, families, neighbors, and reputations.

In some cases individuals or families either held themselves apart from neighborly relationships or were ostracized from an otherwise close neighborhood. For example, Mrs. Preston, born in 1907, whose family kept a shop in Preston, said, "We thought we were better than the rest, but we didn't show it. Because we worked for it, that was the real reason, we've tried and the effort is there. I don't go in anyone's house or have anyone coming in from the neighborhood, but I would do them a good turn."[37] Conversely, as Mr. Rollins, born in Barrow in 1931, remembered, some families were not included in neighborhood mutual aid: "Well, they never clean their windows or it's a dirty house, or they are always cursing and swearing. You know, they are always on the beer, that type of thing, so you don't bother with them."[38] Nonetheless, among informants to this study, close relationships between neighbors were prized and thought to be "normal" in what Standish Meacham, following Robert Roberts, calls the "classic" early-twentieth-century working-class neighborhood.[39] Indeed, the close traditional neighborhoods of informants' childhoods seemed to attain almost mythic proportions in memory and were invariably contrasted with the colder, less attached neighborhoods of the present day.[40]

While houses and neighborhoods were home to all their residents, they were especially important to the women who managed and depended on them. Few Barrow and Lancaster women worked outside the home after marriage, and although the Preston informants were more likely than women elsewhere in England to be employed full-time after marriage, together with other female informants, their identities and reputations were more closely associated with home than with paid work.[41] There can be no doubt that working-class women were subordinate to working-class men. However, it is also true that working-class women were in charge at home and in neighborhoods. Indeed, men essentially ceded control of these spaces to women by their absence. In the workplace during weekdays and at the pub, on the allotment (garden plot), or participating in other leisure interests during nonworking hours, men tended to occupy their

37. Mrs. P2P, 30.

38. Mr. R3B, 44.

39. Standish Meacham, *A life apart*, 46. See also Robert Roberts, *The classic slum: Salford life in the first quarter of the century* (Harmondsworth, Middlesex, 1971. Reprinted 1987).

40. See, for example, Mrs. A3B, 23; Mrs. B11P, 51; Mrs. C2B, 13; Mrs. L1L, 13; Mr. R3B, 43; Mr. R3L, 30; Mr. W7P, 12.

41. In 1911, 35 percent of married women and widows living in Preston were in full-time employment, compared to 11.0 percent in Lancaster and 6.9 percent in Barrow. See Roberts, *A woman's place*, 143. Nationally, "Up until 1931, 13 to 16 per cent of married women were employed," according to Bourke, *Working-class cultures*, 100. Roberts (136–48) and Bourke (126–29) agree that working-class women tended to work to supplement family incomes but preferred to be homemakers if possible.

crowded "castles" only to eat and sleep. Working-class women managed all household resources, including the wages "tipped up" on Friday evening by husbands and older children. Women were also responsible for family reputations, which governed access to the equally important resources of credit and neighborhood mutual aid.

Family reputations depended on factors controlled by women, including demonstrated cleanliness (of front step, net curtains, laundry, privy, yard, and children), chastity regarding sexual behavior and speech (particularly on the part of mother and daughters), temperance (staying out of pubs and consuming only moderate amounts of alcohol at home), appropriate dress, and reciprocal participation in mutual aid activities. Factors controlled by men, including restraint regarding alcohol consumption, appropriate financial support of the family, and minimal violence toward wives and children, were less important, since a good woman could call upon the support of neighbors even if she were married to a no-account man.

Above all, individual and family reputations depended on what people (mainly women) said about each other. Melanie Tebbutt argues, "Gossip seems an appropriate analytical form to apply given the self-enclosed, introspective nature of the working-class neighborhoods which developed between the 1880s and 1950s, and which were characterized by distinct cultural forms and significant degrees of gender segregation. Many working-class women belonged to intimate social networks with strong ties to relatives and neighbors."[42] Their conversations governed neighborhoods, offering reward and punishment to the individuals and families who conformed to or violated the unwritten rules of working-class culture. They also controlled the mutual aid which, before the late 1940s, was the most important support available to working-class households, providing borrowed supplies, playmates for children, jobs for teenagers, sociability and emotional support, and help in times of childbirth, ill-health, and death.

Informal, neighborhood-based mutual aid has a complicated and contested history.[43] For example, the degree to which it depended on reciprocity and calculated expectation of gain is emphasized by Michael Anderson, who argues, further, that such aid was more reliably provided by kin than by neighbors in 1850s Preston. By contrast, Elizabeth Roberts and Standish Meacham consider calculated reciprocity and the primacy of fam-

42. Tebbutt, *Women's talk*, 2.

43. What might be called formal mutual aid—participation in friendly societies—is a related, but different, phenomenon, transcending the geographical boundaries of streets and neighborhoods, and mainly involving men. See, for example, David G. Green, *Working-class patients and the medical establishment: Self-help in Britain from the mid-nineteenth century to 1948* (New York: St. Martin's Press, 1985); David Neave, *Mutual aid in the Victorian countryside: Friendly societies in the rural East Riding 1830–1914* (Hull: Hull University Press, 1991); James C. Riley, *Sick, not dead: The health of British workingmen during the mortality decline* (Baltimore and London: Johns Hopkins University Press, 1997).

ily in mutual aid comparatively unimportant in turn-of-the-century neighborhood cultures, observing that "Working-class attitudes included a clear
duty to help your neighbors, which surmounted other considerations."[44] It
is possible that as neighborhoods became more stable and family resources
increased toward the late nineteenth century, a working-class culture that
prioritized mutual aid strengthened. It is also apparent that while mutual
aid was normative in remembered working-class experience, neither participation nor reciprocity was universal. As we have seen, neighborliness
varied from one area to another; new or "rough" neighborhoods were less
likely than other neighborhoods to develop this resource. Neighbors also
differed in their willingness to exchange privacy for support; at the same
time that helpful neighbors are remembered with affection and gratitude,
nosiness, interference, and destructive gossip were resented and feared.[45]
Upwardly mobile, comparatively prosperous, or self-consciously "modern"
women might distance themselves from neighborhood networks, while
continuing to guard family reputations. Some protection from intrusion
and gossip was offered by the fact that much neighborly interaction and
support took place outside of the home. The donkeystoned front step and
freshly laundered net curtains represented both the household's public
face and a barrier to critical or prying eyes.[46]

Regarding the tension between the needs for privacy, on the one hand,
and support, on the other, Judy Giles argues that increasing attention in
the early twentieth century from a host of middle-class service providers
and researchers encouraged working-class women's value for "keeping
myself to myself"—a tendency Tebbutt explains by the equally strong urge
to protect the family's reputation from the power of negative neighborhood gossip.[47] Tebbutt also points out men's objections to the communication among women that gave women a measure of power, independence,
and support in working-class neighborhoods.[48] I think it entirely possible
that all of these interpretations are valid and underscore both the diversity
in levels of access to and participation in neighborhood mutual aid networks and change in norms regarding neighborliness over time.

Not everyone desired or was welcome to give and receive assistance.
As we have seen, people perceived to be "rough" might be excluded or

44. Roberts, *A woman's place*, 19, quote on p. 184: 184–201; Meacham, *A life apart*, 45–46;
Michael Anderson, *Family structure in nineteenth century Lancashire* (Cambridge: Cambridge
University Press, 1971), 171.

45. See, for example, Bourke, *Working-class cultures*, 142–43.

46. See Tebbutt, *Woman's talk*, 81, for a good description of the weekly ritual of whitening
or coloring front steps by using donkeystones.

47. Judy Giles, *Women, identity and private life in Britain, 1900–50* (New York: St. Martin's
Press, 1995), 101; Tebbutt, *Women's talk*, 93–97. See Behlmer, *Friends of the family*, for useful
discussion of the history of middle-class attempts to influence working-class family culture.

48. Tebbutt, *Women's talk*, 61–62. This situation is reflected in interviews conducted for this
study: see, for example, Mrs. P1P, 63.

exclude themselves from neighborhood networks, although it is noteworthy that even these people, who often were among the poorest in working-class neighborhoods, routinely helped each other. For example, Mr. Boyle, born in 1937 in Preston, remembered that his mother, who was rough by any standard, burning internal doors for firewood and beating her children with the fire poker, depended on friends for help: "My mother, the fire would go out, she had no coal, go down to next door but one, or who she knew, Maggie Hitchin or somebody like that, and borrow a bucket of coal off her. Give her a bucket of coal, and she would come back and start the fire again, you know."[49] However, Mrs. Peterson, born in 1899, who lived in a rough Preston neighborhood, said that her husband objected to her inviting neighbors into their house: "Oh, they [husbands] didn't do in them days, they wanted their homes to theirself. He didn't want me to go in a neighbor's either. He didn't want me to go out anywhere. He just wanted his home. He said that when he had been out at work all day he wanted his own fireside. He didn't want people in. There were a lot that were just the opposite."[50]

At the other end of the respectability spectrum, women with social aspirations or, at least, the means to do without neighborhood assistance, also sometimes kept aloof from neighborhood networks and the nosiness and gossip they bred. Mrs. Critchley, born in Lancaster in 1926, said of her mother:

> She didn't like it, oh no, there were some people who lived across from us and they were never off the doorstep, and my mother used to hate it, I mean when we moved into the second house, the bigger house, we were right across from these people and every time you went out of your front door they were there, you couldn't go in or out without them being there and oh, we all hated it because they just watched everything that was going on, so no, she didn't like it at all. . . . My mother never gossiped with them, I mean, they perhaps gossiped with others, I don't know, but my mother was never one who did a lot of gossiping with neighbors. We never had sort of neighbors coming in a lot and gossiping. I don't think my dad would've liked it, but certainly we never did.[51]

Although this informant's father was a railway laborer and the family lived in a working-class area (Skerton), the fact that Mrs. Critchley went to the Girl's Grammar School and that her mother returned to factory work to help pay her school expenses suggests that her parents had nontraditional aspi-

49. Mr. B11P, 12.
50. Mrs. P1P, 63. See also Mrs. D1B, 32.
51. Mrs. C7L, 5.

rations for her. Certainly, expectation and provision of mutual aid declined after World War II, a change remarked by oral history informants, many of whom were nostalgic for the good old days of neighborliness despite the comparative lack of comfort and prosperity during those times.

MUTUAL AID AND ILL-HEALTH

Informants' comments about neighborhood mutual aid were elicited mainly by the questions, "Did neighbors help each other? If so, what kinds of help did they give?" Almost invariably, responses had to do with support in times of ill-health, which breached the barrier of the front step and admitted neighbors to private family spaces.[52] Mrs. Addison, born in 1892 in Barrow, said:

> The neighbors were far better than what they are today. They were not as clannish. If the next door neighbor was poorly, we would go in and help. We'd do her washing, do her ironing, and we'd take them back and if they wanted any messages going we used to do it. They were always willing to help you. Now today they're more clannish, they seem as if they want to be on their own. . . . When they were ill, they used to get a sheep's head and marrow bone and then two-pennyworth of pot herbs and make a good pan of soup, and some split peas and barley and take them a good bowl of soup in at night. We perhaps used to take them their dinners. . . . I used to be knocked up time out of time when anybody died. They used to come and knock at the door at midnight and say, "Will you come and lay the baby out, will you come and lay so-and-so out?" I used to go and lay them out. . . . We never used to take anything off them, never bothered, but now today everything is altered and the undertaker does all that. . . . The neighbors used to come and ask, if the babies were bad or owt, "Have you got such a thing as a bit of goose grease by you?" I've had it for my own children.[53]

This informant offered both a description and an interpretation of working-class mutual aid. It is clear that the concept of traditional social childbirth, which encompassed the presence and activities of the mother's female relatives and special friends during home-based labor, delivery, and lying-in, could usefully be broadened to a concept of social management of ill-health and death.[54] When Mrs. Addison referred to "neighbors" and

52. In *Friends of the family* (2), Behlmer refers to the importance of the working-class threshold.

53. Mrs. A2B, 23, 40. Mrs. Chase, born in 1887, also did laying out as a neighborly service. See Mrs. C2B, 13.

54. See, for example, Adrian Wilson, "Participant or patient? Seventeenth century childbirth

"they," she was talking about women—understood to be good rather than "clannish" neighbors—who requested, received, and gave assistance with housework, cooking, errands, medicine, and preparation of the deceased for burial. Neighbors helped, not for compensation (required by both undertakers and occupational health care providers), but because it was the right thing to do. "Clannish" neighbors wanted "to be on their own," so were unwilling to either give or receive help—and possibly were only willing to participate in these transactions with kin. Wanting to be alone violated the appropriate roles of both the sufferer and his or her family members, who were expected to be helped and later help in their turn; it also hamstrung the good motives and actions of neighbors and undermined traditional neighborliness.

Just as access to mutual aid was a mark of respectability for working-class families, denial of help could also damage reputations. For example, when in the 1920s Mrs. Peterson had year-old twins ill with whooping cough and a preschooler suffering from measles, she said she managed for quite a while without asking anyone for help: "Because one woman said when I had got them in the pram once, she said, 'Your mother's had you all this while and never asked anybody to help you!' Well, I didn't think I should, that it was my work. This woman come across and one of her sons come across and said, 'Mum, such a thing is on the race today.' They were racing. It was shocking. She wasn't in the house five minutes till he come again for her. She asked if she had to come back and I said no. Fancy him coming about racing. Oh, dear me. I suppose it wasn't her trouble, it was mine, but what a shocking thing."[55] This account of aid provided belatedly, unwillingly, briefly, and ineffectively cast doubt on the respectability of the neighbor providing the help (a mother herself), who thought a horse race was more important than supporting a young mother with sick children. Furthermore, since the informant went on to describe the death of one twin and enforced admission of the other two children to isolation hospital (discussed further in chapter 4), this story compared neighborhood mutual aid and public health intervention, finding both wanting. A possible inference is that appropriately delivered help from neighbors would have been better for both mother and children in a situation where neither isolation nor professional care did this family much good.

While not precluding help offered with no expectation of recompense, informants clearly expressed the normatively reciprocal nature of mutual aid. Mr. Best, born in Barrow in 1897, said:

---

from the mother's point of view," in Roy Porter, ed., *Patients and practitioners: Lay perceptions of medicine in pre-Industrial society* (Cambridge: Cambridge University Press, 1985),129–44; Lucinda McCray Beier, *Sufferers and healers: The experience of illness in seventeenth-century England* (London and New York: Routledge and Kegan Paul, 1987), 186; Judith Walzer Leavitt, *Brought to bed: Childbearing in America, 1750–1950* (Oxford: Oxford University Press, 1986), 4–5, 36–38.

55. Mrs. P1P, 14.

Again, going back to your birth, you've already got four, but the children must not be there when the baby is born. "It's all right, Missus, I'll take your Johnny," and they'd be taken by neighbors up and down the street. It was a known thing, it's going to happen to you, and it's going to happen to me, and that is how the friendliness came, they were all dependent upon each other, no matter what it was. If they were poor and the fellow came out of work and there was no money coming in, "Well, you can have a bucket of coal off me." Sickness brought people together definitely, and that's how everybody seems to know everybody.[56]

This informant expressed the link between shared poverty, need, and neighborliness. Mrs. Arnold, born in 1910 in Preston, said: "If anyone was ill, in those days there was no National Health as you know it today, you had to pay the doctor yourself. If anyone was ill, to try and avoid that large doctor's bill, you would help that neighbor and you would take her food in. My mother would look after that neighbor's children while the father came home from work, and they would go in with a meal for that neighbor that was ill. Things like that. They would do a bit of work in the house. They would wash up for them and tidy up."[57] Again, in this account the sufferer was a woman who would otherwise be in charge of family health and housework. Therefore, the need was great and neighbors offered the most affordable (compared to the physician) and respectable (compared to the Poor Law) alternative for aid. This was particularly true during childbirth and lying-in, when the mother was expected to stay in bed for at least two weeks.

What did neighbors do for each other in times of ill-health? The examples already provided offer a long list of services: cooking, laundry, cleaning, childcare, errands, loans of supplies, provision of remedies, and laying out of the dead. Neighbors loaned bedding and other necessities for a home birth or a bout of serious illness.[58] They also helped with the consequences of illness, which sometimes involved the incapacitation of the breadwinner. For example, Mrs. Melling, born in Lancaster in 1917, said, "There was nothing too good for anyone to do or to give. . . . Any accidents, they'd be there to see what they could do with the child if it was a child, or if it was the husband who'd had an accident, and the husband couldn't work, and the wife had to find a bit of a job, the neighbors would all help and bake, wash, and do anything."[59]

In cases of terminal illness, even the shared public area beyond the front step would be collectively offered to dignify the death and support the family. Mr. Peel, born in 1909 in Barrow, recalled, "You see, if there was

56. Mr. B1B, 27. See also Mrs. D1B, 32, and Mrs. H4P, 39.
57. Mrs. A1P, 34. See also Mr. W3P, 11.
58. See, for example, Mr. H1L, 25; Mr. W3P, 11.
59. Mrs. M3L, 44.

somebody very ill in the street . . . they would close the half of the street where that person was very ill. Say somebody was old and they was going to die, the neighbors would know. And they would close—they would say, 'Now, when you go to play, play down there, not up there.'"[60] When an illness ended in death, neighbors would lay out the dead, as we have seen, and help the family to mourn respectably. Mr. Madison, born in 1910 in Lancaster, remembered:

> It didn't need your own relations to rally round to help in those days, you'd neighbors in your houses helping. . . . The neighbors just rallied round. If there was a funeral and there was a certain piece of black that you hadn't got, somebody would find out and say, "Here, you can borrow that for this afternoon." A pair of black shoes somebody would lend them same size as yours, or even black stockings. Black was black in those days, and they went on wearing it for months after the funeral. People would rally round even in cases like that to lend you that necessary piece of black clothing, happen a black hat or a scarf or something. You didn't need your relations to do it. There was great comradeship, but as I said, everybody was in the same boat and they appreciated this matter.[61]

Mr. Simpkins, born in Lancaster in 1932, remembered that when his father died in 1938, neighbors provided a variety of services, from keeping the dying man and his wife company during his final days and taking up a collection for the funeral, to shaving the corpse's face several days after death when the body was displayed in the family's parlor.[62]

Neighbors helped with home nursing—especially sitting with a sufferer to provide comfort as well as relief to the wife, mother, or other caregiver. For example, Mrs. Parke, born in Lancaster in 1898, remembered: "They [neighbors] would come in and particularly when my father was dying. The neighbors from where we used to live before came up and helped mother. He died of cancer of the throat and he just laid and lingered there. He dropped from quite a nice weight to skin and bone and they didn't take him away. I don't think there was the same drugs then, and he just had to suffer. He got as he couldn't pass anything, and they were very kind, coming sitting up with him at night."[63]

Mr. Eckley, born in Preston in 1895, said of the neighbors when he was

60. Mr. P6B, 25.

61. Mr. M1L, 22.

62. Mr. S7L, 5–6. See Elizabeth Roberts, "The Lancashire way of death," in Ralph Houlbrooke, ed., *Death, ritual and bereavement* (London and New York: Routledge, 1989), 188–207, for a general discussion of older oral history informants' experience and management of relatives' and neighbors' deaths.

63. Mrs. P1L, 39. See also, for example, Mr. H1L, 25; Mrs. C2B, 13; Mr. R3L, 30.

a boy, "They were more sociable. Supposing I had been in bed ill and my granny had been up all night with me, you couldn't go into hospital in them days, the next door lady would probably make my dinner for me and she would come in and wash me like a nurse would. The neighbor across the road would tell my granny to have some sleep and she would stay up with me all night."[64] It is possible that this informant's explanation, "like a nurse would," was an effort to help a much younger interviewer understand bygone practices. As we will see, home nursing was an expected and usual part of an adult woman's responsibilities.[65] It was also one form of paid work available to working-class women and consequently a skill benefiting family members and neighbors after employment had ended. For example, Mr. Rust's mother, who had worked as a nurse at the Royal Lancaster Infirmary in the late nineteenth century before her marriage, later helped her neighbors without compensation.[66]

In addition to nursing care, neighbors provided advice about health and illness. Mrs. Calvert, born in 1919 in Preston, said, "It was like a community, the street, and you would ask suchabody, and they would tell you to give them such a thing. If it was too much, then you would have to send for the doctor; otherwise, it would be asking somebody round the street."[67] Similarly, Mrs. Steele, born in Preston in 1898, when asked, "Who did your mother turn to if she wanted any help with them [children] or any advice?" replied, "She could go to a neighbor or an auntie, unless it was something serious and she would send for the doctor then. Just ordinary things that went on, they just used to advise one another. They would get this for it and get the other for it."[68] Experienced mothers, especially, developed expertise and authority regarding diagnosis and treatment of many ailments and offered advice to neighbors. According to Mrs. Peel, born in 1921, "Mothers know if it's mumps, chickenpox or measles, you know, it's just a natural instinct, isn't it?"[69] Mr. Best, born in 1897 in Barrow, remembered:

> Now, here's a case, Mrs. B[est] in my day came out with a rash all over her face and an old lady friend of mine lived up in Chatsworth Street who'd had a big family, a real mother, looked after the kids and had her own family and so on. My wife says, 'I can't make out what this rash is on here.' 'No, my dear, I can cure that,' she said. 'Go down to Boots [a

64. Mr. E1P, 44.

65. See, for example, Carol Dyhouse, *Girls growing up in late Victorian and Edwardian England* (London: Routledge and Kegan Paul, 1981); Ellen Ross, *Love and toil: Motherhood in outcast London, 1870–1918* (New York and Oxford: Oxford University Press, 1993), 166–69.

66. Mr. R3L, 30.

67. Mrs. C5P, 38.

68. Mrs. S5P, 14. See also Mrs. S2P, 8.

69. Mrs. P6B, 119.

pharmacy] and get so-and-so ointment and put that on. It's a nerve rash
and it will be gone in three days,' and it was. . . . Your mothers used to
cure you, they knew what you wanted.[70]

Mr. Best both expressed his reason for trusting his "old lady friend" and
explained the effectiveness of her advice by referring to her as "a real
mother" who had raised a family and done child-minding. Her experience
was her qualification; however, she had obviously also developed a personal
reputation for competence in health matters. Despite often expressed reliance on "the neighbors," it is clear that in this face-to-face society where
reputations were established and destroyed on the basis of individual
behavior, the reputations of specific women as knowledgeable and successful regarding health problems were very important.

INFORMAL HEALTH AUTHORITIES

While most informants remembered mothers being effective and confident
in dealing with routine health challenges before about 1950, working-class
neighborhoods also had informal health authorities—always women, sometimes unqualified midwives or experts in laying out the dead, sometimes
people who had had some nurse training—who were widely consulted and
respected. The Medical Officers of Health recognized and deplored the
activities of these women. For example, among other factors contributing to Preston's high infant mortality rate, the city's MOH, Dr. Pilkington,
blamed consultation of elderly local women "whose nursing and feeding
arrangements date back to the dark ages, but whose experience of sickness
amongst children—undoubtedly and unfortunately a large one—enable
[them] to pose as an authority on these subjects in the neighborhood."[71]
By contrast, some general practitioners found it more productive to work
with neighborhood health authorities—in part, because of their influence
with working-class families and also possibly because handywomen posed
less occupational competition than qualified midwives or district nurses.[72]
Similarly, neighborhood chemists dealt with both doctors and area residents, including informal health authorities, tolerating and profiting from
a wide spectrum of health behavior. A Lancaster chemist, Mr. Chambers,
who began practicing in 1919, remembered, "We used resin ointment,
which was very good [for drawing boils], but of course the old women
would come in and have some soap and sugar and put that on, which was

70. Mr. B1B, 115.
71. Preston MOH Report, 1896, 10.
72. Dingwall et al., *Social history of nursing*, 162.

efficient. . . . You see, a lot of these things were old witch doctors' business, but witch doctors are very respectable people, I think, and we could learn a lot from them."[73]

Mr. Lane, born in 1896 in Lancaster, remembered, "In Westham Street there was a woman called Mrs. Warrington, and she was a very great help to us, helping people in the street, and there was always one or two like that in every street."[74] Mrs. Masterson, born in Preston in 1913, said:

> If anyone was ill in the neighborhood or anyone died they had what they called a Street Woman. If they were expecting a baby there was a midwife who only came when the baby was being born. You didn't go for prenatal visits, you booked this midwife when you knew they were expecting the baby. This midwife would come and she would deliver the baby and cut the cord and then this Street Lady had to come, you had to pay her, and she would come then and she would see to the mother and the baby and make her food until she got up. . . . Then if anyone died they would send for this lady and her job was to see to the dead person, but you don't see that now.[75]

Mr. Monkham, born in 1948 in Lancaster, remembered:

> And every street had its "lady" who was, say, experienced in these matters; ours was actually the lady across the road that I was telling you has just died, Mrs. Riley. Who had actually had some nursing experience.
> *Interviewer:* Was she a kind of unofficial midwife to the neighborhood, then?
> *Informant:* She was unofficial everything, father confessor, helper, supporter, advisor, nurse, everything was Nana Riley.
> *Interviewer:* Now, what sort of problems would people consult her for?
> *Informant:* Just about everything. There was another lady around the corner who has been long since dead, we used to call her Aunty Viv, although of course she was actually no aunty at all, she was just a very close family friend that we called "Aunty" in that affectionate term. Even Mum and Dad called her Aunty Viv, and she died when she was about ninety-three, and always looked very much the way that old ladies did in the pictures that I have got upstairs. Very leathery wrinkled skin, old-fashioned shawls and clogs, and they were still quite common when I was a child.
> *Interviewer:* How did she get on with the doctor, do you know that?
> *Informant:* I can remember the old doctor very well. I can see his face now. He was actually the father of old Howat, and he actually got

73. Mr. C6L, 6.
74. Mr. L1L, 14.
75. Mrs. M1P, 8.

on very well with her, because she was very well known. He accepted her, but that sort of community matriarch would have a part to play, and unless they were doing something dumb or stupid, he actually saw them, I think, as a very valuable asset to his own care. And they respected his position and if he gave advice, well it would be followed.

Interviewer: So she would be unlikely to say, "Oh, no, that's a funny idea, don't do that?"

Informant: I know some of the old fashioned ones I have come across are liable to do that, in fact professionally I still find that in the medical field now. But not Nana Riley, I found her very sensible. Who of course had the whole wealth of old-fashioned remedies and old-fashioned experiences and opinions of course very often conflicted with doctors, but I think most of them respected him and followed out exactly what they said.[76]

Mr. Norton, born in 1931 in Lancaster, said that his mother had rendered similar services in "maybe two or three streets, that's all. Oh yes, two or three streets. There was probably somebody equally as competent in the next road, yes." She would give advice about "any kind of illness, particularly as far as youngsters were concerned. She diagnosed after looking at the kids, and I don't remember her being wrong, she probably was, but I don't remember her being wrong. And if she felt the doctor was needed, then the doctor was sent for." Mrs. Norton also helped with deliveries and laid out the dead.[77]

Some of these informal health authorities were what Medical Officers of Health called "handywomen"—unqualified midwives who continued to practice after legislation controlled their activities from 1902 and outlawed them altogether in 1936. The MOsH clearly regarded these women as ignorant, unskilled, sometimes immoral, and potentially destructive. In 1910 Barrow's MOH referred to the stereotyped "Sariah Gamp midwife" as part of his report on enforcement of the 1902 Midwives Act. In 1905 the same official, Dr. John Settle, had written:

During the year one registered Midwife lost her license for being drunk when in charge of one of her cases. I have visited most of the others to examine them, their case books and bag of appliances, with very unsatisfactory general results. Few of them understand their rules. Some are unable to write sufficiently to keep a book and few understand the instruments of their calling. When my inquiries are completed, I shall advise my committee as to what should be done to improve the midwife generally.[78]

76. Mr. M10L, 19–20.
77. Mr. N2L, 50, 55.
78. Barrow MOH Report, 1904, 209.

Similarly, Preston's MOH, Dr. Pilkington, reported in 1907:

> Unfortunately, there are a number of women who continue to attend
> confinements without having passed any examination, or even obtained
> the certificate, on the ground of having been in practice before the
> passing of the Act. So long as they do not advertise themselves as
> midwives, this cannot at present be prevented, but it is well that they
> should know that although they may not be liable to the same exami-
> nation and supervision as the certified midwife, any evil consequence
> to either mother or child, resulting from interference, dirt, or want of
> proper care on their part, will be closely enquired into, and if neglect
> be proved, will be severely punished.

Dr. Kuppersmith, a physician who practiced in a working-class area of
Preston between 1928 and 1978, offered a somewhat more balanced view,
which also recognized the tradition for midwifery to run in families: "There
was a mother and a daughter who lived in East Street, and they were a law
unto themselves because they had been in the practice for so long. Before
I came they were very well established. The mother died and the daughter
carried on. There were quite a few of these midwives who were apprenticed to other midwives and never had any training at all. Some of them
were very good, but some of them were very poor."[79] While more will be
said below about professional efforts to reconstruct the image of neighborhood health authorities, it is worthy of remark here that before working-
class people could become fully compliant participants in official health
care, working-class women had to stop serving as informal healers and their
neighbors had to stop consulting them instead of qualified practitioners. It
is not surprising that many physicians, strong believers in both medical science and the progressive political agenda it drove, as well as financial ben-
eficiaries of the trend toward doctor-managed births, had negative views
about unqualified midwives.

Regardless of professional opinions, as I have argued elsewhere, for the
most part working-class women had strong relationships with traditional
midwives and continued to use them long after qualified midwives became
available in their communities.[80] There are a number of possible reasons
for this loyalty including economic considerations (the unqualified midwives were less expensive than their qualified sisters) and social comfort
(in comparison to professionally authoritative and socially superior trained
midwives or general practitioners). In addition, like other informal health
authorities, all unqualified and some qualified midwives participated in

79. Dr. K1P, 1.

80. Lucinda McCray Beier, "Expertise and control: Childbearing in three twentieth-century
working-class Lancashire communities," *Bulletin of the History of Medicine* 78:2 (2004): 379–409.

traditional neighborhood mutual aid networks. Mr. Adderley, born in Lancaster in 1926 and one of eight surviving children, remembered:

> We had to have people like that [midwives] because my mother was always expecting. Now, where we lived at Moorlands we had a woman called Mrs. Oxley, in fact it were her family that introduced us to the Methodist chapel. They were very interested in things like that. Well, she used to be Mother's best friend. . . . And when we moved over Skerton we had a neighbor, Mrs. Huntington, she was around all the time. We used to have a system, we had no telephone, we had a system: we used to bang on the skirting board with the poker and that was just to let them know, come round, you're needed. And the midwife lived directly behind us, so.[81]

How did informal health authorities deal with health challenges? As was also true of physicians regarding most nonsurgical problems before the advent of antibiotics, the main skill they offered was the ability to diagnose and tell people what to do—whether it involved administering a remedy or consulting someone else, such as a physician or a chemist. Both diagnoses and therapeutic recommendations were based on long experience. Their treatments, like those used in most working-class households, tended to be composed of herbs or household substances. Mr. Ford, born in 1906 in Preston, remembered his mother giving health advice: "One or two of the neighbors used to come across if there was anything wrong with their children. She would say what she would give to her own. . . . I know they used to concoct some terrible brews. . . . In those days, you could go to the herb shop. There were three or four in Preston where they sold bark and all that."[82] In addition, echoes remained of traditional magical techniques and powers. Mr. Boswell, born in Barrow in 1920, remembered two women in the neighborhood who helped in times of ill health: Mrs. Knight, the midwife, and

> Mrs. Wall, yes, she used to lay out the dead, she was a witch. . . . Well, she used to read cups, you know, and she was a Welshwoman, Mrs. Wall, and she used to wear a steeple hat. . . . She had been a beauty when she was young, you know, a real beauty, she used to speak Welsh. . . . And they used to say she could put a spell on you. Well, I'll give you an instance, one old gentleman died and she had laid him out and one of his friends was there and he made some remark, and she turned round to him and said, "Have you ever had pneumonia?" He said, "No." "Well, you'll get it." And he did.

81. Mr. A4L, 49.
82. Mr. F1P, 74. See also Mr. V1L, 8.

Interviewer: Would she be called in for things other than laying out the dead, would people call her in if anyone was ailing?

Informant: Yes, sure, she would come and have a look at them, she was quite good with her herbs and that, you know, but she was best for reading the cups, fortune telling, you know.

Interviewer: I see. Who would mainly go to have that done?

Informant: Women.

Interviewer: So was it young women or older women?

Informant: Older women.[83]

Neighborhood health authorities also administered first aid. Mrs. Howard, born in Lancaster in 1931, recalled:

I think she had been a nurse in her time, and she must have left to have a family. . . . But she was the nurse on our street, whether she had ever been a proper nurse, I don't know. But everybody ran for Mrs. Myrtle when anybody was ill. Because I remember two brothers being badly scalded, and she came both times. One had pulled a kettle off the fire onto his legs and I seem to remember her dipping his leg in a bag of flour. . . . I know my sister jumped on a rusty tin once and gashed her leg. "Go for Mrs. Myrtle!" you know, and she used to come back, she used to bring a box with her, and it was full of iodine, cotton wool, and ointments and things. And she used to really make you better, and she used to come and dress it for you and stuff like that.[84]

The strength of such care providers, in part, was their sturdiness in the face of situations that upset other people. Mrs. Shelby, born in 1898 in Lancaster, said about her grandmother:

She was very good and if anybody died she used to go and wash them. I remember two people being pulled out of the canal. I remember a chap went out of his mind and she used to take them up to the asylum then. She would do anything like that. She didn't get anything for it. Doctors used to come for her. They always used to say that she was in partnership with Dr. Todd. He would come and say, "Now Mrs. Woodburn, will you just come so-and-so," If there was scarlet fever and diphtheria, nobody would go but my grandma.[85]

Similarly, Mr. Melling, born in 1906 in Lancaster, answered the question, "Was there anyone in your street or area who helped if anybody was ill?" with the following story:

83. Mr. B4B, 32.
84. Mrs. H5L, 56–57.
85. Mrs. S1L, 7.

My mother used to be asked. She was always around. I always remember
when we were at home and up at Stirling Road, and a knock come in
the middle of the morning, about two o'clock in the morning, Ginny
Darling come across from t'other street, higher up, running across,
"Mrs. M., Mrs. M., come my father's cut his throat." He'd hung himself
on the rack and cut his throat with a razor. So my mother went across,
put a coat on over her nightdress and went across and went for the
policeman and the policeman come and just simply stood there while
he died. He'd cut his throat because he was out of work, a painter, he'd
been out of work and things were bad and they were living off nowt,
near starvation, so it's easiest way out. . . . She wouldn't be called out for
owt, but if there was anybody badly she was ready to help. They were
more neighborly than they seem to be now.[86]

It is possible that informal health experts were sometimes more trusted
than formally qualified doctors and nurses because they shared the financial and living circumstances of their working-class neighbors. The experience of Mrs. Garvey, born in Barrow in 1888, is worth quoting at length
because it contrasts an apparently uncaring, ineffective (female, middle-
class, formally qualified) general practitioner and an empathetic, competent (female, elderly, poor, Irish) neighbor:

Our Jimmy was a very heavy weight, a big boy. There was whooping
cough and he got it. . . . He took an illness and he was a great big boy
about fourteen pounds then and he was nearly twelve month old. He
went down to a young skeleton. I nursed him for three month, night
and day. Then this old lady doctor used to come in. "No change?" "No."
She used to lift his little leg up and let it go down. An old Irishwoman
came in and she said, "Take my advice." She only come for a rest, somewhere to sit at night because the war was still on. She was hiding her
son from going to the war, and she come out of her bed to let him sleep
and walked the streets. She saw a light in my room and she knocked and
said, "Have you got somebody ill? Is your baby ill?" I said, "Yes, very ill."
I was only glad of anybody to come and sit with me. I was sitting in the
parlor nursing this child and I never left him for three month. She said,
"Oh, this baby has got bad bronchitis and whooping cough. I never saw
whooping cough like it in my life, and I've brought up a lot of bairns."
She used to hold him on her arm and rub his little chest. She wouldn't
let a breath of air in, padded round the doors and the windows, and
she said, "Mind you keep the baby warm." I felt, well, all these professional people hadn't done very much for me. My own sister said, "I'm
surprised at you, having that dirty old woman." I said, "Look, . . . that
old woman is not dirty, she is a good old woman." A big Catholic too.

86. Mr. M3L, 10–11.

"Oh, God'll never take your baby from yer." She helped me a lot. My sister said, "Your baby will never get well, you want air." I said, "You leave those windows alone. I'm sick and tired of all you professional people, doctors, nurses, and people coming in. I'm killing my child by putting him in the open air, he can't stand it. He can't breathe, and I'm doing what this old woman tells me and I can see an improvement." Even the doctor gave him up and never come near. Anyway, she [the old woman] told me to get a quarter of best steak. I couldn't afford it, mind you, because my husband was away working, they'd sent him away. I just squeezed the blood out of this steak and gave that child a teaspoon a day. Do you know, the first cry I heard from him was lovely. There was just one night that she gave up hope. She says, "I think you're going to lose your baby." I said, "Oh, how cruel you are. Everybody goes out and leaves me. You all leave me here, but I'm not afraid, I'll nurse him to the end." She says, "I wouldn't leave you, Aggie, but I feel I must go." She shook her head and went into the backyard. I thought, "Aren't people cruel?" But from that day on that child was on the turn. I was eating a bit of bread and he grabbed it. Of course, then I'd to be very careful how I fed him. I was still giving him this teaspoonful of pure blood. Now whether the old woman had told old Dr. McGill, I don't know, but she [doctor] come walking in. I had a house with a parlor and she opened the door. She looked at this little kiddie and his little hands were moving, but he was just a human skeleton. I didn't want anybody to look at him. She says, "Whatever has caused this change?" I looked at her and said, "Well, Dr. McGill, I think it is a change for the better, don't you?" She just picked up his leg like that and let it drop, and said, "I don't know." I said, "Well, I do. It is a change for the better and I've got my baby and that is all that matters to me. You professionals have never been near this door for three weeks, are you waiting to be called for the death certificate?" She said, "To be quite candid, I was." She sat down and told me what this old Irishwoman had told me months ago about this blood. She said, "Who told you about it?" I said, "An old ignorant woman, and I think she is responsible for this child's life."[87]

This story, which had obviously been told many times, contains core elements—whooping cough in infants, which was very common and often deadly; home care for desperately ill children; negotiation of both details of care (e.g., open or closed windows) and appropriate authorities regarding treatment—that document important aspects of early-twentieth-century working-class experience of ill-health. Mrs. Garvey had few resources and little support for dealing with her child, who suffered from a disease in which the whooping stage normally lasted for up to six weeks and caused

87. Mrs. G1B, 14–15.

up to 40 paroxysms a day.[88] By this account, her sister offered no help, but nonetheless criticized both Mrs. Garvey's reliance on the old Irishwoman and her preference of the old-fashioned practice of keeping the windows closed (to eliminate bad air and drafts) to the newer orthodoxy of open windows and fresh air (to prevent and ameliorate illness). The general practitioner was cavalier in her physical examination of the sick baby and callous in dealing with the distraught mother. The old Irishwoman's approach, involving specific advice as well as sustained personal attendance and care of both mother and baby, was ultimately validated by both the doctor, who agreed with administration of blood from a squeezed raw steak to the infant, and the apparent outcome of amateur assistance—the child's recovery.

HOME HEALTH CARE

When asked whether any of his siblings died as children, Mr. Finch, born in Barrow in 1888, answered: "No, we did not. My mother was one of those people who wouldn't allow anything like that to happen. I suppose we were carefully nursed through childish illnesses and, of course, they were all treated at home, different from nowadays when you send the person to hospital and get rid of them. . . . Many people had their own ideas of 'kitchen medicine,' it was generally called. I think with the modern movement in medicine, these things have been done away with."[89] Informants generally remembered their parents—mothers in particular—providing attentive and effective nursing care; indeed, being a good working-class mother was strongly linked to careful management of children's health. Informants' experience to some extent counters Anne Hardy's conjecture that mortality from some contagious diseases—particularly whooping cough and measles—differed according to social class, in part because of the quality of home nursing care, which was not as good among working- as it was among middle-class Londoners.[90] Hardy's argument is based on evidence provided by medical publications and MOH reports and reflects physicians' growing emphasis on isolation and professional advice, either at home or in the hospital, as the best way to limit contagion and the best environment for care. Working-class oral evidence suggests an alternative interpretation of mothers' attitudes and behavior, which involved norma-

88. Anne Hardy, *The epidemic streets: Infectious disease and the rise of preventive medicine, 1856–1900* (Oxford: Clarendon Press, 1993).

89. Mr. F2B, 7.

90. Hardy, *Epidemic streets*, 16–17, 24, 43, 47. Hardy focuses on contagious diseases in late-nineteenth-century London. Thus, it is entirely possible that working-class living conditions and nursing habits were somewhat different from those experienced in working-class Lancashire during the early twentieth century.

tive day-to-day attention to children's health and subsumed both disease prevention and nursing care.

Mr. Finch's approval of home versus hospital care reflects survival of traditional ideas about both the sufferer's well-being and his or her family's obligations to provide care. His somewhat disparaging reference to "kitchen medicine," about which people had "their own ideas" and which, with the advent of "modern medicine," had been "done away with," suggests several realities: before working-class conversion to biomedicine, many remedies were made in the kitchen, usually by women who had had the experience and informal training to support their own ideas about prevention and cure. Those ideas were empirical, in the sense that people perceived the effectiveness of a prophylactic or therapeutic treatment and repeated it if it were deemed successful. Home care was also based on tradition and faith. For example, belief that taking laxatives and keeping the chest warm were necessary for everyone transcended any direct link between these treatments and prevention or cure of any specific ailment. By the time Mr. Finch was interviewed in the 1970s, "modern medicine" had invalidated the theories and practices of working-class people who lacked formal medical qualifications. Therefore, his memories about home care and his retrospective judgment about that care document important changes in working-class health culture.

Working-class attempts to prevent illness harked back to the humoral concepts that had also been common in professional therapeutics well into the nineteenth century. Many informants remember having routinely been dosed in the spring with brimstone (sulfur) and treacle (molasses) to cleanse their blood or, in the words of Mrs. West, born in 1884, "to muck you out, like."[91] Throughout the study period, this was recognized as an old-fashioned practice. Mrs. West remarked that her "old granny used to have it," while Mrs. Hunter, born in Preston in 1931, said, "This is a legacy from my old grandmother, you know."[92] Several families made elderflower wine, which was also thought to be good for cleansing the blood, as was yellow dock.[93]

More common than attention to the blood was the associated emphasis on keeping the bowels open.[94] Mr. Monkham, born in 1948 in Lancaster, commented:

91. Mrs. W3B, 13. See also Mrs. B10P, 3; Mr. G1P, 11; Mrs. H3P, 31, 48; Mrs. M1P, 42; Mrs. M3P, 16; Mr. R3L, 13; Mrs. W4P, 22. Mrs. Winder remembered being given Clark's Blood Mixture and sulfur tablets in spring to clean her blood. See Mrs. W2L, 211.

92. Mrs. W3B, 13; Mrs. H3P, 31. Several families used this remedy more frequently as a general preventive. See, for example, Mrs. B5P, 51; Mr. C1P, 6; Mr. G2L, 9; Mrs. H2B, 118; Mrs. H2L, 16; Mrs. H7P, 29; Mrs. M1B, 16; Mrs. M1P, 42; Mrs. N1L, 2; Mr. P1B, 38.

93. Mrs. R1P, 55; Mr. R3B, 55–56; Mr. W6P, 12.

94. See James C. Whorton, *Inner hygiene: Constipation and the pursuit of health in modern society* (Oxford and New York: Oxford University Press, 2000), for discussion of this obsession in England and the United States during the nineteenth and twentieth centuries.

There seemed to be, I could never understand it as a child, it was this awful preoccupation with the bowels amongst the elderly. . . . And it really, even now after all these years, it strikes me very forcibly that they were always asking about your bowels. And it seemed to me at that stage that if your bowels were okay, you were.

Interviewer: How could you tell if your bowels were bad?

Informant: There used to be all sorts of fascinating things, apart from actually asking you, which under normal circumstances would have been considered bad taste. They were always sticking their tongue out, my dad had a fascination for it. And if his tongue was coated, it was a real indication that his bowels were bad and that he needed something for it. . . . Well, it was considered the first indication of you being out of sorts.[95]

Many informants remembered the most common of all herbal remedies, senna tea brewed from pods or leaves, being administered once a week. Mrs. Ackerman, born in Barrow in 1904, recalled being given "senna tea every Saturday morning. She [Mother] used to make it ordinarily and sit in front of us and put sugar and milk in it as though it was our own tea. 'This is funny tea, Mam,' we'd say. 'Get it down, get it drunk,' and that was it, senna tea Saturday mornings."[96] Other informants remembered taking licorice powders, castor oil, California Syrup of Figs (an over-the-counter patent remedy), and foods including All-Bran, prunes, and cabbage water to make their bowels work.[97] Mrs. Horton, born in 1903 in Lancaster, recalled, "They had California Syrup of Figs. I used to like it that much I took nearly a bottle full once. I remember m'mother telling us about it, it was for worms and it cleared me, took the whole bed away. I've always had a laugh o'er that. . . . Always got a dose of working medicine. She used to keep that up."[98] Her reference to "working medicine" harks back to an older understanding of what it is for a medicine to *work*—not necessarily to cure, but to have an expected effect: laxatives were quintessential working medicines. Mrs. Jenkins, born in 1932 in Barrow, remembered: "The one thing I didn't agree with, which people know better now, about once a week I got a purge. Oh, it was a fruity one, sometimes chocolate laxative and sometimes a fruity one. I've forgotten the name of it now, but I used to hate it. . . . I think that was if you were actually constipated, they would give you Syrup of Figs or something."[99] Informants remembered having been given suppositories or enemas as children. Mrs. Sykes, born in 1927,

95. Mr. M10L, 60–61.

96. Mrs. A2B, 37, 65. See also, for example, Mrs. D2B, 12; Mrs. D3P, 15; Mrs. N1L, 2.

97. Mrs. B5P, 51; Mr. G2L, 9; Mrs. J1B, 62; Mrs. L5B, 45; Mr. M10L, 60; Mr. N2L, 52; Mrs. R4B, 75; Mrs. W2L, 188; Mr. W5L, 48.

98. Mrs. H3L, 61.

99. Mrs. J1B, 61.

remembered that for constipation, "Well, I know what she used to do to us, she used to stick a piece of soap in, like a suppository, yes."[100] Similarly, Mrs. Ruthven, born in 1936, said her mother occasionally gave her an enema:

> Well, I think it was soapy water, because she had a kind of a horrible rubber bulb with a nozzle that she squoze it into my back passage, which was disgusting. She didn't do it very often, but she did on occasions.
> *Interviewer:* How often did she expect your bowels to move?
> *Informant:* Every day, and I had a chart at one point that I had to tick if I had been, this was when I was older.[101]

Related to concern about keeping the bowels healthy was the effort to protect children from drafts and damp, thought to cause a variety of ailments and ever-present in Britain's chilly climate and working-class homes where the main (sometimes the only) source of heat was the range in the living room. Mrs. Peterson, born in Preston in 1899, reflected, "I used to live in a little house down the lane here, and it was cold going in the kitchen and we only had a little room to live in and a kitchen and then going upstairs at night, it was shocking. I think a lot of children would have lived longer if they had had warmer houses."[102] This concern sometimes governed parents' decisions about housing. Mrs. Hampton, born in 1887 in Barrow, remembered her family moving into "a new house and more modern, a bathroom and what have you. Then we weren't there very long because my mother thought it was very damp, which it was and still is, and we left there."[103] Some parents also thought it important for children's clothing and bedding to be warm and dry. Mrs. Jenkins, born in Barrow in 1932, remembered: "My dad was very very strict. Everything had to be aired about ten times over, and the best place to air them, which we always did before we put clothes on, was in the oven next to the fire. . . . It was the old-fashioned fire with the oven and everything was aired in there in winter, of course in summer you didn't need to as much. But when the fire was on everything got aired in there before you put it on. Bedclothes and everything."[104]

Parents' concern about damp and chill also influenced the ways informants dressed as children. Mrs. Wilson, born in 1900, reflected on the threat haunting many mothers in the early twentieth century: "I think tuberculosis worried her more than anything. She was always sure we had dry feet if our feet were wet and to dry our stockings and sit by the fire until we were all dried up."[105] Certain garments were particularly associated with

100. Mrs. S3B, 74.
101. Mrs. R4B, 76.
102. Mrs. P1P, 70.
103. Mrs. H3B, 37.
104. Mrs. J1B, 62. See also Mrs. B10P.
105. Mrs. W1B, 16.

disease prevention. Mrs. Critchley, born in 1926 in Lancaster, remembered: "You'd to always have a vest [undershirt] and keep well wrapped up. And when I was a child I always used to suffer from leg ache a lot, I realize now it was rheumatism, this has been a thing in our family, there had been a lot of rheumatism. And the doctor said to keep me in long black woolen stockings and not to wear Wellingtons [rubber boots] because they draw your feet and make you worse, so that was one thing. We'd always to keep well wrapped up, plenty of woolens and things, you know."[106] Her account illustrates a link between the informal health culture of home and neighborhood on the one hand, and the general practitioner's authority on the other, which in this case validated the traditional approach.

By contrast, Mr. Morris, born in 1933, viewed his parents' similar ways as different from up-to-date medical practices: "But they were great believers in the old-fashioned nursing. You don't go out into the cold if you have got a cold and you put your hat on. . . . Well, I always had a vest on and a pullover. I always wore boots, actually; initially, when I was younger, because they believed that shoes weakened your ankles. Probably totally wrong, I don't know, but that's what they were like, they believed in the old-fashioned ways."[107] Mr. Rollins, born in 1931, recalled having been very thin as a child: "You must always wrap up and, you know, wrap a scarf round your neck three times and have it pinned diagonally across your chest. . . . I had a raincoat obviously and a cap, but we didn't have Wellingtons or anything like that, just an outer coat and a cap."[108] Mrs. Lucas, born in 1950, remembered wearing a scarf, hat, and Wellingtons, sometimes with extra socks, in the winter.[109] It was particularly important to keep the chest warm. Many informants remembered having worn a liberty bodice—a tight-fitting undervest worn beneath other clothing to protect the chest from cold.[110] Along the same lines, Mrs. Hill, born in 1903, said, "I would be about seven or eight and low necks came in, they stopped having the collars and things. They said it would cause pneumonia, that it would kill folks off with having low necks. One person in our street happened to die with it, and they said it was through having those low necks."[111]

Diet and mothers' responsibility for family health were closely linked. According to Elizabeth Roberts, informants consumed a lot of potatoes and bread, much of it homemade. They also ate vegetables, often in soups,

106. Mrs. C7L, 56.
107. Mr. M12B, 45.
108. Mr. R3B, 52. See also Mrs. L5B, 45.
109. Mrs. L5B, 45.
110. Mrs. C8P, 89; Mrs. J1B, 62; Mr. K2P, 93; Mrs. L3L, 63; Mrs. L5B, 45; Mrs. P5B, 38; Mrs. T4B, 73. Liberty bodices were routinely worn by children into the 1960s and are still marketed by at least one company, Woods of Morecambe, a seaside community adjoining Lancaster.
111. Mrs. H8P, 38.

stews, and casseroles, as well as salads, fish, cheap cuts of meat, and offal.[112] Household finances affected the quality and variety of food; families with larger incomes ate better than poorer families, while periods of unemployment directly influenced diet. This is not the place to join the debates over the extent to which women and children ate as well as men, or whether working-class women were successful household managers—although certainly these issues affected family members' health.[113] Instead, we will briefly explore the extent to which oral history informants perceived a connection between food, illness, and health.

Informants believed that food prepared from scratch was healthier than canned food. Mr. Lane, born in 1896, remembered, "There wasn't a lot of tinned food in those days because there was a certain amount of fear about being poisoned with the tin. Don't touch the tin, don't scrape the tin, and just empty it out and all that kind of thing."[114] Mrs. Hancock, born in 1893, said her mother also believed that "canned stuff . . . would poison you." She cooked over "the open fire, and my mother wouldn't have a stove. She had a chance of a gas stove, but she wouldn't have it. She said that it poisoned people."[115]

Informants also linked quantity and quality of food with illness—particularly rickets and tuberculosis. Miss Coyle, born in 1903, suggested that some parents made poor dietary decisions that resulted in children with rickets: "We had some that lived in one of our houses on the Marsh that had them. They all had them, they were all bow-legged. . . . I don't know as they were poorer than anybody else. They used to get out a lot all over the place, by what they told us. They'd sooner buy fish and chips than make a proper meal. M'mam and dad used to play hamlet [make a fuss] and say, 'If only they'd get a bit of neck-end, some potatoes and some carrots and make a pan of hash instead of going for fish and chips they'd do a darned sight better.'"[116]

Mr. Danner, born in 1910 in Preston, speculated that public health provision, which included inexpensive or free foodstuffs, helped to eradicate this condition: "Rickets was absolutely rife and I, as a youngster, you used to be told that people who were bandy-legged were good footballers. I don't know why that ever came about, but you would see these kiddies with the terrible bent legs, and since my children, I don't know of any child

---

112. Roberts, *A woman's place*, 151–61. For general information about British eating habits, see Derek J. Oddy, *From plain fare to fusion food: British diet from the 1890s to the 1990s* (Rochester, NY, and Woodbridge, Suffolk: The Boydell Press, 2003).

113. See, for example, Laura Oren, "The welfare of women in laboring families: England, 1860–1950," in Mary Hartman and Lois W. Banner, eds., *Clio's consciousness raised: New perspectives on the history of women* (New York: Harper Torchbooks, 1974), 226–44; Roberts, *A woman's place*, 163–68; Walton, *Social history*, 293.

114. Mr. L1L, 10.

115. Mrs. H1B, 2.

116. Miss C2L, 17.

that's bandy-legged. They introduced better standards, orange drinks, and there's more care for milk and things, if you couldn't afford it."[117]

Like rickets, tuberculosis was both blamed on poor diet (associated with poverty) and treated with food. Mrs. Musgrove, born in 1886, recalled, "There was a lot of it [tuberculosis], but it was mainly in poorer families, undernourished families. The whole population was half starved unless you were a tradesman. You were living on the borderline, and TB killed them off."[118] Mr. Madison, born in 1910, contracted tuberculosis when he was nine or ten, and was sent to a sanatorium in Helmsley. His treatment consisted of

> lots of fresh air and food that I'd never had before because they kept their own pigs, hens, and they had a few acres of land which was tilled for turnips and vegetables.
>
> *Interviewer:* What would you have that you didn't have before?
>
> *Informant:* Porridge, milk, sugar—lots of it every morning. Bacon more often than you'd get it at home only because of the fact that it couldn't be afforded. . . . A cooked meal on a plate rather than a jam cake to run out to school with. So you really got something in your stomach that you really needed so it might have boiled down to lack of food, a sort of mild malnutrition bringing on the tuberculosis which was called consumption in those days. The place where they found it out was Middle Street which is still there today, but the place isn't. There you went to a doctor and spit into a can and they examined it and that determined that you had this complaint. But I think that came about from the fact that one didn't get the food.[119]

Similarly, when Mrs. Smith's brother (born in 1895) developed tuberculosis as a teenager, their mother "fed him on eggs and sherry, egg flip, and it took a lot of hard work to do it. He used to take cod-liver oil and malt and he stayed off work six months."[120] Open-air schools, built in Preston and Barrow during the interwar period, were intended to reduce undernourishment and prevent diseases including tuberculosis and rickets among frail working-class children.[121]

An important link between official medicine and working-class health

117. Mr. D2P, 34. See also Mr. C2B, 23; Mr. L1L, 16.

118. Mrs. M3L, 32.

119. Mr. M1L, 36. See also Mr. B11P, 4. Dr. K1P, who started practicing medicine in Preston in 1928, said, "No, there was nothing. No treatment was any good whatever [against tuberculosis]. They used to give them fresh air treatment, go to Switzerland, but it had very little effect. . . . Good food and rest in bed: that was the most important thing. The fresh air used to have some health-giving factor" (9).

120. Mrs. S2B, 27.

121. See, for example, John Welshman, *Municipal medicine: Public health in twentieth-century Britain* (Oxford: Peter Lang, 2000), 125, 188–89, 204. Mr. D2P and his sister went to an open-air school, as did Mr. B11P and Mr. S4B.

culture was the regular use of cod-liver oil, sometimes mixed with malt, to prevent disease and preserve health. Introduced into British therapeutics as a remedy for tuberculosis in the 1840s, its use was almost universal in informants' households.[122] According to Mr. Williams, born in 1900 in Preston, it was part of an annual preventative regimen: "Mother was very keen on our health and we used to have a course of sulfur tablets every February. Every Friday night our bowels were assessed and according to whether we were severe or not, we had different kinds of treatment for it. We had caster oil if it was serious, senna pods, we had our choice. We had cascara and a few things like that. All through the spring we used to go out to school with a spoonful of cod-liver oil and malt. And Parish's Chemical Food, we had that in the early part of the year to build and cleanse."[123] Younger informants remember being given cod-liver oil every day. Beginning in the 1920s, together with milk for infant formulas, orange juice, and vitamin products such as Virol and Minadex, cod-liver oil, with or without malt, sometimes formulated as "emulsion," was provided at little or no cost by child health clinics. By the 1930s, informants were given cod-liver oil at school—a practice that continued after World War II. Mrs. Britton, born in 1936 in Lancaster, remembered:

> The only medical precaution I remember my mother taking, at school children had to line up to be given emulsion, it was revolting, it was made from cod-liver oil, and it was awful and evil smelling. And if your parents had told the school that they would give you the equivalent at home, then you could get out of this. And my mother in the end promised to give me this malt extract of cod-liver oil, well cod-liver oil mixed with malt, and it hid the taste of cod-liver oil. And every morning I had a great big spoonful of this shoved down my throat, mother was the sort of person, if she had promised the school she would do it, she would make sure it was done.[124]

Mrs. Rowlandson, born in 1945, even remembered her father being given cod-liver oil tablets at work:

> My dad used to get Haliborange, no they weren't Haliborange tablets, but they were like cod-liver oil tablets from work, now when he used to

---

122. See, for example, Mr. B2B, 38; Mrs. B4L, 63; Mrs. C7L, 55; Mrs. C8P, 89; Mrs. H3P, 48; Mrs. J1B, 62; Mr. K1B, 12; Mr. L3B, 47; Mrs. L5B, 44; Mr. M10L, 53; Mr. M12B, 45; Mr. M14B, 40–1; Mrs. P3L, 49; Mr. P5B, 48; Mrs. P6B, 118; Mrs. R3P, 57; Mr. S4B, 64; Mrs. S6L, 23; Mr. W3P, 29; Mr. W5L, 48; Mrs. W6L, 80; Mr. W7B, 41; Mrs. W7P, 43. The on-line *Oxford English Dictionary* indicates that cod-liver oil was "Recommended in 1783 by Dr. T. Percival as a cure for chronic rheumatism, but app. not taken up. Introduced into medical practice on the continent in 1825, and into English practice in 1846–7, as a remedy for consumption."

123. Mr. W3P, 28–29. Parish's Chemical Food was also mentioned as a preventive medication taken by girls when they started to menstruate. See Mrs. B2B, 42.

124. Mrs. B4L, 63.

work at Dick Kerr's [Preston engineering works] at it was called, they used to give the men these oil tablets. . . . And they used to give them those, they were for the men really to keep them working. So that they don't get colds and flu. But he never used to take them, so he used to bring them home—he used to get a week's supply—and bring them home and we used to take them, you see. So we had his vitamin tablets. But they were horrible.[125]

This evidence indicates that cod-liver oil made the transition from remedy to periodic health-maintenance routine to daily preventive, ultimately helping to pave the way for regular vitamin usage.

Informants remember family members having a good deal of knowledge about common health problems and remedies. Indeed, some kept notes about cures. In answer to the question, "Who sort of was in charge when someone was ill?" Mrs. Wheaton, born in 1933, answered, "Oh, my grandmother was always there, she was never ill." To the question, "Did she have any special cures for you?" Mrs. Wheaton responded, "Oh yes, I've got a book in there with them all written down, from everything from piles to whitlows to everything, and we had a cupboard with all sorts of stuff, there was one bottle that was dead poisonous, but that was used in tiny little bits."[126] In addition to being a "natural" and normative aspect of motherhood, home management of health problems was sometimes interpreted as a rational response to the high cost of calling the doctor. Mr. Best, born in Barrow in 1897, said, "Somebody the other day was talking about that, they said the doctor. . . . 'Oh, m'mother was the doctor.' You had a family of six or seven children, and remember you'd no doctor, you'd no Social Security to pay the rent or the doctors, so it was up to you to know what to do. That is where you get all the old remedies from. And of course, again, one mother would tell another one how to bake. She'd also say, 'Your little girl has got mumps, you want to get so-and-so and put on that,' and so it went. You learnt one off the other."[127] Fathers sometimes also had opinions on health matters. According to Mr. Gordon, born in 1879 in Lancaster, his mother made health care decisions, "But my Dad had a doctor's book, a big thick doctor's book. And that used to get referred to such a lot, it was a very welcome book."[128] Mr. Burrell, born in 1931, explained that his home was equipped to deal with health challenges: "Oh, we had a first-aid box, and there was allsorts in it, sort of things like iodine, lemon and ipecacuanha and linseed oil . . . goose grease."[129]

Informants' families obtained patent remedies, medicinal ingredients, and other health aids such as leeches from local chemists' shops. They also

125. Mrs. R1P, 54.
126. Mrs. W5B, 50. See also Mrs. S3B, 72.
127. Mr. B1B, 114.
128. Mr. G2L, 46.
129. Mr. B2B, 37.

made their own remedies from household materials such as bread, onions, sugar, soap, cinders, and the ever-present goose grease. Particularly important were poultices and plasters used to warm congested chests, as counter-irritation, or to "draw" skin infections. Almost all informants remembered their mothers saving goose grease from the Christmas fowl and applying it to the back or chest.[130] Mrs. Addison, born in 1902, said: "We used to have a plaster put on our chest made a heart shape of brown paper and mother used to rub either goose grease on it or tallow, real tallow candles, and she would warm that and you had that on your chest. . . . She'd leave that on for a day or two and if it didn't get any better you got another one slapped on you. You'd get one on your back."[131] Mrs. Brayshaw, born in 1947, remembered having croup as a child: "The various treatments for this ranged from rubbing of the chest with goose grease and then for a covering of red flannel to be affixed, the drinking of hot treacle water or lemon, to the fastening of a slice of fat bacon round your neck."[132] Mr. Kennedy, born in 1930, remembered goose grease being used as a preventive: "Goose grease on your chest all winter, and then she used to get brown paper and we used to wear two vests. We had a bodice on, a vest with a little liberty bodice, but then before that she used to cut some brown paper and we used to wear it like a little jacket underneath, all soaked with goose grease or on a bodice for your chest with your liberty bodice on."[133] Some informants remembered goose grease being taken internally.[134] All remembered its unpleasant odor.

Other household materials were also used to treat common ailments. Mrs. Dorrington, born in 1905 in Preston, remembered, "For gathered fingers, it was sugar and soap poultice. We would wrap it in a rag round the finger and bandage it all up."[135] Bread poultices were also used to relieve infections. Mr. Ingham, born in 1930, said, "My father used to, if you had cuts or bruises and cuts that had gone septic or boils, well then my mum and dad used to do their own poulticing of the wounds, yes. . . . It was either bread, bread poultice made by two layers of cloth with the bread in and then castor oil on the outside, that was only to stop it burning. And they used to pack it tight and it used to draw the poison out. . . . Oh yes, it used to work, and then of course there was just the kaolin poultice, which was similar."[136] Many informants recalled hot onions or potatoes being applied

130. See, for example, Mr. B2B, 37; Mr. B4B, 30; Mrs. C2B, 18; Mr. C4L, 11; Mrs. D1P, 39; Mr. E1P, 42; Mrs. F1L, 50; Mr. F1P, 70; Mr. G1P, 10; Mr. K1B, 12; Mr. K1L, 17; Mr. L1L, 15; Mr. M1L, 40; Mr. M3L, 10; Mrs. O1B, 55; Mr. Q1L, 14; Miss T4P, 32; Mr. W3P, 29; Mrs. W5B, 50;

131. Mrs. A3B, 40.

132. Mrs. B10P, 3.

133. Mr. K2P, 93.

134. See, for example, Mr. B4P, 30; Mrs. C2B, 18; Mrs. F1L, 50; Mrs. H8P, 37.

135. Mrs. D3P, 7. See also Mrs. L3P, 35; Mrs. M1P, 41.

136. Mr. I2L, 38. See also Mr. B2B, 39; Mrs. L1P, 39; Mrs. T2L, 80. The on-line *OED* defines kaolin as "A fine white clay produced by the decomposition of feldspar, used in the manufacture

to aching ears or inserted in socks and wrapped around sore throats.[137]
They also remembered cough mixtures made of ingredients including tur-
nips, treacle, onions, sugar, black currant jam, and whiskey.[138]

In addition to the use of household substances in remedies, there was
a strong tradition in Lancashire for use of herbs, which were grown, collected, or purchased from herbalists.[139] Miss Thompson, born in Preston in
1912, said:

> I can always remember my dad's mother. . . . [S]he used to make nettle
> soup. . . . [S]he believed in nettles and others believed in knitbone
> [comfrey]. Another thing my mother used to do when we were off
> color, she used to say, "You want some isinglass in milk." Now, isinglass
> when you bought it, people confuse isinglass with water glass. Now,
> water glass was something you dissolved in buckets and preserved eggs
> in it. Isinglass was white fine fish bone to look at and you dissolved them
> in milk and she used to tell us that her Sunday School teacher told her
> it went to the weakest part of the body.[140]

Mrs. Dent, born in 1908 and also from Preston, remembered her grandfather favoring use of herbs and poulticing, particularly as an alternative
to surgery: "He said, 'Now look, there's always something in all the flowers
and there's always something as God sends in hedgerows as can cure. It's
a good remedy for something!' Same as knitbone, as I told you before. It's
the finest thing you can use."[141] Mrs. Lodge, born in 1922, also recalled her
grandparents mixing and applying herbal medicines:

> My grandfather, you'll have seen him with these little boxes to grind
> herbs. We always had one of those, and my granddad used to collect
> herbs, and always do, he used to call it rubbing stuff, you know for
> aches and pains. He always did his own rubbing stuff. And different
> remedies for different things. He was very, very good at it, and as I said,
> my grandma, although she wasn't a nurse, she used to look after all the
> children in the family, you know, while their mothers went to work. And

---

of porcelain; first employed by the Chinese, but subsequently obtained also in Cornwall, Saxony,
France (near Limoges), United States, etc."

137. See, for example, Mrs. A2B, 65; Mr. B4P, 30; Mrs. F1L, 51; Mr. F1P, 70 (his family always
used the left sock); Mrs. H6L, 84; Mrs. H7P, 29; Mrs. N1L, 15; Mrs. O1B, 55; Mrs. T2L, 80; Mrs.
W5B, 50.

138. See, for example, Mrs. A3P, 4; Mrs. B2B, 43; Mrs. C8P, 87; Mr. G2L, 9; Mr. K2P, 198; Mrs.
L3B, 71; Mr. M1L, 25; Mrs. M3P, 16; Mrs. M5L, 15.

139. See, for example, Mrs. D2P, 12; Mrs. H2P, 5; Mrs. H7P, 28; Mrs. L3P, 35; Mrs. R1P, 54–5;
Mrs. R3B, 55–6; Mrs. S3B, 72; Mr. S7L, 80; Mrs. T4B, 74; Mr. W3P, 29; Mrs. W4P, 43; Mrs. W6P,
50.

140. Miss T1P, 42.

141. Mrs. D1P, 23, 39.

she used to, if anyone was sick in the street, they used to come for her. And she wasn't educated.[142]

Use of herbal remedies was considered an inexpensive alternative to consulting the doctor; however, informants also claimed herbs could yield superior results. According to Mrs. Huddleston, born in 1916:

> It was my father really, it was all herbs. He had a herb book and whatever was wrong with us, mother would go to town to the herb shop and they were always brewed and given to you. The doctor then, it was all paying for the doctor. . . . For the cold it was elder blossom and peppermint that I always remember. It was brewed and oh, it was bad. It had an awful taste. It was boiled in a pan in muslin, but by gum, it shifted that cold in a night. As soon as we came from school or work it was on top of this oven brewed ready and you took a cupful of that with a cupful of treacle in it and to bed. It would sweat it right out of you. Then you were right for work the day after. You weren't as ill with it because this elder blossom, it sweated everything out of you, but you went to bed soon enough as soon as you came home. . . . It was herbs for everything.[143]

Mrs. Lewthwaite, born in 1920, said, "Mother was great believer in herbs, really. Even to her last day, she used a lot of comfrey, it's for all sorts of things, bathing swellings, or you can drink it as tea or you can have tablets. It's very good."[144]

A few informants described use of magical cures. Red flannel, worn as a plaster or a belt, was thought to have special salutary properties—perhaps heat, associated with both the soft fabric and the red color. Mrs. Masterson, born in 1913 in Preston, compared adult use of preventative red flannel belts to the pervasive use of belly-binders for newborn infants:

> In those days, I remember, a lot of elderly people, men as well, they had like babies in those days. When they were born they used to put what they called a binder. . . . They had like a string through. Well, the elderly people used to make those themselves. They would go on the market and get this red flannel and make these broad belts. They always wore them and it was to keep them warm, you see. If they had these pains and that, it would be the red flannel belt. They all had them on. They were old-fashioned remedies, you know.[145]

Similarly, Mrs. Winder, born in 1910 in Lancaster, remembered: "I used to do a lot of coughing and well they thought at one time that I was going

142. Mrs. L3P, 34.
143. Mrs. H7P.
144. Mrs. L3B, 71.
145. Mrs. M1P, 42

to be consumptive. They used to rub m'chest with camphorated oil, and I had a little vest sort of thing that went over the back and round the front, made out of red flannel and tied round the waist. This was soaked in camphorated oil. Oh, I used to stink like a polecat. I used to hate the stuff, but it was very effective."[146] Several informants recalled their mothers rubbing a sty with a golden wedding ring—perhaps in association with the proprietary Golden Eye Ointment.[147] However, unique to Lancaster was a spring thought to have curative powers. Mrs. Nance, born in 1899, discussed this matter with her son, born in 1928:

> *Mr. Nance:* I'll tell you another well-known thing, spring well water. You know where the garage is on Morecambe Road near the Catholic school, between the social club and that garage there used to be a well. A spring well as we used to call it, and it used to come from there and out into the [River] Lune. It was only like a trickle and there was always watercress. That water, a lot of the older people same as my granddad, always believed in that water. They used to go and get bottles of it and keep it for winter for bathing sore eyes.
>
> *Mrs. Nance:* I've a niece now who is fifty-four and she was born with a bent leg and they said that it would never come right. I used to have to get bottles of that water, and m'brother used to rub it down and they always said that that straightened her leg. Old people in that area were big believers in that water. Mrs. Kirkby used to go down for two or three bottles a day. She was seventy or eighty year old and you'd see her going first thing in a morning and then last thing at night with the bottles. She used to drink it, wash in it. If they had sore throats, they used to gargle with the water and then put a stocking round with a warm potato.[148]

As these examples indicate, home care was not limited to children. Throughout the life course, health was maintained and ill-health dealt with at home when possible.[149] We will be considering traditional neighborhood- and home-management of childbearing in chapter 6; however, it is important to note here that almost all working-class births and postpartum care took

146. Mrs. W2L, 59.

147. Mrs. O1B, 55; Mrs. P6B, 123.

148. Mrs. N1L, 15. A Lancaster chemist, Mr. Chambers, born in 1896(?), also remembered waters of this spring being used as an eye lotion and for bathing sore legs. See Mr. C6L, 6–7.

149. See Peregrine Horden and Richard Smith, eds., *The locus of care: Families, communities, institutions and the provision of welfare since Antiquity* (London and New York: Routledge, 1998), particularly the Introduction, 1–18; and Peregrine Horder, "Household care and informal networks: Comparisons and continuities from antiquity to the present," 21–70, for discussion of both institutional and charitable care available to the poor and the observation that "self-help and domestic care constitute the great submerged ice sheets of the history of health, as also of the history of poverty in general. We perforce devote most of our attention to the visible peaks and ridges of documented medical practice and institutional support. Yet we also have to find ways of reminding ourselves how small a proportion of the whole subject is actually in view" (23).

place at home before the 1920s. Equally, until after World War II it was usual for people with acute serious illnesses as well as the elderly, disabled, chronically ill, and the dying to be cared for at home. The interviews contain instances of people receiving institutional care—particularly surgical cases and victims of contagious diseases, who were treated at local infirmaries and isolation hospitals; sufferers from mental illnesses who were sent to asylums; and older adults who went to workhouses in their final years.[150] However, these examples are rare and often involved compulsion or pressure from public health or medical authorities; it was more common for the ailing to be looked after at home, whatever the toll on the caregiver and his or her family. Indeed, taking responsibility for home care and avoiding the shame of institutional care (especially in the workhouse) for elderly or disabled relatives was clearly linked with a woman's or family's respectability. Mrs. Arnold, born in 1910, expressed this association:

> There was just Auntie and Cousin Lily next door and then we had Grandma with us. Then she had a seizure and there was four children of us and as my mother said, we kept being born one after the other, and she had this seizure when she wasn't quite 71 and she was 77 when she died. She was in bed all that time. It paralyzed her all down one side and she could get out of bed with her good side but couldn't get back. So my auntie next door took her and she had her in the front room in the bed downstairs and my mother looked to her in the daytime and Auntie looked to her at night. . . . I think you thought it was your duty in those days. None of our relatives have ended up in homes or anything. My mother lived with my eldest sister over thirty years and as I say, my eldest sister is 70, no 71, and mother is 99 this year and she has got to be constantly watched but we wouldn't dream of putting her away, I would put myself in the cemetery before that.[151]

Similarly, Mrs. Crest, born in 1897, looked after her elderly aunt and mother in her own home. "The nurse said I was a credit because my mother, she hadn't a bed sore. I used to be a slave to keep her comfortable, well you do if you are a decent sort of person." She also looked after her mentally handicapped brother until shortly before his death.[152] Occasionally, elder care was traded for housing. Mrs. Yardley, born in 1927, having lived in a rented room with her husband and newborn daughter (Mrs. Paulson, born 1948), moved in with her blind great-aunt and looked after her for 16 years before her death.[153] However, this arrangement also supported the family's reputation.

Several informants remembered their mothers being chronically ill when they were children—a situation that posed special challenges, since

150. See, for example, Mrs. C3P, 48; Mrs. A4L, 21; Mr. F2P, 6–7.
151. Mrs. A1P, 4. See also Mr. D2P, 63; Mr. I2L, 76–77.
152. Mrs. C3P, 3, 48.
153. Mrs. Y1L, 44–45; Mrs. P3L, 6–7.

mothers generally took responsibility for family health care. Often grandmothers stepped in to help. Mrs. Ralston, born in 1889, remembered, "We went to live in m'grandma's house in Rodney Street, and that was where my mother died. She was thirty-nine. She'd been in hospital and had her breast off, and then half a breast off. When we were living at that house, my father had rheumatic fever again. We'd to live and there was seven of us to keep."[154] In other cases, the family muddled along with children caring for each other and their mother. Mrs. Yardley recalled that her mother was always ailing:

> Well, she always had asthma and things, and then when she had the nervous breakdown she got worse. . . . Well, I can't really remember a lot about it, but I know she had one because we had gone out and she was lighting the gas mantle, you know, old fashioned, and it set fire and after that she was never right.
>
> *Interviewer:* Well, how did the family manage the breakdown, did she have to go into hospital?
>
> *Informant:* No, I don't think she went in hospital. Her nerves all went, her nerves all just went really, you know. And then she got all right after, apart from her asthma and bronchitis and things, that was very bad. She had that, as long as I can remember she had that until her dying.

Mrs. Yardley's brother missed a lot of school to stay home and look after their mother.[155]

The Fleming's experience, old-fashioned for the post–World War II period, exemplified traditional home-based care. In 1935 at age 14, Mrs. Fleming and her extended family including her parents and her older sister (Nanny) and Nanny's husband moved into a four-bedroom house in Lancaster. Mrs. Fleming stayed there after her marriage in 1941 and raised her six children (all born by 1950) there. She and Nanny (who remained childless) cared for the children and also for her parents until they died at home: "Fortunately, they were just senile, they were just tired, if you understand. I was really glad there was nothing really wrong with them. Because they had all had hard lives in them days, hadn't they?" They also looked after Nanny's husband, whose care was more difficult:

> Well, he had an ulcer on his face and he went [to] Christies [Hospital, in Manchester] then. It was terrible having them taken off, and he never recovered, and he had kind of a stroke. Oh, it's really rotten to talk about it. He used to like do his business and he would have it in his pocket and all sorts. And you had it all to clean up. . . . For the last

154. Mrs. R1B, 5, 28.
155. Mrs. Y1L, 8. See also Mrs. B2P, 33; Mrs. P1L, 58.

eighteen months he only breathed.

Interviewer: Did he stay at home though?

Informant: Oh yes, she wouldn't let him go away.

Interviewer: So she looked after him?

Informant: Well, she did in a way, she was working so she looked after him when she came home at night, but it was to me.

Interviewer: It was to you, so everyone was still living in the same house?

Informant: Yes, and my six children as well. . . . Oh yes, shocking it was. Washing, and I had no washing machine. I was washing for twelve.[156]

Despite—or perhaps *because* of—the difficulty, working-class women's obligation and capacity to provide care, in addition to being important components of their traditional identities and roles, fostered their confidence about dealing with health matters. Mr. Ford, born in 1906, commented: "I don't know that my own mother would want advice from anyone! She would more often give it than want it! There was nobody to turn to, only relations. They all had such big families! They had a wealth of experience in bringing children up and babies being born. More so than what they have today. If a baby had a tummy-ache or anything like that, they didn't run to the doctor. We are the same! If you are brought up like that, we don't run to the doctor every five minutes. We should know ourselves with our own ideas!"[157] In matters of health, as with traditional capacity to make do and mend family clothing and household furnishings (e.g., peg rugs), working-class women's lack of resources made them resourceful, and their lack of support from formally qualified "experts," combined with experience and practice, spurred their competence and self-reliance.[158]

That working-class homes were the primary environments for illness and care affected relationships between medical professionals and family members. General practitioners, midwives, and nurses were invited into sufferers' homes and negotiated treatment and care arrangements with the women who would implement them. Consequently, power dynamics were very different in home than in institutional settings—a factor that influenced medical pressure for hospitalization and provision of a growing range of clinic-based services. For example, in 1913 Dr. H. O. Pilkington, Medical Officer of Health for Preston, argued that hospitalization for contagious diseases protected the public from the spread of infection allowed by careless family members who were unable or unwilling to enforce isolation rules at home. In addition,

156. Mrs. F1L, 13, 14, 53–55.
157. Mr. F1P, 73.
158. See, for example, Roberts, *A woman's place,* 128, 151.

Apart from this, and as regards the great majority of cases in a manu-facturing town like this, it is certain that it is to the patient's advantage that he should be removed to some institution, where he will have greater air space, and stricter cleanliness than at home, and where he will have the benefit of that attention to all those matters—great and small—which combined together go to form a system of careful and efficient nursing. And it is in the convalescent, as well as in the acute, stage of the illness that the constant observation to which a hospital patient is subjected does so much good, since if it does not always pre-vent, it at any rate ensures the early recognition of those after effects so frequently met with in the treatment of infectious diseases. A mild case of Scarlet Fever may be followed by Nephritis, Enlarged Glands, or Ear mischief, Cardiac failure, or Paralysis may attack the patient who has apparently recovered from Diphtheria, whilst the mistaken kindness of his friends, by supplying solid food at too early a stage, may bring about the death of the Typhoid convalescent. But in Hospital, where a patient is under constant observation, and where the temperature is regularly and frequently taken, the first appearance of these after-effects is at once noted, and immediate steps can be taken to deal with them.[159]

Here Pilkington rejected the long tradition of amateur home care in favor of professional institutional care, using worst-case scenario rhetoric that became common for a variety of conditions, including childbearing. This type of argument was increasingly accepted by local policymakers, middle-class ratepayers [property-tax payers] and voters, and, ultimately, working-class people, who began to view hospitals as safe and homes as unsafe places to be ill, and doctors and nurses as competent and mothers and grannies as incompetent care providers. The status of professional care rose among working-class people, while that of home care declined. Thus, Mrs. How-ard, born in 1931 in Lancaster, remembered it being a sign of poverty for children to walk around with cotton wool in their ears.[160]

The flipside of growing working-class dependence on professional and institutional medicine in the mid-twentieth century was women's reduced confidence in their own ability to manage health and ill-health within their households. For example, Mrs. Boyle's first baby, born in the mid-1950s, cried constantly. Her mother-in-law, with whom she was living while her husband finished his national service, advised her to take the infant to the doctor to see whether there was anything "internal" wrong with him. The general practitioner checked the baby thoroughly, found nothing wrong, and advised Mrs. Boyle to wrap him warmly, turn the radio up, and put him out in the yard in his pram between feeds. Her mother-in-law agreed with

159. Preston MOH Report 1913, 6, 25.
160. Mrs. H5L, 1931.

this advice. The child health clinic nurse stopped by, checked on the baby, and advised Mrs. Boyle to "keep doing that."[161] There are many elements of this situation that might explain Mrs. Boyle's inability to cope—a difficult mother-in-law on whom Mrs. Boyle was dependent, shared living accommodation that complicated the challenge of managing a noisy infant, and first-baby jitters. However, it is indisputable that in the 1950s Mrs. Boyle sought and acted on much more advice from professionals than her counterpart would have done a generation earlier. In this case, the physician's and health visitor's recommendations were more culturally than medically dictated and were probably similar to what working-class neighbors would have suggested in an earlier period. However, the status of the health care professionals was quite different from that of the neighbors; furthermore, their authority stemmed from their credentials rather than from their personal reputations in the neighborhood—a development that characterized the transformation of working-class health culture after World War II.

An important factor that had strengthened working-class faith in biomedicine by the post–World War II years was increased perceived effectiveness of medical interventions. When asked if she gave her daughter traditional home remedies, Mrs. Owen, born in 1916, responded: "If something happened to her, I used to take her to the doctor's and get the *proper* thing. . . . Well, I let Mum goose grease if she [daughter] has a bad chest. I used to say, that child's got a bad chest, and out would come the jar of goose grease. An earthenware jar with a piece of brown paper with a rubber ring round, and she would come down and rub her back and front. In the end, I took her to the doctor and he gave me some antibiotics and it cleared up in no time."[162] Mrs. Owen straddled the divide between traditional working-class health culture and working-class conversion to the emerging national culture of biomedicine.

THE CONSTRUCTION OF "OLD WIVES" AND PROFESSIONAL AUTHORITY

The early years of the period under consideration witnessed parallel growth in attention to working-class health issues, the professionalization of public health, and pressure on working-class people to use formal medicine.[163]

---

161. Mrs. B11P, 46.

162. Mrs. O1B, 58.

163. See, for example, Jane Lewis, *What price community medicine: The philosophy, practice and politics of public health since 1919* (Brighton, Sussex: Wheatsheaf Books, 1986); David Armstrong, *Political anatomy of the body: Medical knowledge in Britain in the twentieth century* (Cambridge: Cambridge University Press, 1983); Ann Hardy, *Health and medicine in Britain since 1860* (Houndmills, Basingstoke, Hampshire: Palgrave, 2001); Helen Jones, *Health and society in twentieth-century Britain* (London and New York: Longman, 1994).

Spurred by the rhetoric of national degeneration, fed by fears of imperial decline, and encouraged by developments in the new field of bacteriology, upper- and middle-class reformers, policymakers, and service providers emphasized the importance of changing working-class domestic behavior to reduce infant mortality rates and improve the fitness of potential workers and soldiers.[164] Necessarily, the focus was on working-class women who were responsible for all matters relating to household health. Furthermore, because of the linked influence of neighborly support and older women on working-class health care, the effort to change behavior included discouragement of mutual aid and demonization of informal health authorities. Jane Lewis argues:

> It was ironic that in prescribing middle-class ideas of responsible motherhood, child and maternal welfare policies often discouraged already existing patterns of mutual aid between women. For example, the health visitor competed with the grandmother and neighbors for the role of adviser, and the local authority-approved home help and the trained midwife with the "handywoman," who was proscribed by law but highly valued by working-class women, because she both delivered the baby and looked after the family. The leaders of working women's organizations also had occasion to deplore the patronizing attitudes which child and maternal welfare workers often exhibited towards their clients.[165]

As Lewis indicates, the effort to transform working-class health culture was local, carried forward by health authorities including Medical Officers of Health and the health visitors who were appointed in Barrow, Lancaster, and Preston in the years before World War I. Their accounts blamed mothers for most morbidity and mortality in working-class families. For example, in Barrow, where infant mortality rates began to drop in the 1880s, the Medical Officer of Health who had written in 1884, "More young children lose their lives from the ignorance and mismanagement of mothers than from any other cause," wrote in 1888, "Young children are peculiarly susceptible to insanitary influences, and an improvement in their death-rate not only points to better feeding and nursing, but also to better sanitary regulations and fewer nuisances."[166] While all MOsH worked to improve public and domestic sanitation, they agreed that without change in work-

---

164. As Behlmer points out in *Friends of the family* (31–62), such attempts to influence working-class family norms was not new in the early twentieth century, but grew out of religious "district visiting" dating back to the eighteenth century and became institutionalized in occupations such as district nursing and health visiting.

165. Jane Lewis, *The politics of motherhood: Child and maternal welfare in England, 1900–1930* (London: Croom Helm, 1980), 20–21.

166. Barrow MOH Report, 1884, 201; Barrow MOH Report, 1888, 193.

ing-class mothers' behavior, infants and young children would continue to die unnecessarily.

What did health authorities think were working-class mothers' main deficiencies? In 1896 Dr. Pilkington of Preston reported: "There are few people with less knowledge or experience of household duties than the ordinary factory girl, and as a consequence she becomes a wife and mother knowing little of the duties required of her, and content, as regards the management of her children, to follow the example of her parents and the customs of those amongst whom she lives."[167] According to this MOH, ignorance and adherence to community traditions contributed to working-class mothers' difficulty in keeping their children alive. In addition, he blamed infant deaths on female employment, early marriage, failure to breastfeed, unsanitary preparation of feeding bottles, infants sharing parents' beds, maternal drunkenness, consultation of informal female neighborhood health authorities, and the practice of buying burial insurance for children, "by which the death of a child brings monetary gain to the parents."[168] Preston's infant mortality rate remained stubbornly high, even compared to other Lancashire cotton towns.[169] Dr. Pilkington's negative views of working-class women arguably reflect both frustration and fear that his employers might hold him responsible for the city's poor health record.

Although not as voluble as Pilkington, the MOsH for Barrow and Lancaster agreed that working-class mothers' ignorance caused unnecessary sickness and death.[170] As we will see in chapter 4, they also viewed relationships among neighbors as potentially dangerous, sometimes contributing to the spread of contagious diseases. In 1900, while advocating the expansion of local isolation hospital facilities, Barrow's MOH wrote:

> There can be no question that a case of scarlatina removed from a working man's house with a large family to a well-conducted Isolation Hospital is much less likely to affect others than if left at home. . . . There was no doubt a great amount of gross carelessness on the part of mothers in allowing their infected children to run about and mix with healthy children. . . . I tried to get evidence against some people in Worcester Street, but the neighbors refused to give any evidence to be used in Court, so that the attempt failed. In all cases parents were personally warned against allowing their infected children to mix with healthy children during the six weeks, but I suspect this had very little effect in

167. Preston MOH Report, 1896, 10.
168. Preston MOH Report, 1898, 7; Preston MOH Report, 1899, 14; Preston MOH Report, 1900, 13; Preston MOH Report, 1902, 10–12; Preston MOH Report, 1906, 8–9; Preston MOH Report, 1911, 10–11.
169. Walton, *Social history,* 310.
170. Lancaster MOH Report, 1919, 18; Barrow MOH Report, 1912, 240, 282.

most cases. Isolation would alone place an infected child in a position of safety as regards other children.[171]

The contrast between public health authorities' value for isolation and working-class mothers' regard for neighborliness and mutual aid is apparent. Since disease and prevention were handled in working-class homes and neighborhoods, health authorities were obliged to challenge working-class health culture there.

With Medical Officers of Health nationally, local MOsH agreed that one potentially successful approach was appointment of "Lady" health visitors—a description that reflected the class implications of "ladies" encouraging working-class mothers to adopt middle-class behavior but also suggests the ironic effort to replace traditional neighborhood health authorities with a new kind of health advisor to working-class households.[172] According to Barrow's Dr. Settle in 1907, "We have no female officer, either as Health Visitor or School Nurse, to advise the poor people at their homes—to keep them clean, advise as regards the baby and the children generally. I am sure a great deal could be done in this direction to improve things."[173] Preston appointed its first health visitor in 1902, Lancaster in 1903, and Barrow during World War I.[174] Health visitors began by calling on new mothers and babies as soon as possible after birth. As time went on, they expanded their activities to visiting sufferers from notifiable contagious diseases and expectant mothers.

In 1910 Lancaster's Medical Officer of Health was concerned about "wasting diseases" among infants, in which he included

premature birth, congenital defects, injury at birth, want of breast milk, starvation, atrophy, debility, marasmus. . . . This is, in my opinion, work which is best attempted by the quiet talks of the Lady Health Visitor with mothers. I do not consider lectures and pamphlets to be of very much use. No doubt a card of instructions, which can be hung on the walls of the dwelling, and is sufficiently ornamental to be pleasing to the

171. Barrow MOH Report, 1900, 192–93.

172. Lancaster's annual reports of the Medical Officer of Health for some years included reports of the "Lady Health Visitor." See, for example, Lancaster MOH Report, 1907, 25–26. See also Celia Davies, "The health visitor as mother's friend: A woman's place in public health, 1900–14," *Social History of Medicine* 1:1 (1988): 39–59; Dingwall et al., *Social history of nursing,* 173–203.

173. Barrow MOH Report, 1907, 199. The need for Lady Visitors was reiterated in Barrow's 1909 MOH report, 251.

174. Preston MOH Report, 1902, 12; Barrow MOH Report, 1917, 249; Michael Winstanley, "The town transformed, 1815–1914," in Andrew White, ed., *A history of Lancaster 1193–1993* (Keele: Keele University Press, 1993), 181. Preston and Lancaster were early participants in this national trend, since, according to Dingwall et al., *Social history of nursing,* 185, it was only in 1904 that an Interdepartmental Committee called for "national provision of a 'health visiting' service."

eye, will do a certain amount of good, but it is to the quiet influence of the lady Health Visitor that I chiefly rely for an improvement.[175]

Dr. Pilkington recognized the challenges associated with this approach, writing in 1901:

> The consideration of the subject of Infantile Mortality brought up the question as to the advisability of increasing the Sanitary Staff by the appointment of certain Female District Visitors, whose duties would be, under the control and supervision of the Medical Officer, to visit houses in the poorer parts of the town, and by advice and practical example endeavor to raise the standard of cleanliness and sanitation. Their services would be especially useful in giving instruction as to the management of children, particularly during time of illness, and in abolishing those insanitary living conditions which are so frequently the result of ignorance and want of care. But the value of such instruction depends entirely upon the spirit in which it is received, and in hope that its reception may be beneficial it must be given with tact, in a kindly manner, and with consideration for those shortcomings which too often have become habitual. Anything like ill-judged or unnecessary interference with domestic matters would be unwelcome in the home of a Lancashire operative; whereas a little judicious help, given during the trying time of sickness, would be gratefully acknowledged and received.[176]

Pilkington's doubts about the reception of health visitors by working-class mothers were borne out by early experience in the study communities. Lancaster's Lady Health Visitor reported in 1910 that she had visited 2,258 infants in their homes:

> Some of the facts that these . . . visits have shown me are still not understood, are the difference between clean and unclean milk; fresh air and poisoned air; muffling up and exposing a child, and real warm clothing; neither is the fact that a child should be taken out at least once every fine day readily understood; an evening's entertainment in some badly ventilated room, or a gossip at the front door with the child in a draught between back and front doors is frequently considered as good as a walk in the open air; healthy babies are very often dosed with some preparation at regular intervals, quite regardless of the fact that the child requires nothing at all of the sort; many infants always sleep between two adults, and remonstrance is generally laughed at—"the

175. Lancaster MOH Report, 1910, 22.
176. Preston MOH Report, 1901, 17.

Health Visitor is a crank, a silly thing." On the other hand, there are some splendid mothers who achieve a great deal by sensible judgment, and are delightful to meet and cooperate with.[177]

It is clear that the health visitor's advice had class-related resource implications: access to clean milk, fresh air, and real warm clothing together with leisure and energy for a daily walk were more common among middle- than among working-class women. The health visitor's comments also reveal a cultural divide, including disdain for working-class women's leisure activities ("an evening's entertainment in some badly ventilated room, or a gossip at the front door") and approval of women who display "sensible judgment" by taking her advice—as opposed to the apparently more typical working-class opinion that "the Health Visitor is a crank, a silly thing." Further in her report, the health visitor made clear the fatal consequences of noncompliance: "I am quite aware that a supply of clean milk is not everything; dirty beds, clothes, floors, and general surroundings are all very conducive to the spreading of a disease of this kind [infant diarrhea], and are repeatedly pointed out, and the reckless exposure of all the family food to flies in the summer is deplorable. One often sees food left on the table from meal to meal, and the less perishable kinds, such as bread, butter, and sugar have their permanent place on some tables, thereby getting infected from flies."[178] She went on to speculate that scarlet fever would be less prevalent and dangerous if "it were possible to secure the more cordial cooperation of parents in the disinfection of articles of clothing, etc., which may possibly have been in contact with the sick person."[179] Leaving aside the question of the "correctness," from our vantage point, of her health knowledge and recommendations, there can be no doubt that while this health visitor was altruistically motivated, she also helped to construct and perpetuate an image of the ignorant, willfully careless, working-class woman—the problem for which she was expected to be the remedy. Embodying, as she did, the physical and social surveillance exercised by institutionalized public health, as well as displaying a patronizing and superior demeanor, it is not surprising that a number of oral history informants remembered resentment of the health visitor, referred to by one woman's mother-in-law as "an interfering busybody."[180]

While there were variations in the extent to which public health authorities blamed working-class women for their family's problems, the same

177. Lancaster MOH Report, 1910, 26.
178. Lancaster MOH Report, 1910, 26.
179. Lancaster MOH Report, 1910, 26.
180. Mrs. J1B, 64. See also, for example, Mrs. C2B, 18; Mrs. H3P, 31; Mrs. H4P, 6; Mrs. M11B, 9. For further discussion of the relationship between public health authorities, social reformers, and working-class people, see Judy Giles, *Women, identity, and private life*, and David Armstrong, *Political anatomy of the body*.

cannot be said for officials' views that informal health authorities, often called "handywomen," represented the most dangerous aspects of working-class health culture. While more will be said about traditional midwives in chapter 6, it is worthy of remark here that the characteristics Charles Dickens gave Sarah Gamp—drunkenness, carelessness, and enthusiastic willingness to attend either "a lying-in or a laying-out"—were extended by health officials to handywomen, who, in addition, were portrayed as old, illiterate, dirty, meddlesome, and unteachable.[181] Their midwifery activities were regulated by the 1902 and subsequent Midwives' Acts. Yet, it was difficult for authorities to enforce the law, and there was nothing to keep handywomen from serving as monthly nurses (who helped mothers and their families during the lying-in period), laying out the dead, or offering advice. According to Dr. Pilkington in 1918, in Preston, "There still remains an astonishing predilection for the members of the old school, many of whom possess only the merest rudiments of general education. This due to their 'motherly' character, and to the fact that they are bound by long acquaintance, and in some cases by relationship, with the members of their clientele."[182] This observation indicates the MOH's awareness of the position of informal health authorities in working-class neighborhoods and his eagerness to uncouple health care from its traditions in those neighborhoods. The handywoman was coming to represent the destructive "old wife" and the "tales" she told, which countered valid biomedical practice. Many of the local health authorities' activities—health education, health visiting, clinic services—were directed at providing alternatives to old wives' tales and undermining the power of handywomen in working-class communities.

As public health providers struggled against working-class health care traditions, they were also trying to raise the scope and status of their own occupations.[183] Beginning with the establishment of MOH positions in the study communities in the late nineteenth century, and continuing with the steady addition of responsibilities (e.g., isolation hospitals, school medi-

181. Charles Dickens, *Martin Chuzzlewit* (Harmondsworth: Penguin, 1968. First published in 1843–44), 378. The on-line *OED* defines a gamp as "An umbrella, esp. one tied up in a loose, untidy fashion." Joan Mottram argues that public health authorities who favored midwife registration tended to portray "handywomen" as gamps, while general practitioners who thought that registered midwives would compete with them for patients were more tolerant of unqualified midwives; see Mottram, "State control in local context: Public health and midwife regulation in Manchester, 1900–1914," in Hilary Marland and Anne Marie Rafferty, eds., *Midwives, society and childbirth: Debates and controversies in the modern period* (London and New York: Routledge, 1997), 134–52. For MOH descriptions of "handywomen," see, for example, Barrow MOH Report, 1904, 209; Barrow MOH Report, 1906, 200; Barrow MOH Report, 1912, 242; Lancaster MOH Report, 1912, 70–71; Lancaster MOH Report, 1920, 28; Lancaster MOH Report, 1926, 42; Preston MOH Report, 1904, 17; Preston MOH Report, 1905, 33; Preston MOH Report, 1908, 14; Preston MOH Report, 1918, 12.

182. Preston MOH Report, 1918, 12.

183. See, for example, Lewis, *What price community medicine;* Anthony S. Wohl, *Endangered lives: Public health in Victorian Britain* (London: J. M. Dent & Sons, 1983), 166–204.

cal inspection, clinics) and personnel (e.g., health visitors, school nurses, school dentists) in the early twentieth century, the success of local health departments depended on their ability to make positive visible changes. Thus, the same narratives that disparaged working-class traditions, behaviors, and people praised and credited the efforts of public health providers. For example, in 1916 Dr. Pilkington reported a dramatic reduction in infant deaths from diarrhea in Preston, which he attributed mainly to "improved general sanitation and to the work of the Health Visitors in connection with the notification of births and the supervision of infants and young children at the various Maternity Centers. Slowly . . . but still gradually and steadily, information is being spread as to the correct method of nursing and feeding young infants."[184] Similarly, in 1921 Barrow's MOH wrote: "This fall in the infant mortality rate is more than a coincidence, and is, in my opinion, attributable to the supervision, treatment, and educational work done by the Medical Officer in charge of the work (Dr. Wallace), and her staff of Health Visitors. It should be noted that very simple skilled advice given to a young mother will, in many cases, save the life of a baby."[185] These examples suggest that the image and professionalization of public health depended, in part, on the inability of working-class women to manage effectively the health of their families.

As public health services proliferated in the study communities, other types of formal health care providers, including general practitioners, dentists, and hospitals, became increasingly viable alternatives to traditional self-care for working-class people. Favored by both governmental policies and local self-help vehicles including friendly societies and hospital schemes, official health care—at least for workers and children—challenged working-class health culture in the early twentieth century. The following chapter will consider working-class access to, use of, and attitudes regarding formal health care provision in the study communities before 1948.

---

184. Preston MOH Report, 1916, 8.
185. Barrow MOH Report, 1921, 338.

Chapter Three

❦

"We know what's good for you"

*Formal Health Care Provision
in Barrow, Lancaster, and Preston*

The availability and the utilization of medical services are quite different matters. Despite conventional presumptions that morbidity and mortality are due to lack of formal health information and care, that health and longevity result from professional medical treatment, and that "patients" will automatically welcome these services if they are offered, the evidence shows rather that people seek, accept, and reject available health care resources at different times in different places and for a variety of reasons. Local conditions, social class, ethnicity, gender, economic realities, and culture affect people's choices about how to deal with birth, illness, injury, disability, and death. Furthermore, national studies can be vague or misleading about the use of medical care, implicitly offering urban as representative experience. For example, while many residents of large English cities, including Manchester and London, used inpatient hospital care during the second half of the nineteenth century, people living in smaller communities or rural areas became accustomed to hospitalization much later and were hospitalized for somewhat different reasons.[1] Furthermore, while some

---

1. See, for example, John V. Pickstone, *Medicine and industrial society: A history of hospital development in Manchester and its region, 1752–1946* (Manchester: Manchester University Press, 1985); Marjorie Levine-Clark, *Beyond the reproductive body: The politics of women's health and work in early Victorian England* (Columbus: The Ohio State University Press, 2004); Lara Marks, "Mothers, babies and hospitals: 'The London' and the provision of maternity care in East London, 1870–1939" in Valerie Fildes, Lara Marks, and Hilary Marland, eds., *Women and children first: International maternal and infant welfare 1870–1945* (London and New York: Routledge, 1992), 48–73; Andrea Tanner, "Come all, cure few: The diseases of the in-patients at Great Ormond Street Hospital, 1852–1900," unpublished paper delivered at the Social Science History Association conference, November 2005, Portland, Oregon.

scholars argue that there was an oversupply of general practitioners in late-nineteenth- and early-twentieth-century Britain, consultation of physicians was by no means universal or routine, with many people preferring self-treatment or advice from alternative practitioners and chemists.[2] The decision to seek medical attention in working-class Barrow, Lancaster, and Preston before the mid-twentieth century was influenced by factors including financial resources, beliefs about appropriate ways to manage health and illness, and issues associated with social status.

In 1880 the study cities offered a range of formal health care services typical of Lancashire cities and large towns.[3] Each had a voluntary hospital that dealt mainly with accident and surgical cases; indoor and outdoor provision of medical care for paupers under the Poor Law; general practitioners who mainly attended the ailing at home; and chemists, who offered advice and sold medical ingredients, patent remedies, and prescription drugs in shops. In addition, each city possessed a new public health service that by 1920 would expand to include isolation hospital, health visiting, and infant welfare clinic services. There were private dentists who, before the advent of school dentists in the early twentieth century, mainly treated members of the middle and upper classes. There were nurses and midwives with various types of educational attainment, occupational training, and qualifications.[4] And in Lancaster, the County Asylum (established in 1816) admitted people with mental illnesses, while the Royal Albert Asylum (opened in 1864) housed what were then called "idiots and imbeciles in the Northern Counties."[5] There are many excellent studies of professional and institutional medicine.[6] This chapter will not replicate their

2. See, for example, Anne Digby, *The evolution of British general practice 1850–1948* (Oxford: Oxford University Press, 1999), 23–39; Anne Hardy, *Health and medicine in Britain since 1860* (Houndmills, Basingstoke, Hampshire: Palgrave, 2001), 17, 21.

3. For comparative information about hospitals in Lancashire communities, see Pickstone, *Medicine and industrial society.*

4. See Anne Witz, *Professions and patriarchy* (London and New York: Routledge, 1992), for a feminist discussion of the gendered nature of the professionalization of medicine, which effectively excluded female occupations such as midwifery and nursing. See Hilary Marland and Anne Marie Rafferty, eds., *Midwives, society and childbirth: Debates and controversies in the modern period* (London and New York: Routledge, 1997), for comparative international perspectives on the professionalization of midwifery. See Celia Davies, ed., *Rewriting nursing history* (London: Croom Helm, 1980), for diverse viewpoints reinterpreting the standard Whig interpretation of the history of nursing in Britain. See Robert Dingwall, Anne Marie Rafferty, Charles Webster, *A social history of nursing* (London: Routledge, 1988), for contextualization of nursing, midwifery, and health visiting in health care more broadly construed. This study also very usefully critiques the conventional idealized account of Florence Nightingale's role as visionary, champion, and implementer of trained nursing.

5. Michael Winstanley, "The town transformed, 1815–1914," in Andrew White, ed., *A history of Lancaster 1193–1993* (Keele: Keele University Press, 1993), 159–61.

6. See, for example, Anne Digby, *Evolution;* Ivan Waddington, *The medical profession in the Industrial Revolution* (Dublin, Ireland: Gill and Macmillan Humanities Press, 1984); Rosemary Stevens, *Medical practice in modern England: The impact of specialization and state medicine* (New

approaches and source materials. Rather, it will provide an alternative perspective on this history by focusing on working-class relationships with and attitudes toward chemists, general practitioners, and hospitals dealing with physical ailments (including medical specialists and hospital nurses), leaving discussion of public and school health services and midwifery for later chapters. While several oral history informants experienced mental illness and handicap within their families, in-depth discussion of these challenges is beyond the scope of this book.

CHEMISTS

In addition to managing health and illness at home and relying on neighborhood mutual aid for advice, household help, and assistance with nursing, working-class people typically consulted chemists, who offered advice and first aid, provided preliminary diagnoses, and sold medical ingredients, patent remedies, and prescription drugs.[7] Within the memory of older informants, some chemists also pulled teeth.[8] The many oral history accounts of interactions with chemists are explained, to some extent, by chemists' increasing numbers and availability; as Anne Hardy points out, the number of shops licensed to sell patent medicines grew from about 10,000 in 1865 to more than 40,000 in 1905.[9] The chemist bridged traditional working-class and biomedical health cultures, supporting self- and home care and, at the same time, interpreting biomedical information for customers and referring sufferers to general practitioners and hospitals.[10] It is worthy of remark that the boundary between pharmacy and medicine was more porous in the early years of the study period than it later became, with many general practitioners dispensing medication, and some chemists having formal medical or surgical training. However, as tradespeople living behind or above shops in working-class neighborhoods, chemists presented less of a social class barrier than did physicians.[11] Indeed, the relationship between shopkeeper and customer

Haven: Yale University Press, 1966); Pickstone, *Medicine and industrial society;* Brian Abel-Smith, *The hospitals 1800–1948: A study in social administration in England and Wales* (Cambridge, MA: Harvard University Press, 1964).

7. According to Anne Digby, *Evolution,* "British sales of patent medicine increased from half a million pounds in the mid-nineteenth century to five million by 1914, with a particularly rapid growth occurring from the 1870s. The sufferer's growing predilection for self-medication was shown clearly by the fact that expenditures on patent medicines increased twice as fast as real wages" (228).

8. See, for example, Mr. C6L, 4; Mrs. A3B, 40; Mr. W3P, 30.

9. Hardy. *Health and medicine,* 21.

10. Stuart Anderson and Virginia Berridge, "The role of the community pharmacist in health and welfare, 1911–1986," in Joanna Bornat, Robert Perks, Paul Thompson, and Jan Walmsley, eds., *Oral history, health and welfare* (London and New York: Routledge, 2000), 48–74.

11. Stuart Anderson, "'I remember it well': Oral history in the history of pharmacy," *Social*

may have appealed to laypeople because it lacked both the class and professional power of the doctor, on the one hand, and the deference and passivity of the "patient," on the other. Nonetheless, oral history evidence shows that chemists' training and expertise gave them authority, while their prices—affordable by comparison with general practitioners' fees—attracted low-income consumers.

Mrs. Masterson, born in 1913 in Preston, recalled:

There were a lot of chemist shops. There would be three or four in every district; perhaps in every street there would be one. We would go for ointments and for earache and toothache. It would be cloves for your tooth and olive oil for your ear and they had a special bottle for your throat. If you were ill and didn't feel well, you would tell the chemist your symptoms and he would make a bottle up of his own. You bought the bottle from him. The chemists were really useful in those days before this insurance scheme [the National Health Service] came. I think they did good work.

Interviewer: Why do you think people went to the chemist as opposed to going to the doctor?

Informant: I suppose they would have to pay for the doctor and it was expensive, where at the chemist it wasn't. You would get a bottle for 3d or 4d, perhaps 2d if it wasn't too much. Then there was a lot of olive oil used in those days and linseed oil. They used to mix them. Then there were special ointments and different things.[12]

This informant's account emphasized the accessibility and moderate cost of chemists' advice and wares. Other interviewees also focused on the chemist's knowledge and skill. Mr. Grand, born in Lancaster in 1904, said:

I remember Mr. Shattock and he had his shop on Prospect Street which is now a launderette, at the bottom of Eastham Street. Everybody went to Mr. Shattock, and people would go and get his advice and quite often medicine from him in preference to going to the doctor because he was much cheaper. He was only a chemist, and I'm told, but I don't whether this is true, I think my mother told me that Mr. Shattock would have been a doctor or would have been a surgeon, but he couldn't do the cutting up of people's bodies. He was an extremely clever man. People used to go in there and take the children in and he would look at them and say, "Oh yes, this child has got so-and-so. Take this bottle," and it would be just coppers as against it might be a shilling at the doctor's. Children, if they cut themselves

12. Mrs. M1P, 50.

at all, used to run into Mr. Shattock's shop and he'd put a bandage on and probably never get paid for it.[13]

Several other Lancaster informants echoed similar recollections of the Shattocks.[14]

Mr. Norton, born in 1931, emphasized another Lancaster chemist family's expertise and effectiveness:

> There was a chemist on the corner of Cable Street and North Road called Cuthbert's. And it was a father and son, as I remember, and even into my early twenties, we still went to Cuthbert's for advice on various problems. And he made us up some potion that always seemed to work.
>
> *Interviewer:* Why was it that you preferred the chemist to the doctor?
>
> *Informant:* No waiting room, no long-winded detail and explanations. We could mention to Cuthbert, and I don't think he was ever confronted as a chemist by an original illness, everything he treated somebody had had before. And he produced these bottles you would describe as snake oil and it worked. Whether it was a tummy problem or whatever, and I remember one occasion I traveled by rail every day to Preston and I got an infection, just inside the hairline on the back of my head. And this was spots and that kind of thing, and I kept scratching the thing and making it worse, not realizing. And I decided that I would go and talk to Cuthbert and he immediately recognized what was the cause of it, before I had told him, and he said, "You know, are you traveling by train?" "Yes." "It's been a dirty headrest," and he gave me a bottle, and within two days it had literally cleared it.[15]

This account indicates the longevity of the chemist's importance to working-class health culture; even after the advent of the National Health Service and decline of financial barriers to consultation of physicians, some people continued to view the chemist as the first step in primary care.

However, it is also clear that the chemist's reputation was measured, to some extent, by his likeness to the physician. As we have seen, Mr. Shattock of Lancaster "would have been a doctor," but could not stand doing surgery.[16] Similarly, Mrs. Hocking said her mother relied on a chemist who had trained to be a doctor, but his "health let him down."[17] According to Mrs. Peterson of Preston, born in 1899, her chemist Mr. Gore was "as good

13. Mr. G1L, 15.
14. See, for example, Mr. F1L, 30; Mr. H3L, 15; Mr. V1L, 4; Mrs. W2L, 59.
15. Mr. N2L, 53–54. See also Mrs. F1L, 51; Mrs. L5B, 47.
16. See also Mrs. W2L, 59–60.
17. Mrs. H6L, 84–85.

as a doctor. We would go and ask what he advised and we would get something for sixpence and it were wonderful instead of going to the doctor."[18] Sometimes the chemist was viewed as more effective than the physician. Mrs. Hill, born in 1903 in Preston, said, "We had one of the best chemists there were up here, and he is retired now, but sometimes he could do better than the doctor could."[19] Mr. Vales, born in Lancaster in 1908, remembered that Mr. Shattock dealt effectively with a disease that defeated general practitioners: "One of the prevalent scourges of young children was whooping cough. Highly contagious, and he produced a remedy and working people got to know the symptoms and whip round to old Shatters and spend about sixpence or nine-pence for this. He'd got the nearest thing that was ever known in those days, it didn't actually cure it, but it arrested it and eased that terrible whooping."[20]

It is clear that in the face-to-face society of working-class neighborhoods, chemists' shops, often involving multiple generations of the same family, developed personal relationships and reputations with customers. Many informants remembered and mentioned a particular chemist's name. As we have seen, Lancaster informants talked about the Shattocks and the Cuthberts. Mrs. Burrell from Barrow recalled Mr. Last; Mrs. Peel and Mrs. Sykes from Barrow referred to Mr. Murray; Mrs. Crest from Preston named Mr. Emmot; Mrs. Hocking from Lancaster remembered Mr. Spencely.[21] Mrs. Crest, originally from Oldham but living in Preston, said:

> In fact, we used to go to Penny Street, it was Mr. Collins who had the chemist's and he was from Oldham was Mr. Collins and, of course, how you get to chatting to people, and he was ever so nice and he would give advice on things if there was anything I would ask him, sore throats, or things like that. Err, but he was a real gentleman. I always remember one time, I think it must have been Phil that was ill, and all of a sudden he had to have this medicine and they hadn't got it in, and he [the chemist] even brought it round for me. He was ever so obliging was Mr. Collins. So, yeah, he was nice; now, whether we'd built up this relationship with being from the same town, I don't know.[22]

Mrs. Crest, who was born in 1897, said she was never taken to the doctor when she was ill as a child. Rather, "There was a chemist across the road and my grandmother would go to the chemist if I was ill, which wasn't very often. . . . The chemist was a Mr. Emmot and he was a terrible talker."[23]

18. Mrs. P1P, 72.
19. Mrs. H8P, 51.
20. Mr. V1L, 4.
21. Mrs. B2B, 40; Mrs. C3P, 14; Mrs. H6L, 51; Mrs. P6B, 122; Mrs. S3B, 72.
22. Mrs. C3P, 18–19.
23. Mrs. C3P, 14.

Since an important part of the social life of working-class communities—
particularly for women—involved chatting in local shops, the participation
of chemists in neighborhood conversations enhanced their reputations
and business success.[24]

Chemists were proud of their relationships with working-class customers. Mr. Chambers, who joined his father in 1919 in a Lancaster chemist's
shop, said:

> Mine was a cash business and I was often urged by my accountants to
> buy other businesses in town. They'd say, "Look, if you had the busi-
> ness you'd have names on your books that you'd be proud of." I said,
> "I'm not proud to have any name on my books. The people I'm proud
> of are these people, for instance the mill girls and the men from the
> loco sheds who come in, plonk their money down, and there it is, all
> finished. I'm satisfied, they're satisfied, no booking." The young ones
> don't know us now, but their mothers and grandmothers do. We can't
> walk into town without being stopped many times.[25]

One reason for chemists' popularity was their uncritical support of traditional theories of disease causation, home remedies, and informal health
authorities. Mr. Hope, another Lancaster chemist who qualified in 1930,
provided a commonsense yet scientific-sounding justification for a popular therapy: "Goose grease is goose grease, you could buy it. That was for
chests and sore throats, there was no Vick or anything like that in those
days. It would be goose grease and camphorated oil, the vapors came up
as well. The theory behind putting goose grease was that it was near to the
natural grease of the body and it was absorbed, it sort of took the things
in with it."[26] The chemist Mr. Chambers remembered making a humoral
treatment: "Blisters. Let me see, how shall I describe it, a counter-irritant
to apply to the skin to bring the inflammation up to the surface and then
it would raise a blister and draw the inflammation from inside." When
asked, "What was in these blisters?" Mr. Chambers responded, "It was the
Spanish blistering fly, and that's another product. . . . These flies were little
green beetles ground up, and if put on the skin as an ointment or anything
like that, they would raise a blister." Mrs. Chambers, who helped in the
shop, remembered, "We used to use a lot of antiphlogistics in those days
for pneumonia." Mr. Chambers explained, "Yes, that's kaolin poultice, and
put it on the chest back and front and, again, it's the counter-irritant."
He commented further, "A lot of the old remedies, they were really old

24. See, for example, Melanie Tebbutt, *Women's talk? A social history of 'gossip' in working-class
neighborhoods, 1880–1960* (Aldershot, Hants., Scolar Press: Brookfield, VT: Ashgate Publishing
Co., 1995), 61.
25. Mr. C6L, 13.
26. Mr. H10L, 9.

grandmother's remedies, and they were based on something scientific. You see, . . . a lot of the old things were based on logic and experiences over the centuries, and they were proved right. . . . There used to be their own little recipes that they would bring in. They'd have a pennyworth of oil of peppermint, a pennyworth of oil of aniseed, a pennyworth of paregoric." In response to the interviewer's question, "What was paregoric?" Mr. Chambers said, "It's a camphorated tincture of opium that was given for babies in those days. Quite all right in small doses."[27]

This account raises the issue of chemists' sale and lay use of opiates during the period under consideration. Perhaps the most notorious issue associated with this matter was the administration of "infant cordials" to babies to keep them quiet.[28] Dr. H. O. Pilkington, Medical Officer of Health for Preston, linked this practice to maternal employment and child-minding done by handywomen.[29] However, the oral evidence indicates that use of infant cordials was common and adopted by many working-class people, particularly before World War I. Mrs. Dorrington, born in Preston in 1905, commented:

> For babies, you bought some stuff at the chemists that you could dip their dummies [pacifiers] in to keep them quiet while you got on with your work.
>
> *Interviewer:* What was it called, do you know?
>
> *Informant:* Foster's Cordial.
>
> *Interviewer:* And did your mum have it for you?
>
> *Informant:* Everybody had it, it was the only way they could have their work done and go to work. I don't know what was in it. . . . The old-time chemist's shop or herbalist used to have these three glass jars, one was red, one was green, and one was blue, and we used to get it. I have been for it for my youngest sister at a shop near St. Mary's Church in Friargate. Then they were all done away with and the modern chemist came in.
>
> *Interviewer:* So it was still there after the First World War if your sister had it?

27. Mr. C6L, 4, 6, 22. According to the on-line *OED*, an antiphlogistic is a "medicinal agent allaying inflammation." In *The therapeutic perspective: Medical practice, knowledge, and identity in America, 1820–1885,* 2nd ed. (Princeton: Princeton University Press, 1997), John Harley Warner explains that the dominant therapeutic approach among early-nineteenth-century American physicians could be characterized as a heroic antiphlogistic depletive approach "premised on the belief that most prevailing diseases were overstimulating; while in principle diseases could be either sthenic (*sthénos* = strength) or asthenic, nearly all those the physician encountered were sthenic, tipping the patient's vital balance to a dangerous overexcited condition. The task of treatment was to lower the morbidly animated patient to a healthy, natural state. Sthenic conditions were associated with an inflammatory or phlogistic . . . state; therefore therapy that sought to quench morbid elevation was commonly called antiphlogistic treatment" (91).

28. Anthony S. Wohl, *Endangered lives: Public health in Victorian Britain* (London: Dent, 1983), 34–35.

29. Preston MOH Report, 1900, 13. See also Preston MOH Report, 1896, 10.

Informant: Oh yes. She had it on her dummy like everybody else, and she is 61 now.[30]

Mrs. Maxwell, born in Preston in 1898, was less approving:

I looked after a little boy who was drugged. There used to be a chemist down Marsh Lane and this was when I had two children. This boy was . . . was a proper crybaby and she used to go to this shop and get this Infant's Cordial so that they could sleep at night. When she went to work and I took the child to look after and I used to wheel the child out in his pram he used to look drugged. Somebody once asked me if they gave that child anything. When I said that he had some Infant Cordial they said that it had opium or something like that in. They have stopped it now. I think there was a shop in Friargate too, where you could buy it. It was their own. Forrest, Livesey or something, Forrest Livesey's Infant Cordial, and it was in their own bottle.

Interviewer: But he survived?

Informant: Oh yes. It stopped after a time, it was only while she was working and her husband was on nights. It was to keep this child sleepy because he was a crybaby. . . . It was just stopped after that as there was trouble over it. I think it was opium or something that was in it. The shop has gone now and they used to make it up. It must have been within the law or they wouldn't have made it.[31]

Chemists' sale of opiates over the counter was, indeed, legal, although both the law and cultural norms regarding the sale and use of these substances changed after passage of the Dangerous Drugs Act of 1920, which regulated the import, export, and manufacture of opiates and also limited the amount of morphine, heroin, and cocaine that could be contained in patent medicines.[32] However, while the trend during the twentieth century was to increase the role and power of physicians and limit the discretion of chemists regarding the sale of dangerous drugs, chemists retained a good deal of control over these transactions. Mr. Hope, a Lancaster chemist, mentioned paregoric, a camphorated opium tincture often used to soothe infants, as an example of a remedy that had been requested by older customers but was no longer called for: "Even the young pharmacists, I could guarantee that I could take you to ten pharmacists that have qualified in the last five or six years and I could ask them what paregoric was and they wouldn't have a clue." When asked by the interviewer, "But there was no legal restriction on paregoric?" Mr. Hope responded, "Not in the old days."

30. Mrs. D3P, 7.
31. Mrs. M3P, 38–39.
32. Stuart Anderson and Virginia Berridge, "Opium in 20th-century Britain: Pharmacists, regulation and the people," in *Addiction* 95:1 (2000): 29.

He went on to say, "That was going out by then, but as long as they kept the child quiet, and they were mainly paregoric, which you could buy. You could go into any pharmacy and buy two-pence-worth of paregoric and no questions asked. If anybody came in today and asked for five pence of paregoric today, they wouldn't get it because I wouldn't dream of selling it today." The interviewer asked, "I suppose it would be illegal now?" Mr. Hope replied, "Oh yes, to sell it as such. I mentioned All Fours before, there's nothing to stop me selling that made up ready for consumption as long as you sort of disclose what is inside and the percentage of the paregoric and the date and everything."[33] This account reveals the chemist's ambivalence regarding sale of some preparations containing opiates; he apparently thought paregoric was safe but had stopped selling it, partly because of changes in the law, partly because it was no longer requested, but also probably because of a declining popular consensus about whether its use for infants or minor ailments was appropriate. This change was also reflected in the comments of working-class informants. Mrs. Fleming, born in 1921, remembered that her mother

> used to make some cough medicine, and it were gorgeous, but you can't do it now. It was butter, sugar, vinegar, black treacle and, I don't know whether you have heard? We used to call it paregoric. . . . And old-fashioned fireplaces had a shelf, you know, above, and it used to be in a basin covered up until it had all melted down. And that cured your cold. . . . I went for it once when our Pat [her daughter, born in 1942] had a right bad cough, and I thought, "I'll try this." And the chemist nearly booted me out of the shop.[34]

In addition to potentially addictive drugs, women asked chemists for substances they hoped would induce abortion. While procuring abortion had been made illegal in 1861, the law was unenforceable. According to Barbara Brookes, "Abortion was impossible to police, and, because of the frequency of the act and popular sympathy with the practice, juries were reluctant to convict."[35] As we shall see in chapter 5, before the mid-twentieth century, abortion was a common birth control method among working-class women; the chemist's shop was a usual source of the agents used for this purpose. However, since these agents could often be applied to more

33. Mr. H10L, 2–3, 10. Mr. Hope's recipe for All Fours contained laudanum, aniseed, paregoric, and peppermint, which, mixed with treacle, was used as a cough mixture. Mr. Kennedy, born in Preston in 1930, remembered his mother keeping a cough remedy with this name in the house (Mr. K2P, 198). As we have seen, the chemist Mr. Chambers remembered selling paregoric. In addition, he commented that in the "very old days before my time" opium in solid form ("a little knob") had been sold for toothache (Mr. C6L, 3–4).

34. Mrs. F1L, 49.

35. Barbara Brookes. *Abortion in England 1900–1967* (London, New York, and Sydney: Croom Helm, 1988), 22.

than one health problem and women were loath to ask for an abortifacient, chemists had difficulty determining the reason for a purchase. Mr. Hope recalled:

> Quinine was controlled for several reasons, because it was one of the things that they used to take to produce an abortion. . . . There is what was known as ammoniated tincture of quinine which was sold for colds and could still be sold as we have some in the cellar, but nobody ever asks for it at all. . . . We used to sell quinine powder in 4½ d and 8 d packets, a white envelope, and it was labeled, quinine sulphate powder.
>
> *Interviewer:* Everyone knew what it was for, did they?
>
> *Informant:* Well, it didn't have on, "for abortions," but allegedly they weren't buying it for that, it could have been for a cold, 90 percent of it would be.

Mr. Hope also remembered selling slippery elm bark, which was inserted into the cervix, where it swelled, thus stimulating an abortion.[36]

As we have seen, customers often asked chemists to diagnose and treat minor ailments. Anne Digby points out, "The prescribing or counter-prescribing chemist was ubiquitous and was widely resorted to, especially by the poor."[37] However, chemists also referred sufferers to physicians. Mr. Burton, born in the 1890s in Preston, said, "I remember being taken to the chemist often and my symptoms being listed and the chemist prescribing! If it wasn't too serious, the chemist would do." Mrs. Burton added, "But he would give you advice and if he thought it was the doctor, he would tell you to go."[38] Mr. Chambers explained, "You see, people didn't go unnecessarily to the doctor in those days. . . . We were the first filter, as it were. The trouble was that we had to do things that are not really proper for a chemist. We had to do a bit of diagnosing in our own way and be responsible for it." He was often asked to diagnose children: "It might be just nettle rash—very often it was measles and teething trouble, a little feverishness, constipation, or something like that, the usual childish ailments, but we had to be very very careful in case there was little yellow spots behind the throat, and then right to the doctor. That threw a responsibility onto us that was not really ours, and which wouldn't be permitted now." However, he also maintained, "I think we didn't do much harm, and I think we saved a lot of petty worries from doctors."[39]

Working-class informants were aware of the chemist's screening function. Mr. Cranston, born in 1884, said, "The chemist in those days was

36. Mr. H10L, 11–12.
37. Digby, *Evolution*, 35.
38. Mrs. B5P, 50.
39. Mr. C6L, 2–3.

looked upon more as a doctor's assistant in a way."[40] Mrs. Peterson, born in 1899, said about chemists, "They were as good as a doctor. They wouldn't carry on letting go for things again if it wasn't right. After once or twice if it didn't do, they would tell you to go to the doctor. It would be their fault, wouldn't it, if anything went wrong? But it was grand just to know what to do."[41] According to Mr. Thomas, born in 1903, "There was always the chemist. He was the be-all and end-all, apart from the doctor. If they didn't want to trouble the doctor, they went to the chemist. The chemist was a local man and the chemist knew the faults and the whims of every person around the chemist shop."[42]

In addition to the other services, chemists offered advice and first aid for injuries. For example, Mr. Cranston hurt his hand at work:

I was working overtime one time and I was new on the job and I was doing some yarn testing and instead of having my eyes on what I was doing one time, I was turning a handle of a measuring machine to measure the amount of yarn and I must have looked the other way and put my hand out and my finger went through between the cog wheels. They were pretty badly torn and made a mess of my finger end, burst it and so on. Anyhow I wrapped a handkerchief round and got to the chemist as soon as I could. He said, "Well, I can't do anything for you." Except he gave me some sort of disinfectant and told me to take it home and mix it with hot water and dip my finger in it. So I did that and I went the following day to the First Aid Room, they had started a First Aid Room at Horrockses then, and I told the nurse what had happened and she said it was the best thing that could have been done, to have put it in hot water and this disinfectant.[43]

This account is interesting because the informant depended entirely on the chemist and factory nurse for advice and treatment; unlike some contemporaries, he did not go to the hospital. The chemist Mr. Chambers remembered a similar scenario: "A man fell off his bike and he was smoking. He was a retired art master and he was coming into town and . . . they called me across. He'd been taken into what was a coffee tavern across the way and his pipe had gone up and gone through the palate. It was very awkward and he was very shaken. He couldn't smoke a cigarette of course, he couldn't suck. It would heal up in time."[44]

An important reason working-class people consulted chemists rather than doctors was price. Mrs. Burton said, "We used to have to pay for the

40. Mr. C1P, 77.
41. Mrs. P1P, 73.
42. Mr. T2P, 65.
43. Mr. C1P, 77.
44. Mr. C6L, 15.

doctor, you know! I thought they [chemists] had as much in their heads as the doctor had!"[45] Physicians were aware of the cost issue. Dr. Kuppersmith, born in 1900, who practiced in a working-class Preston area, commented: "They [patients] used to try home treatments quite a lot. Especially before the National Health Service came, they couldn't afford the doctors' fees so they would go to the chemist to get home remedies, you see. . . . The chemist was the unofficial practitioner. Some of them were very well versed in home remedies."[46] Chemists recognized their advantageous market position. Mrs. Winder, born in Lancaster in 1910, said: "I know Marjorie Simpson, Marjorie Shuttleworth, when her little boy was little he always had a cough, and they used to get the medicine off the doctor and it was always that red stuff. She once asked the chemist at Skerton. . . . He said, 'Instead of going to the doctors, I can let you have the same thing for about half price.'"[47]

Mrs. Burrell, born in 1931 in Barrow, said, "If you went to your doctor you had to pay your doctor for a consultation, but if you went to the chemist, I mean you would get six-penn'orth for your cough, that was the bottle then." When asked, "Did you have a feeling that you were getting different kinds of medicine from the chemist than you would have gotten from a G.P.?" Mrs. Burrell answered, "No, I think it would be all the same, knowing afterwards when I went to work in the chemist, it would be the same, but you would pay a lot more through the doctor."[48] Particularly before the advent of antibiotics in the mid-twentieth century, this observation was probably accurate. The chemist Mr. Chambers commented, "There isn't anything you can give for scarlet fever, really, or chicken pox, you've just to wait for nature to take its course, warmth and rest are the things. Mind you, if any complication comes, then it's a case for the doctor. I'm talking about years ago." He said, further, "There was no penicillin in those days, none of these antibiotics at all, all we could do was aspirin and whisky or hot lemon and go to bed and hope for the best."[49] However, beginning with the sulphonamides in the 1930s, effective remedies for infection became available, and after 1948 the National Health Service removed the financial barriers to formal medical care. This reduced working-class dependence on chemists as primary care practitioners. Mr. Hope observed, "Counter-prescribing is not as prevalent as it was . . . because of the Health Service, there's no doubt about that."[50]

45. Mrs. B5P, 50.
46. Dr. K1P, 11.
47. Mrs. W2L, 60.
48. Mrs. B2B, 40. See also Anne Digby, *Evolution*, 228.
49. Mr. C6L, 11, 15.
50. Mr. H10L, 1.

DOCTORS

In 1880 Barrow, Lancaster, and Preston each had well-established medical communities composed mainly of general practitioners.[51] Physicians, usually middle-class in origin, had long figured among nineteenth-century civic leaders and local social elites.[52] It should not be presumed, however, that all doctors were successful and wealthy. With growing numbers of general practitioners and increasing efforts to extend professional medical services to working-class patients who could ill afford advice and treatment, many doctors had trouble earning an income that matched their social status. Fees were either too high to attract patients more accustomed to informal or self-care, or too low to support the physician and his family. Furthermore, low-income patients, who tended to call the doctor only in a crisis, were often unable to pay the bill. As Ann Digby writes, "The fact that doctors during the late nineteenth and early twentieth centuries had targeted working-class areas as an important area for professional expansion undoubtedly increased their vulnerability to bad debts. General practitioners could therefore expect to treat between one in ten and one in twenty patients without remuneration."[53]

Physicians developed creative ways to collect fees. In the study cities, it was common for a "Doctor's Man" to collect installments of a family's medical debt on a Friday afternoon when workers were paid and brought their wages home. In Preston, as in some other larger cities, there were "six-penny doctors," who charged sixpence for an examination and an additional equivalent sum for a bottle of medicine.[54] Some physicians ran prepayment schemes into which families paid a fixed amount per week for treatment.[55] General practitioners affiliated with a friendly society ("club practice") could depend on receiving payment, however moderate, to cover members' care. Similarly, doctors were paid by local Poor Law Guardians to treat paupers. And, after implementation of the 1911 National Insurance Act, panel physicians (affiliated with this program) were compensated

---

51. See Waddington, *The medical profession*, for discussion of the development of general practice in nineteenth-century Britain.

52. John G. Blacktop, *In times of need: The history and origin of the Royal Lancaster Infirmary* (no publisher, no date), 10; Pickstone, *Medicine and industrial society*, 65; Peter Williamson, *From confinement to community: The moving story of 'The Moor,' Lancaster's county lunatic asylum* (publisher unclear, 2000[?]), 6; John Wilkinson, *Preston's Royal Infirmary: A history of health care in Preston 1809–1986* (Preston: Carnegie Press, 1987), 38–39; Nigel Morgan, *Deadly dwellings: Housing and health in a Lancashire cotton town. Preston from 1840 to 1914* (Preston: Mullion Books, 1993), 25; J. D. Marshall, *Furness and the Industrial Revolution: An economic history of Furness (1711–1900) and the Town of Barrow (1757–1897) with an epilogue* (Barrow-in-Furness: Barrow-in-Furness Library and Museum Committee, 1958), 322–23, 377; Dr. A5L, 30.

53. Digby, *Evolution*, 41, 110.

54. Ibid., 101.

55. See, for example, Mr. A4L, 51; Mrs. N1L, 68.

for treating covered workers.[56] Regardless of these systems, however, GPs serving working-class neighborhoods encountered challenges to status and purse that ensured continuing diversity in local medical communities.

While it had long been usual for upper- and middle-class families to consult physicians, late-nineteenth-century working-class residents of Barrow, Lancaster, and Preston did so rarely, and usually only for selected problems including serious injury, perceived danger of death, or suspicion of notifiable infectious disease. Indeed, it is worthy of remark that although oral history informants generally wished to present themselves in the best possible light to the interviewer and also associated consulting physicians with modern, and therefore good, behavior, few born before 1920 remembered their families regularly calling the doctor. Of course, this is a complicated issue because self-reliance was also considered admirable and, conversely, many people who said they rarely saw a doctor also remembered having the same family GP throughout their childhoods.

The most important and frequently mentioned barrier to calling the doctor was financial. While people who belonged to friendly societies and, after 1911, workers eligible for National Health Insurance were entitled to care that was free at the point of use, few women or children were covered.[57] Since women tended to be family health care decision-makers and also managed family incomes, oral history informants remembered extreme conservatism about calling the doctor and inevitable anxiety about paying his bill. Mr. Madison, born in 1910 in Lancaster, explained: "A doctor medical-wise was absolutely out of the question. If you was ill, you was ill, and your parents doctored you. Maybe sometimes in ignorance and by the time they'd found if it was something different it was too late because you paid your own doctor's bill. You paid him seven-and-six to come and see you, seven-and-six a visit. So much if he prescribed a bottle of medicine, and then you paid his fee what he put on the top, so people used to avoid sending for the doctor. You had to be really desperate."[58] Mr. Melling, born in 1906, said similarly, "We used to get doctors' bills, but never much. You only went when you were dying to the doctor's."[59] Mrs. Wilson, born in 1900 in Barrow, remembered a lot of tuberculosis when she was young: "They had it well under control in the 1920s, but, of course, people would ignore the warning, they were always this way inclined, 'We'll try this before we call the doctor,' and they would just put off calling the doctor. I think it was because

56. See, for example, Hardy, *Health and medicine*, 17–20, 45–46.

57. See, for example, Helen Jones, *Health and society in twentieth-century Britain* (London and New York: Longman, 1994), 26; Digby, *Evolution*, 242. See also Mrs. S1L, 10; Mrs. M10B, 11; Mr. H1L, 51; Mr. G1P, 14; Mr. G1L, 14; Miss C2L, 17; Mr. C1B, 15.

58. Mr. M1L, 40. See also Mrs. A2P, 18; Mrs. B2P, 33; Mr. B9P, 28; Mr. C1B, 14; Mrs. C2P, 6; Mrs. D2B, 12; Mr. F1L, 29; Mr. G1L, 14; Mr. H1L, 14; Mr. H3L, 58; Mrs. L3P, 118; Mr. M1L, 21; Mrs. N1L, 2; Mr. P1L, 47; Mrs. P2P, 26; Mrs. S3L, 24; Mr. T1P, 36; Miss T2B, 26; Mr. W3P, 29.

59. Mr. M3L, 10.

they had to pay, and it was a big bogey to them having a doctor's bill and you didn't like calling the doctor knowing you couldn't pay him."[60]

Few working-class families were able to pay a doctor's bill in a lump sum. Thus, many doctors employed collectors who, like other creditors, called at working-class homes on Friday, before wages had been spent. Mrs. Mallingham, born in Barrow in 1896, remembered, "You were never out of the doctor's debt. . . . They had collectors and you paid sixpence or a shilling a week for doctors' treatment, because if you had the doctor you had to pay for him."[61] Dr. Kuppersmith said: "Of course, the doctors used to do their own dispensing in those days. . . . They used to run up bills, these patients, and doctors would have collectors to collect so much a week, 3d or 6d a week some paid, or a little more. At one time I had three collectors going round collecting at the weekend from patients. . . . They used to pay 3/6d for a visit and then 3/6d for the medicine. So it used to cost 7/-d."[62] Most informants simply referred to the "Doctor's Man" or, more rarely, "Woman." However, Mr. Madison said more specifically, "Again, a retired policeman could always get a job going collecting doctors' bills and there was no messing about it. 'It's about time you paid something off, never mind you've got nothing. It's about time you paid summat.' That was the attitude. 'I'm sorry.' 'Never mind about sorry, you've got to find it.'"[63]

Another barrier to consultation mentioned by informants was difference in class status. Working-class people generally viewed doctors as being members of a social elite. For example, Mr. Rust, born in 1890 in Lancaster, classified physicians with local gentry, commenting about the early twentieth century, "There wasn't above thirty cars in Lancaster. There was Dr. Mannix, Lord Ashton [mill-owner] had two—a Lanchester and a Rolls Royce, Dr. Varley, Dr. Dean, they'd cars at Ellel Grange, Lord Sefton had a car, and I don't think there was anybody else. All the doctors had cars."[64] When asked toward the end of an interview, "How did they treat you, the few [people] that you met who weren't working-class?" Mr. Cranston, born in 1884 in Preston, responded, "I met very few. I can't think of any except, perhaps, the doctor. I had occasion to deal with the doctor once or twice. . . . The doctor and the vicar, you could call those probably middle-class, and I can't think of anybody else outside those two who might be termed middle-class."[65] Mr. Best, born in 1897, said his father was a coachman for "the three main doctors" in Barrow. He recalled, "Doctor was 'Yes Sir, No Sir.' You mustn't say anything to the doctor. You mustn't ask him

60. Mrs. W1B, 22.
61. Mrs. M6B, 13.
62. Dr. K1P, 3.
63. Mr. M1L, 40.
64. Mr. R2L, 15.
65. Mr. C1P, 73.

why he hadn't come this morning."[66] Perception of a class barrier persisted. Mrs. Howard, born in Lancaster in 1931, commented, "It was quite posh to have the doctor call."[67] Mr. Norton, born in Lancaster in the same year, said that the doctor "was a distant character that was held in some reverence and we didn't particularly want to see him, because obviously when we went to see him it was a reflection of trouble. That was no disrespect to him as an individual, but the best relationship and our family—as in most working families—you know, was distant."[68]

Not all doctors were perceived as equally socially remote. For example, Mrs. Sanderson, born in 1892, remembered: "Dr. Hamilton used to have a daughter and a son. They had ramrod backs and used to be right stately and they never used to speak to you. Old Dr. Aitken, it didn't matter what you ailed if you went to him. He used to say, 'Give them a good dose of Gregory Powder.'"[69] Other Lancaster informants also remembered Dr. Aitken, who founded the Dalton Square practice in 1903. Mrs. Horton, born in that year, suffered with sore feet as a child. "The doctor was old Dr. Aitken, and he never sent her [mother] a bill in for me. 'The poor wee lassie,' he used to say. He was right Scotch. But he was a grand old doctor. He didn't send a lot of bills in, I'll tell you."[70] Mrs. Britton, born in 1936, remembered a younger member of the Dalton Square practice, Dr. R. G. Howat, who practiced in Lancaster from 1922 to 1962:

He was quite a character. . . . Well, he was a self-educated man. He left school at eleven years old and went to work in a chemist's shop as an apprentice. . . . But old Dr. Howat brought me into the world and he often used to tell my mother, he used to come and sit in the pub, you see, in the back room, in the living room, drinking whisky with my mother and father, and he'd sit there for an hour or two at a time. God knows what his patients were doing; they must all have been sat there waiting for him to turn up. And he would tell you all these tales.[71]

66. Mr. B1B, 55.

67. Mrs. H5L, 58.

68. Mr. N2L, 53.

69. Mrs. S3L, 24. Another informant, Mrs. Scales, born in 1896, also remembered Dr. Hamilton, saying, "He used to come in a coach, in a carriage and pair, but he was the Mayor of Lancaster, you know, Dr. Hamilton, but he died in the Moor Hospital [insane asylum]" (Mrs. S4L, 33). According to the chemist Mr. Chambers, Gregory Powder, a laxative, "was a mixture of rhubarb, ginger, and light magnesia. It was a very horrible thing, and you'd a job to mix it unless you used hot water to wet it, or otherwise you'd chase it round a cup for ages. I had an apprentice and he was a very grand young man, but his first week he went home and told his mother I'd asked him to wrap packets of Gregory Powder up. He said, 'Mother, it's like wrapping wind,' and it was, you know. Of course, there's a knack in it, you know. It was so light it would float away and cover him" (Mr. C6L, 8).

70. Mrs. H3L, 65–66. See also John H. Chippendale, Andrew L. Paton, and Sandy Clark, *100 years of the Dalton Square Practice* (Lancaster: Privately published, 2003).

71. Mrs. B4L, 99–100.

Similarly, Mr. Carson, born in 1902, recalled: "Our doctor was Dr. Dean and he was one of the good old lads and if the old man [father] was ill, he used to say, 'It's all right, Mrs. C., give him plenty of hot milk. Have you a drop of owt to put in?' He used to prefer brandy or a drop of rum, just to warm up, get him into a sweat. 'Keep him there for about three or four days, and then if he wants to get up, he can do. Keep him on a rather light diet and he'll be ready for work.' It was just commonsense to sweat the fever out of you."[72] These accounts suggest that socially accessible doctors were those who were prepared to chat (or drink) with working-class people outside the sickroom, validate traditional therapeutic approaches, and consider family finances when composing their bills. However, physicians who did not maintain a serious professional demeanor also risked their reputations in working-class communities. For example, Mr. Perkins, born in 1900, remembered:

> I lived in Westmorland Street for a period and the wife scalded her leg and I went for Dr. Miller and he came up. He'd just come to Barrow at that particular time and he'd got a motor bike, a Federation he'd got from the Co-op. He was only a youngish chap and he come and knocked on the door. He come in and I had an engine on my table. "Hello," he said, "Are you interested in bikes?" I said, "Aye." He said, "Come out here and look at mine, what do you think of this?" He took me outside and said, "Go and have a ride on it and see." He hadn't even seen the wife then.[73]

Along the same lines, a few informants remembered incompetent or drunken GPs.[74] Some observed the poverty of doctors in the old days compared to more recent times. For example, Mr. Sage, born in 1896, said, "In those days a doctor was more humble than they are today, and the GP came round on his bicycle."[75] However, generally speaking, physicians were considered socially remote.

Just as what might be called the "common touch" could ease the doctor-patient relationship, it is clear that better educated or upwardly mobile people were more likely both to maintain social relationships with and consult physicians. Mr. Southwort, born in 1915, whose mother had been a teacher before marriage, said his mother "was very close to the doctor. Dr. Mooney, the father and two sons, were prominent Catholic doctors in Preston, and Mother's mother had been a close friend of old Dr. Mooney's wife, and so this connection carried on. Mother never hesitated to go straight to the doctor."[76]

72. Mr. C1L, 36.
73. Mr. P1B, 73.
74. Mr. M2B, 21; Mr. D2P, 42, 45; Mrs. P1P, 16; Mr. T2P, 74; Mr. W6L, 26.
75. Mr. S1B, 27.
76. Mr. S4P, 35.

Regardless of their social ease or discomfort with doctors, working-class people faced increasing pressure from many directions to consult GPs, who had influence over a growing range of activities and resources including employment, friendly society membership, sickness benefits, school attendance, military service, and (eventually) council housing and preschool places.[77] Some medical examinations, including school, pre-employment, or military inspections, were free and arranged by someone other than the person examined. Other consultations, such as the one required when a schoolteacher sent a child home with a suspected contagious illness, often involved both action and payment on the part of the child's parents.

As we shall see, before 1948, some families paid for medical services through membership in a friendly society. However, society admission required a medical examination. Mr. Best, born in 1897, remembered:

> Every one of my family then were Oddfellows, in the Oddfellows Friendly Society. I was the only one who never passed into the Oddfellows. My sister took me by the hand to the doctor and we had to pass a doctor in those days to go into a friendly society who then for a penny per week provided you with a free doctor. My sister took me to Dr. Thomas in Dalkeith Street, right opposite the Trevelyn Hotel, who was the family doctor. He looked after us all and brought us into the world and he said to my sister, I remember going. My sister took me by the hand and the doctor said, "Well, what do you want?" The doctors were very severe in those days. "My mother has sent us to see if you'll put Bert into the Oddfellows." He says, "You can take back and tell your mother he should have drowned when he was young and I'm not going to do it."[78]

Similarly, Mrs. Hunt, born in 1885, said:

> M'father was in and m'brother got in. He was in Sons of Temperance, but they never did have me. I remember once mother taking me—Dr. Carmichael and Dr. Stark had been in partnership in Ramsden Street. I'd been ill through the wintertime and I suppose mother thought perhaps a change of doctor. Having no more sense, I suppose she took me to Dr. Stark and he gave me the once-over and said that he didn't think that if Dr. Carmichael wouldn't pass your daughter as I would, did you? Mother said, "No I didn't really think when I came." I never got into a Society.[79]

77. See Digby, *Evolution*, 247–58, for a useful discussion of the physician's growing gate-keeping activities.

78. Mr. B1B, 15.

79. Mrs. H2B, 59.

These accounts indicate both the power of club doctors and the conflict of interest inherent in their roles.

Public health legislation also forced people to consult doctors. As contagious diseases became "notifiable" after 1889, a physician's diagnosis was necessary, either to free the suspected victim from further suspicion or to govern the terms of the sufferer's isolation, either in home quarantine or in hospital.[80] Therefore, ailments such as scarlet fever, diphtheria, and measles were among the most frequently mentioned as conditions for which the doctor was called; working-class parents were afraid *not* to consult a GP. Mrs. Maxwell, born in 1898 in Preston, when asked, "When you were young, when would you call the doctor in?" responded, "Oh, spots, or be poorly. Measles was a notifiable disease. You had to bring them in for measles."[81] Another informant supported this statement. When asked, "Did you ever have the doctor for your children?" Mrs. Warton, born in 1899 in Preston, replied:

> My daughter went to school with the measles and I didn't know. She came home and I asked her what was wrong. She said that her teacher said she had measles. I said it was only a rash and to go back and tell her. It ended up she sent her home again, so I went to see her. I told her it was only a rash, but she said she thought it was measles. I went to the doctor and he said she did have the measles, but that they weren't severe. He told me to keep her warm. I couldn't keep her warm as she was playing and she had children running in the house. This is the only complaint she ever had. I never knew my boy to be ill. Some children are always ailing, aren't they?[82]

This account reflects both a common traditional, casual attitude about "childhood diseases" and an equally common basis for tension between professional health care providers and working-class mothers—issues that will be further discussed in chapter 4.

Physicians enforced vaccination laws and served as gatekeepers for employment. Mr. Grove, born in 1903 in Preston, said:

> You weren't allowed to start work unless you had passed the doctor. It was funny, this passing the doctor. It shows how ridiculous it were. You had to be vaccinated, he looked at your teeth and he looked at your head. Them were the three things as he passed you for. I remember a

80. A system of notification was in force in Preston from 1879, but it was not until enactment of the Infectious Disease (Notification) Act in 1889 that such systems were instituted in Barrow and Lancaster. See Anthony S. Wohl, *Endangered lives,* 136.

81. Mrs. M3P, 35. See also Mrs. H3P, 49; Mrs. M1B, 17; Mr. T3P, 65; Mrs. A1P, 40.

82. Mrs. W1P, 41.

boy that were passing and he smoked, he was only 12. It was the town
doctor, old Dr. Brown. He had him with a mirror and he was taking all
the brown off his teeth, they were that bad. He was doing that to see if
his teeth were sound or not. . . . You had to go and be vaccinated before
they would allow you to go in the mill. My oldest brother and sister, they
had never been vaccinated as babies and they had to go to the doctor
before they could start work in the mill.[83]

Similarly, Mrs. Black, born in 1916 in Preston, remembered, "I was vaccinated, you had to be. You wouldn't get a job unless you were vaccinated. I
don't know whether you went to the doctor's or whether the doctor did it
at work because the doctor would come round every so often at work and
you have to go and visit him."[84]

Doctors examined children leaving school for employment. According
to Mrs. Steele, born in 1898 in Preston, who began half-time work as a
weaver at age twelve, "Yes, he [the doctor] would come to the school and
examine our chest and ears and see if everything was all right."[85] Doctors
also influenced the type of work people did. Mrs. Hunt, born in 1885,
recalled, "I wanted to be a confectioner but the doctor put his foot on that
and said that I wasn't strong enough for the long time that I'd have had to
work." She became a dressmaker instead.[86] Similarly, Mrs. Ackerman, born
in 1904, remembered: "All I wanted to do was nursing, but I didn't get
the chance. The doctor was attending my dad and they didn't want me to
go nursing. It was old Dr. Coffey at the time, and anyway I didn't pass the
doctor. . . . Whether I had a medical or whether he said that I wouldn't be
fit, I just can't remember . . . but I didn't get nursing."[87]

Wage earners required a physician's approval to stay home from work
and receive sick pay. In answer to the question, "Did you have a piano?"
Mrs. Winder, born in 1910 in Lancaster, remembered a situation that, in
addition to illuminating social class relationships, suggested both popular
notions about the way doctors set fees and the GP's role in policing malingering:

We had a piano and we learned to play, but none of us made much of it.
It stood in the living room. My brother hadn't been working very long
and he was in bed with flu and a young doctor came who was a locum.
He'd just qualified, and he walked in and played on the piano as he

83. Mr. G1P, 89. See also Mr. N2L, 17. As we will see in chapter 4, many informants'
families were opposed to smallpox vaccination, and, thus, children were not vaccinated until the
procedure was administered by educational, employment, or military authorities.

84. Mrs. B2P, 33. See also Mr. G1P, 89.

85. Mrs. S5P, 35.

86. Mrs. H2B, 65.

87. Mrs. A2B, 7.

went past. He said, "My word, a piano, another bob on your visit." . . . Of
course, then you paid for every visit. He said to my brother, "You'll
need a certificate." My brother said, "No, I don't need a certificate for
the first three days." He said, "Oh, you're one of the wealthy ones, are
you." Mean actually. My brother should have had it but he didn't think
the first three days counted. He was working as chief clerk in the Town
Clerk's office. But this young doctor was a bit sarcastic about him not
needing a certificate.[88]

A physician's hasty judgment could have more significant consequences
than merely causing offence. Mr. Norton, born in 1931, told the terrible
story of his father committing suicide by drowning himself in the Lancaster
Canal. "He was off work ill, again that was an event because we never knew
that before and I'm told that the doctor had told him that there was nothing wrong with him. Well, now, to a guy that proud . . . I don't think he
could have taken it. It went down very very hard. I think he got up early
one morning and left home and that was that."[89] This account illustrates
both the growing professional authority of physicians and their power over
the patient's self-image and reputation.

In addition to their role vis à vis employment, doctors also could exempt
children from school attendance. Mr. Simpkins, born in 1932, stayed home
from school for a year at about age twelve, "Because I had a doctor who
believed that I had a grumbling appendix, that was an appendix that flared
up every so often. And because he didn't want me doing sport or any vio-
lent exercise or anything like that, then he signed me off school. And then
he gave me a certificate to say I hadn't to go to school, it was as simple
as that."[90] Mrs. Dent, born in Preston in 1908, remembered a physician
excusing her from school at age 13, not because of illness but because her
mother was worried about her chastity. "My mother took me to Dr. Rose,
she was a woman doctor and I had started with my periods, and she got
me exempt from school before I should have been. . . . She exempt me as
she said it wasn't safe for me to sit with the lads and that."[91] This account
suggests the extension of the physician's authority from strictly medical
matters to social and moral issues.

Physicians served as gatekeepers for military service—a function that
was highlighted by widespread anxiety over national degeneration, jump-
started during recruitment of volunteers for service in the Boer War.[92] As
with other types of screening, informants remembered their premilitary
examinations cynically. Mr. Martin, born in 1892, recalled that his brother

88. Mrs. W2L, 60.
89. Mr. N2L, 68.
90. Mr. S7L, 47.
91. Mrs. D1P, 60.
92. See, for example, Hardy, *Health and medicine*, 40. Jones, *Health and society*, 22.

was turned down by the doctor who had examined him for the friendly society to which his family belonged. "He [doctor] said, 'You'll soon be up the hill.' It turned out that he [brother] joined the Yeomanry, the Territorials that same year with two of his pals. The other two didn't get passed, but he did. He did two camps with the Yeomanry, went to France in 1915 and was there until early 1918. He never ailed a thing."[93] Mr. Middleton, born in 1898, said of a Barrow physician, "It was in the papers that he'd been arrested because he'd had a bit of a collision and he was tight, drunk round the corner. He was a terrible fellow. You could see he'd pass anything for the army. He'd pass anything for money. He was all right of a man, but he was a bit rough I thought. He was out in France all the time in the first War."[94] Mr. Eaton, born in 1902, remembered: "I wanted to join the RAMC and I passed the eye test and I'd to see the doctor the next day and he noticed that scar where I'd had the operation and he said, 'I'm sorry I cannot pass you unless you go in hospital and have a piece of skin grafted on.' Instead of that I went from the old Drill Hall and I joined the Territorials and I passed. I was in there for nearly twelve years. I was working in the yard, in the Gun Shop when the 1939 war broke out and of course I was called up."[95] These accounts indicate both the physician's influence regarding military service and some informants' low regard for professional medical authority—at least in this context.

Nonetheless, doctors could influence award of important benefits. Mrs. Winder, born in 1910, remembered the family GP, Dr. Gibson, getting compassionate leave for her father, who was then serving in France during World War I, when her mother and two siblings became ill during the 1918 influenza epidemic.[96] Mrs. Smith, born in 1895, remembered: "My husband [a veteran] wasn't getting a pension, he had malaria and he used to be off ill with it. He wouldn't have a pension and Dr. Livingstone saw this, it was a thing in the *Mail* and it asked if anybody was in the Westmorland and Cumberland Yeomanry, had they anything. . . . He sent him to Tommy, head of the Legion. He said, 'Just go and tell him that I've sent you.' He got him a pension for seven shillings a week."[97] Of course, physicians also negatively affected benefit determinations. Mrs. Young, born in 1915, said, "I've worked in nursing and I've heard the consultants say, 'Don't put this person down for compensation, they're going to die within six to twelve months; they won't benefit from the compensation, and I don't see that the relatives should get it.'"[98] In addition, physicians influenced other decisions, including (once it was available) allocation of council housing. Mr. White-

93. Mr. M1B, 90–91.
94. Mr. M2B, 21.
95. Mr. E1B, 7.
96. Mrs. W2L, 75.
97. Mrs. S2B, 42.
98. Mr. Y1P, 3.

side, born in 1940 in Lancaster, remembered that before the advent of the National Health Service, "Our doctor then was Dr. Daniels, he was off King Street, and I always remember him being a good fellow, him. . . . I remember he used to always be writing letters on my mam's behalf, when we was after getting moved, you know. Because, as I say, she was on the housing list for about seventeen years, because I have heard them talk about it, you know. He was always a good fellow, was Dr. Daniels, yes."[99]

In addition to seeking doctors' intervention in official matters, working-class patients also began to rely on them for personal advice. For example, Mrs. Masterson, born in 1915, lost her husband during World War II. She worried about her fifteen-year-old daughter dating a nineteen-year-old boy. "I had no husband to discuss it with, and she had only just left school and she met him at the works annual dance. . . . I didn't dissuade her, but I had a talk with our family doctor who is like a friend and you can speak to him. He said to leave it and it would maybe peter out and if not, then they were made for each other."[100] Similarly, Mrs. Read, born in 1927, asked the doctor for advice when her daughter did not like a new school. The doctor recommended that the child be returned to her old school and volunteered to call the headmaster himself.[101] These accounts suggest that among working-class people, from the interwar period the GP was taking on a paternalistic role that might previously have been filled by a clergyman or domestic servant's master.

In the late nineteenth and early twentieth centuries, the most common reason for working-class families to consult a general practitioner was for serious illness or injury. Because of the barriers discussed above, consultation was often delayed—a matter that concerned both physicians and family members, particularly when the sufferer died. Mrs. Hill, born in 1903 in Preston, remembered:

> My mother died with it [pneumonia] anyhow, but there wasn't much cure for that then. My mum, she was only 53 and she was only in bed two days, but she had knocked about with it, and never said, because there was such a crowd of us. When I went to school and the others went to work, she would just go to bed and get up and make the meals for us coming in. When the doctor came, he said that we should have brought him a week before. He said it was too late. She fought for her breath like a demon, but she only lasted three days. The doctor came again and he said, "Send this child up to my surgery in Newhall Lane and I'll give her something." He gave them to me and he said, "Here you are. See that she gets them. It's either kill or cure." She was dead

99. Mr. W5L, 47.
100. Mrs. M1P, 47.
101. Mrs. R3P, 90–91.

in four hours. She fought the whole time and when she was dead the bed was wet through when she died. She did fight, bless her. . . . [T]hey sent for her sister and when she came, Auntie Nellie told us we children had better go to bed because mum was unconscious then and it was frightening to see her fighting for her breath. We just seem to have got to bed when we heard Auntie Nellie shouting that she had died and we all came down.[102]

This account reveals much about self-help, home care, and responsibility shared between physician and laypeople; with the mother ailing, only a schoolgirl and (belatedly) a female relative were available to make decisions and provide care. There was no suggestion that the patient be hospitalized, despite awareness that she was in danger of death. The GP, consulted only when the seriousness of the woman's illness became obvious, was both irritated and fatalistic about the probable outcome of treatment.

Similarly, when asked, "Did your mother have the doctor very often? Do you remember him coming when you were children?" Mrs. Masterson, born in 1913, said:

Not very often. The only time I remember the doctor coming, she took us to the doctor mind, but the only time I remember him coming was when he came to my father when he died. As I say, he was an engineer and a piece of steel pierced his neck as they were doing a job. It caused poisoning and he broke out in those big carbuncles and it poisoned his system. He was only a week, stayed off for the week's annual holidays, and he was dead the following Friday. This doctor had gone away and never told the other doctor to come and see him. Well, it was too late when he was sent for. I always remember, in his coffin, all his arms were bandaged and all his neck was covered in these huge boils. I remember mother boiling bread in a big pan, bread in water. And making big bread poultices. There wasn't a lot of ointments and that. But they really believed in a bread poultice.[103]

Again, the doctor's attentions were belated and not positively remembered; by contrast, the informant emphasized her mother's knowledge, effort, and competence—despite the negative outcome.

As these examples make clear, regardless of the ailment's severity, the doctor's primary workplace was the sufferer's home. Before World War II, even surgery—particularly tonsillectomy—was often performed in private homes.[104] Mr. Parke, born in 1894, recalled:

102. Mrs. H8P, 38.
103. Mrs. M1P, 41.
104. See, for example, Mrs. A1P, 38; Miss A3P, 4; Mrs. C1B, 15; Mrs. C3P, 15; Mrs. H1B, 14; Mrs. L3P, 148; Mrs. P2P, 26; Mrs. S1B, 28; Mrs. S5P, 13; Miss T4P, 40.

I had my tonsils out at home in front of the bedroom window. I'll never forget it as long as I live.

Interviewer: Did you have an anesthetic?

Informant: No. He clipped something on them and then he had an instrument with a wire on the end which went up there like a hook. Here was the shutter and a hole in there and he had his thumb in there. That went down there and the tonsil was put in there. He put his tweezers on it and brought this down and pulled. He did both at the same time. It was just as if somebody was tearing m'throat. It hurt really shocking.[105]

Mrs. Anston, born in 1900, also remembered her daughter having this operation at home.

Joyce had her tonsils out when she was young, she had scarlet fever. This was my eldest daughter and the other was only about seven months old, so she had to go into hospital. Then when she came out she had to have her tonsils out. She had them out at home. She had it done on the table.

Interviewer: Did they give her an anaesthetic?

Informant: Yes.

Interviewer: And did you have to help?

Informant: No.

Mrs. Anston requested that the surgery be performed at home, since the child had just come out of Isolation Hospital at Deepdale. The doctor gave her instructions about preparing for the procedure:

He asked me to put a sheet up outside for the light, you prepared the table and you had to scrub up the sink and that kind of thing. . . . He brought another doctor. There were two doctors.

Interviewer: And how did you feel when it took place, a bit apprehensive?

Informant: I said, "She's not gone under yet!" He said that I could stay until she was properly under. He lifted her hand up and her eyes weren't closed. I said, "Her eyes aren't closed," I could tell that they were sort of glazed. He called her by her name and there was no response and he said, "She's all right now. Now, you go wait in the other room." I had a friend who had done some nursing who came in and stayed with me and then she carried her upstairs after. As soon as she called out, "Mummy!" she said I could go up.[106]

105. Mr. P1L, 77.
106. Mrs. A2P, 34.

Mrs. Clarke, from Barrow, had surgery at home in about 1912:

I can never remember having the doctor until I was twelve years of age, but the operation was done on the kitchen table at Buccleuch Dock Road. The nurse came and the doctor and I've so much of my rib taken, it's cut from here and down my back, and it was done on the kitchen table. The nurse came and attended to the wound for seven weeks, it was dressed. They gave me an anaesthetic. All that had to come in during the housework and the older ones coming in for their meals. I always remember mother saying, we had a very nice long table, that the doctor said, "Mrs. T. this is ideal for the job, you couldn't have had a better table." There was no talk of going into hospital and it was just done at home. . . . There was no walls scrubbed, everything had to be clean and I remember mother saying that the nurse said, "Well you've got everything just right." They had a bucket at the end to hold the blood, I can remember her saying it. The operation was done on the kitchen table by Dr. Reed. . . . We were fortunate we never had the doctor very much. My sister had an operation at home as well and that was in St. Andrews Street. She had her tonsils taken out and that was done at home.[107]

Mr. Grove, born in 1903 in Preston, remembered a procedure done at home:

Our oldest boy, he had to be circumcised and the doctor said that he would do it at home. He did it on the table in Harrington Street and I had to assist him. It should have been three guineas for the fee, but he would have had to bring another doctor and it would have been a guinea for him. So he got his own two and I assisted him and it saved us a guinea. . . . He would say, hand me this and hand me that, like. Bring hot water and that.
    Interviewer: It must have been very upsetting?
    Informant: He was experienced, like.[108]

At home, the surgeon shared decision making and agency with lay caregivers. It was also difficult for him to exclude relatives and friends from the operating room—something that was already an established hospital rule. It is noteworthy, however, that a GP informant remembered socioeconomic factors affecting the decision about whether or not to operate at home. Dr. Kuppersmith said:

107. Mrs. C1B, 15. This account includes a rare reference to home nursing services, probably provided by a district nurse. See Dingwall et al., *Social history of nursing,* 174–203, for a useful discussion of trained home nursing.
108. Mr. G1P, 13.

I remember giving an anaesthetic for Mr. Sumner who was the ear, nose, and throat specialist, on the kitchen table he was removing the tonsils and adenoids. I used to give the anaesthetic for him from time to time.

Interviewer: When they had the tonsils and adenoids out at home, did you ask for any special precautions in the way of hygiene?

Informant: Very often it was a better-class home. We wouldn't do it in one of the slum areas, the Ribbleton Lane area. It would be a better-class home where they could provide the facilities. You would have a nurse in attendance and hot and cold water and everything laid on.[109]

However, the range of backgrounds of lay informants who remembered home surgery suggests that either the surgeon's criteria for deciding whether or not to operate at home changed over time or that physicians differed regarding this decision; both alternatives are likely.

Consultation of general practitioners became more common as time went on, although strict periodization of this trend is difficult, since a few informants' families routinely called the doctor in the earliest years of the study period, while some other families strongly relied on self- and home care after World War II.[110] This decision was influenced by financial and social factors. We will first consider the financial support that arguably paved the way for first, behavioral, then cultural change in working-class experience of professional medicine.

As Anne Hardy points out, "Working people's access to orthodox medicine was greatly improved during the course of the nineteenth century by the emergence of the insurance principle," in the form of friendly societies.[111] Related to the self-help movement, these organizations, which generally offered social activities, sick pay, funeral benefits, and the services of a "club" physician, were formed beginning in the late eighteenth century.[112] By 1898, according to James Riley, "4.2 million people, mostly workingmen, belonged to registered friendly societies in the United Kingdom, compared with the no more than 1.6 million who belonged to labour unions. . . . Even in the years after 1910, when labour unions were thriving and friendly societies were fading, working people belonged to friendly societies in larger numbers than to any other secular organization."[113] Elizabeth Roberts writes that in 1900, "about a sixth of Barrow's population (and about one-sixth of the [interview] sample), belonged to a friendly society, ensuring

109. Dr. K1P, 4–5.
110. See Digby, *Evolution,* 139–44, for discussion of development of the twentieth-century GP's surgery.
111. Hardy, *Health and medicine,* 17.
112. Pickstone, *Medicine and industrial society,* 65.
113. James C. Riley, *Sick, not dead: The health of British workingmen during the mortality decline* (Baltimore and London: Johns Hopkins University Press, 1997), 16.

free medical attention for each insured member. There were rather fewer members in Lancaster and Preston."[114] As indicated above, friendly societies rarely covered children and women and did not necessarily accept all the members of a family; thus, they influenced working-class health culture less than might otherwise have been the case. Nonetheless, oral history informants whose family members belonged to friendly societies remembered consulting GPs more often than those without such coverage.

Mr. Best, born in 1897, who twice served as the District Chief Ruler of the Rechabite Order (a temperance society) in Barrow, explained: "In those days a child could join the Rechabites for a halfpenny per week, and it was my duty in those days to collect that money and pay it into a common pool which all the friendly societies, Forresters, Oddfellows, all pay this halfpenny into a common pool which was divided out by a man called Mr. Cryer who then paid the doctors in turn for the services for the children. Each society had what they called their own doctor."[115] According to Mr. Sage, born in 1896 in Barrow:

> I'll tell you what most people relied on, they were all in the friendly societies. The friendly society's constitution was the forerunner of the Health Service, and did provide a very good beginning and it worked very well.
> *Interviewer:* When you belonged to a friendly society, did you feel you could call a doctor a bit more often than if you weren't in one?
> *Informant:* Oh yes.
> *Interviewer:* They'd come for nothing would they?
> *Informant:* Oh, they were in the contract. . . . I think a lot of families found it wise to be in a friendly society for medical cover because they couldn't afford. One memorizes there was the private patient in those days and of course he sent his bill in and of course the GP had his debt collector. . . . We'd a chap who was a doctor . . . and he lived in Hartington Street just opposite the King's Hall there. . . . This is going back well over seventy years, and he was the GP for the area, and he used to knock about a bit on his push bike.[116]

Mrs. Ackerman, born in 1904, said that as children she and her siblings were members of a friendly society. "We had a free doctor. I'm saying free doctor, we were in the Rechabites. Paid in the Rechabites Club so that we could go to the doctor when we wanted to. I don't remember a lot about going to the doctor's, but I know our doctor was free." Her parents were

114. Elizabeth Roberts, *A woman's place: An oral history of working-class women 1890–1940* (Oxford: Basil Blackwell, 1984), 163–64.
115. Mr. B1B, 16.
116. Mr. S1B, 27. See also Mrs. M11B, 6; Mrs. O1B, 57; Mrs. W2B, 12; Mrs. W2L, 112.

not members.[117] Mr. Hunt, born in 1888, remembered, "M'father was secretary of the Sons of Temperance in Barrow for years. It was a Sick Society as well. You got about seven shillings a week sick and you got a free doctor."[118]

As this example indicates, friendly societies offered more than medical services. When asked, "Did your father belong to a friendly society?" Mr. Carson, born in Lancaster in 1902, said:

> Yes, the Oddfellows, and I'm still in it. It was the greatest thing, that, and a lot more of them such as Rechabites. They've all been very, very good things because it was a kind of social atmosphere and they brought people together. There were lots of interesting discussions, which didn't do anybody any harm. They never got political, and I think generally all round it was good for the country. The Fellowship of the Oddfellows is one of the greatest things in England today. . . . You used to pay your subscription, now was it once a week or once a month? I go once a year now. . . . You used to get sick benefit. When I first joined, I used to pay three-pence a week and if you were off ill you used to get about fifteen bob or a pound, which was a lot. It was more than half your wages.

This informant explained how the sick benefit was administered: "One of the committee men known as the Sick Visitor used to come round with the dole. It used to run about nine, ten, or twelve bob according to how good a member you were. If you were always off, it used to dwindle down. M'father wasn't a poser and he wasn't a sick man and if he was off with influenza due to an epidemic he used to get sick pay."[119] This account suggests both the personal honor system that kept friendly societies going and controls against malingering administered by members.

There is some question about whether doctors offered the same quality of services to club patients as they did to their fee-paying private clients.[120] Mr. Martin, born in 1892 in Barrow, recalled that his family belonged to the Forrester's. "We could never understand when we went for the medicine, some people had it wrapped up in polished paper, we called it toffee paper. It was white paper all neatly wrapped up, and ours wasn't. We couldn't make out why our medicine hadn't wrapping, and the reason was we were

117. Mrs. A2B, 65.

118. Mr. H2B, 81.

119. Mr. C1L, 25, 36. See also Mrs. C7L, 51; Mrs. H1B, 14; Mr. R3B, 50. Mr. Rust, born in 1890, describes his father's activities as a Sick Visitor for the Oddfellow's (Mr. R3L, 76). According to the on-line *OED*, a "bob" was a shilling.

120. See, for example, Digby, *Evolution*, 19, for discussion of the negative impact of first club, then National Health Insurance panel practice, on the normative quality of care provided by GPs.

club patients and the others private patients."[121] Supporting this perspective, Mr. Finch, born in 1900 to a comparatively prosperous, small (three children), upwardly mobile family (father was a postman and mother had been a servant at 10 Downing Street before marriage), remembered that his mother "was treated herself by a doctor as a private patient, and I know at the time she died we were paying a pound a week for the service, but that wasn't by any means unusual, but it would be looked on now as a drain on the family purse." When asked, "Did the family belong to a friendly society?" he responded, "No, we got by with the doctor's scheme and the money wasn't large, so I think we got our full value out of it, and, of course, the advantage again was that when we went to a doctor for medicine, he knew us in an intimate sort of way medically because he had brought us into the world."[122]

To minimize the expense of consulting a GP, like residents of other large towns some Preston families used "six-penny" doctors, so-called because they charged sixpence a visit. Mr. Brown, born in 1896, remembered, "There was a sixpenny doctor and if you ailed owt you had to go to him, sixpence a time."[123] When asked, "I am never too sure about this sixpenny doctor: did it mean he only cost sixpence a week or did you pay him sixpence a week, do you know?" Mr. Malvern, born in 1901, explained, "We paid him sixpence when we went. You paid sixpence a week if you had run up a bill for a long illness." Otherwise, "It was sixpence a visit or sixpence for a bottle of medicine."[124] Again, there was a perceived quality difference between the six-penny doctors and the GPs who charged considerably higher fees to private patients. Mr. Grove, born in 1903, remembered:

> Now, for your wife and children, you had to pay a doctor for that. They had a man come round and he collected for the doctor. It was so much for a visit, so much for a bottle. He mixed the medicine in them days. When you were ill, you went to the doctor and he gave you a bottle of medicine. I think if the doctor did a visit in them days it was 3/6d. Then it would be about half a crown for a bottle of medicine. He put all that down and for every pound that you owed him he would put 3/d on because he had to pay a collector for collecting it. So you paid for the collector as well.
>
> *Interviewer:* When you paid sixpence a week, you were really paying off a debt, you weren't sort of putting an insurance in?
>
> *Informant:* No. We were paying off a debt. We had one doctor in town and called him the six-penny doctor. When you went there you paid 6d and that was you done with. But he wouldn't give you medicine

121. Mr. M1B, 17. This account is repeated on page 90 of the transcript.
122. Mr. F2B, 7–8.
123. Mr. B8P, 5. See also Mrs. B5P, 20; Mrs. C3P, 15; Mrs. P2P, 71; Mr. R1P, 36; Mr. W3P, 29.
124. Mr. M2P, 143.

or anything like that.[125]

Some informants remember GPs running what amounted to a private club practice for which families paid a small sum every week. According to Mr. Finch, born in Barrow in 1900: "There was a penny a week, I think, that several practitioners in the town had in these insurance books, and I think it did enable them to get some money in that they would otherwise have missed. We can hardly believe today that often people used the services of a doctor did not pay. It was rather lax, I thought, because I always felt conscientious about full services rendered and am rather strict on that."[126] It is noteworthy that Mr. Finch viewed this arrangement as financially good for both patients and practitioners and also believed that it enhanced the quality of medical care by fostering long-term care relationships.

The very poor who needed professional attention and were unable to pay, but were willing to accept charitable services, sought help from the Poor Law Guardians, who, in turn, contracted with local doctors to provide treatment. Mrs. Ball, born in 1888, was raised by her grandmother after her mother's death and her father's progressive alcoholism. She described the process for obtaining medical relief in Lancaster during her childhood:

> If you wanted a doctor you went for a recommend. You'd to take the recommend up to the Infirmary and then they would send a doctor down.
>
> *Interviewer:* Would this be from the Guardians?
>
> *Informant:* It must have been. "Sally, go down there and get a recommend for your Grandma." I'd go in this place and this little old man would come. "Please, I want a recommend for m'Grandma." "Who's your Grandma?" "Mrs.—." "Where do you live?" "On Aldcliffe Lane." "What's the matter with Grandma?" "Don't know. She's ill." The old fellow would come out with a written paper. "Take this, Love." Then you used to go in the Infirmary and sit and then there was a little place over there that door shut. If you wanted any medicine you used to have to go there and put your bottle down.
>
> *Interviewer:* Did you have to pay for the doctor?
>
> *Informant:* No, I don't think so. It would be recommended because we hadn't money to pay. Dr. Bromley used to come. . . . It was him that come when I scalded that leg . . . when I was scalded by the teapot.[127]

Similarly, Mr. Lane, born in Lancaster in 1896, remembered hard times in his adult household. "You went to the Relieving Officer and you got a

125. Mr. G1P, 10.
126. Mr. F2B, 7.
127. Mrs. B1L, 40. See also Mrs. H3L, 61.

chit to go to the doctor's with. The doctor was Dr. Mather at the Pointer, facing what is Dr. Frankland's now. The Relief people would pay."[128] Mr. Lane's left-wing politics possibly reduced for him the shame others might have felt about accepting charity. However, as we shall also see below in the discussion of hospital treatment, there is no doubt that Poor Law relief of any kind carried a social stigma and even affected people's willingness to use non–Poor Law services such as hospitals and public health clinics.[129] For example, Mr. Boyle, born in 1927, said his mother would not have taken her babies to a child-health clinic because "it was all linked somehow with welfare. It wasn't quite the same thing as the workhouse, but the same sort of tradition of public help for individuals, it used to be avoided if you tended to keep your self respect and all the rest of it. . . . She would rather have been seen dead, I think."[130]

An important step toward reducing working-class resistance to consultation of general practitioners came with the 1911 introduction of National Health Insurance (NHI) for workers paid less than £160 per year. Targeting mostly men, who were viewed as the main family breadwinners, NHI, according to Helen Jones, "did nothing for most married women, young workers between the ages of fourteen and sixteen or children when they were ill (presumably on the assumption that the man of the family would bring home a family wage sufficient to provide for their medical needs.)"[131] National Health Insurance, implemented in 1913, to which workers, employers, and the government contributed, offered sick pay, disability, tuberculosis sanatorium, and medical benefits. It also paid for the services of a registered midwife for the wives of insured workers.[132] Structured along the lines of friendly society club practices, patients joined the panels of affiliated GPs.[133]

Oral history informants suggest that NHI, often called the "Lloyd George" scheme, increased consultation of physicians among male wage earners.[134] Miss Thompson, born in 1912, remembered, "They used to call it Lloyd George because it was Lloyd George that brought the first free doctor out."[135] Mr. Burrell, born in 1931, said of his family, "Well, we were

128. Mr. L1L, 12. See also Mrs. M3P, 24, who applied to the "Town Hall" for assistance in paying for midwifery services when her son was delivered by a qualified midwife, but her husband had run out of NHI benefits.

129. Hardy, *Health and medicine*, 19–20. For further discussion of study informants' views on charity and public poor relief, see Elizabeth Roberts, "The recipients' view of welfare," in Joanna Bornat, Robert Perks, Paul Thompson, and Jan Walmsley, eds., *Oral history, health and welfare* (London and New York: Routledge, 2000), 203–26.

130. Mr. B9P, 10.

131. Jones, *Health and society*, 27.

132. Hardy, *Health and medicine*, 26–27.

133. See Digby, *Evolution*, 306–24, for discussion of the impact of NHI on general practice.

134. See, for example, Mr. C1B, 15; Mr. C1L, 10; Mr. C3L, 14; Miss M4L, 12.

135. Miss T4P, 39.

on what you call a doctor's panel, and I think this was paid for through installments through work, possibly. I know when the doctor came there was no cash to be paid." He remembered the doctor coming "quite frequently."[136] Nonetheless, informants recognized the program's limitations. When asked whether his family benefited from NHI, Mr. Grand, born in 1904, said, "Yes, but that didn't pay anything like the family. It only covered the man."[137] Mrs. Shelby, born in 1898, similarly recalled, "Women like that [housewives] didn't come under the health insurance. I had a bill for eight pound to pay when my mother died. There was nothing for women in those days."[138] Even male workers saw some drawbacks to the Lloyd George scheme. Mr. Grove, born in 1903, remembered: "You had a card and by the time we started work there were two. One for unemployment and one for National Health. You only paid about 6d for one stamp and 8d for the other. You started work at twelve, but you didn't start paying that until you could get the free doctor [at age 16]. Then when you got twelve months' stamps on you would have free doctor and you could claim off them for being off sick." However, the same informant praised the maternity benefit offered by NHI: "Previous to 1911, the midwife was anybody that could do it. Some charged 5s. or something like that. Then it come 1911 and there was a grant of 30s. for every child that were born. Then they compelled them to have a registered nurse. Now, her fee was 30s., so the patient was not better off. But you got better treatment because you had a fully trained nurse instead of an amateur."[139]

Informants whose families consulted doctors remembered diverse relationships with GPs. In some cases, their memories are imbued with nostalgia for a possibly mythologized past. For example, Mr. Best, born in 1897, said:

> The doctor when he came into your house, the family doctor, and he got to know your mother. . . . He knew all about your mother, and she'd nothing to hide from the doctor. The doctor would come in and she'd say, "What can I do now doctor, little Willy has got a cough, somebody has got ringworm, somebody has got earache." It depends on the doctor and the attitude, and he'd say, "You want to give them some steamed fish, cut out sweets." The doctor was the doctor and he was the adviser and knew all about the house and what you were doing, whether your husband went out to the pub. He knew all about you, so in my early days of the family doctor, I was the last of the family. In those days, and it is done today, you couldn't have the doctor unless you put your child or baby into a club. You went into a friendly society for halfpenny per

136. Mr. B2B, 13.
137. Mr. G1L, 14. See also Mr. H1L, 51.
138. Mrs. S1L, 10.
139. Mr. G1P, 7, 67. See also Mrs. D3P, 67.

week and for the halfpenny a week the society paid your doctors bill if
the child had to go to the doctor. That was the attitude, that the doctor
was everybody in those days.[140]

This account reiterates the importance of the friendly society in providing
access to the doctor in the first place. It also emphasizes the significance of
the GP's familiarity and long-term associations with family members, which
were often considered more significant than medical knowledge or skill.

Younger informants especially remembered special relationships with
doctors. For example, Mr. Kirby, born in 1921, said, "Our doctor was very
good, a very nice gentleman, and I used to play with his son. We didn't
live far away, and they had a surgery in Albert Street, and that doctor was
marvelous. He used to come and see me when I had that pneumonia. He
really did attend, a proper family doctor."[141] This account suggests a social
comfort level absent from most informants' experience. It also emphasizes
the physician's regular and personal attention. Mrs. Hunter, born in 1931,
recalled liking the family doctor when she was a child. She praised him, in
particular, for answering the telephone himself and coming quickly when
he was called. "Mind you, he was a unique doctor, bless him, there'll never
be another. . . . Our doctor was Dr. Rigg, his father had the previous practice."[142] Mr. Lewthwaite, born in 1950, said, "Dr. Healey, our GP, was a husband and wife team and I'm sorry really that the situation is not the same.
I mean, they more or less saw me into the world, I suppose, from being,
although I was born at Risedale [maternity hospital], they would have seen
me from a very early age, and you phoned for the doctor."[143] Mrs. Thornbarrow, born in 1949, said, "Well, I think there was a healthy respect for Dr.
Liddel and all the rest of them. . . . I remember being trooped off to the
doctor's fairly frequently for sore throats and all this, that, and the other.
So, I mean, they weren't averse to going to the doctors or taking advice."[144]
As was true of chemists, informants who had good relationships with doctors emphasized individual, face-to-face familiarity and interaction, as well
as intergenerational family continuity.

Some informants remembered generous GPs waiving or reducing fees
for poor families. Mrs. Lincoln, born in Preston in 1900, said:

We had a Dr. McDade in Ribbleton Lane, he was a Scotsman . . . swear,
but he was a good doctor. There were four of us down with measles
once, and I can remember this to this day, coming in, "How's so and so
today?" When we all recovered, I remember my mother saying, "How

140. Mr. B1B, 55. See also Mrs. M1P, 41.
141. Mr. K1B, 12. See also Mrs. H5L, 113; Mrs. L2L, 58–59.
142. Mrs. H3P, 88.
143. Mr. L3B, 47.
144. Mrs. T4B, 74.

are we going to pay this bill?" He said, "Don't bother about the bill, sixpence a week will do." That's how we paid that big bill of twenty or thirty pounds, at sixpence a week. He was a hard case but he was a good doctor. He never used to bother about payment from his patients.[145]

Mr. Warwick, born in 1931, said, "The first doctor I had was Dr. Ruxton, he delivered us. Delivered me, and my mother thought the world of him, you know, even when he murdered his wife, she still wouldn't have a word said against him. Primarily because he used to take pity on the poor, he would treat you for nothing, wouldn't he."[146]

Other informants remembered negative experiences with physicians. Some, as children, were frightened by the doctor's appearance. Mrs. Arnold, born in 1910, said, "Well, our doctor, he had a white beard, he was a big man, and I think we were a bit afraid of him. We didn't like to have the doctor."[147] Mrs. Wheaton, born in 1933, was scared of the family doctor because he was very tall.[148] More important, however, were issues of competence and professionalism, which influenced individual and family opinions of physicians generally. For example, Mr. Ackerman, born in 1904, remembered that his mother lost her last baby, "due to breast feeding. The medicine prescribed by the doctor for Mother killed the baby. . . . It is one of these mistakes that GPs make. They still make them, I suppose."[149] Mrs. Norton, born in 1909, looked after her mother-in-law, whose eyesight was failing, "And the doctor persuaded her that if she'd go and have one eye that was very bad operated on, it would strengthen the other. She said, 'Are you quite sure, Dr. Daniel?' and so he said, 'Oh yes.' Well, she had this operation, and, God bless her, she went blind. She said, 'I can never forgive him for asking me to have that operation.'"[150] Similarly, Mr. Ritter, born in 1894 in Lancaster, recalled, "After she [mother] come out of the Infirmary, she was made stone deaf. The doctor cut a goiter in her neck. She said that it was like guns going off, and she went stone deaf. She never heard m'younger sister speak."[151] Mrs. Peterson, born in 1899, called a doctor when her infant son developed complications after a stay in Preston's isolation hospital. The doctor did not respond promptly, and when he came to the house, he had been drinking. "He sent a fellow for

145. Mrs. L1P, 3. See also Mr. G7P, 84; Mr. W6L, 26.
146. Mr. W6L, 26. Dr. Ruxton became notorious because in 1935 he murdered his wife, Isabella, and their maid, May Jane Rogerson; dismembered their bodies; and disposed of them in rural Scotland. Ruxton, of Parsee heritage, was hanged at Manchester on May 12, 1936. Other Lancaster informants also mentioned him. See, for example, Mr. H1L, 14; Mrs. H2L, 17; Mr. N3L, 11; Mr. C6l, 19.
147. Mrs. A1P, 40.
148. Mrs. W5B, 50.
149. Mr. A2B, 73.
150. Mrs. N4L, 3.
151. Mr. R1L, 12.

the money. . . . This fellow come, and I said, 'I'm not paying for my son. He could have died, my baby, through his neglect. He come here at 10 o'clock at night and he were drunk!" This informant also lost her young daughter on the evening of the same day she had taken her to the doctor for an upset stomach.

> He gave her some medicine and her tummy was swelling up a bit and she kept having diarrhea. . . . She had had one lot of medicine. When she went to bed at night, I could feel her jumping. I had hold of her hand, and I thought it was cold. I didn't know. She had to be in bed with us as we were that poor we hadn't a cot then. She was in the middle and he had hold of her hand at the other side. She were jumping away like this and all at once he said that we have to get up. And do you know she had died in bed holding our hands like that. It was a shocking thing. It took me a long time to come round.[152]

In some families, chronic illness may have stimulated more consultation of physicians than occurred in healthier families. For example, Mrs. Parke, born in 1898 in Lancaster, remembered, "My brother was a weakling, and he only did about a third of his schooling. He was more often under the doctor than he wasn't."[153] Mrs. Struck, born in 1897, said she saw the doctor a lot when she was little. "Oh yes, up to being seven they'd spent a hundred pound on me. That was an awful lot of money, m'Mother said, in those days. I had every blooming ailment that ever came."[154] Mrs. Winder, born in 1910, remembered seeing the doctor often when she was a child:

> Yes, I had bronchitis as a little one and the doctor seemed to be always coming. We were only saying the other day that mother used to say that he used to come every day for about a week and then every other day. She used to say, "Oh, I wish he wouldn't keep coming," once I started to be better, but of course they kept coming because every time they came it was half a crown, half a crown a visit and half a crown for a bottle of medicine.
> *Interviewer:* It would take her ages to pay it off?
> *Informant:* They used to nearly die when the bill came because they only sent them monthly or quarterly, but I know mother sort of used to have a fit when the bill came. Every three months I think you used to get your bill. She used to say, "Oh, another doctors bill." By the time you'd paid it, you'd had a few more visits and you knew there was another one.[155]

152. Mrs. P1P, 9, 16.
153. Mr. P1L, 47. See also Mr. G1L, 14.
154. Mrs. S5L, 13. See also Mrs. S4L, 33.
155. Mrs. W2L, 144. Half a crown was worth 2 shillings and sixpence in old (pre-1970)

Some families called the doctor more frequently after delaying professional treatment had had a negative result. Mrs. Critchley, born in 1926, had an older brother who died of appendicitis. "He'd been eating green apples and he started having stomach pains in the night and my mother thought it was colic so she was giving him hot water bottles and things, well it wasn't till the following morning, she wouldn't send for the doctor in the night because she didn't like to call the doctor out." After this happened, her mother changed her consultation pattern: "Well, after Tommy died, she became very worried and nervy, and she would call him [the doctor] out more, because I've told you she didn't call him at first for Tommy because she thought it was colic. And then of course he died. So it made her much more nervous. But she would call the doctor for things like sore throats if it was tonsillitis, because Peggy had tonsillitis and that turned into rheumatic fever, and she was ill for a long time, so she became very frightened of sore throats. Those kind of things really, mainly."[156]

However, consultation of general practitioners was combined with informal home care, even among younger informants. Mrs. Read, born in 1927, said that as a mother, "If I was worried about anything, I would see my Mum, you know. If I thought they were ill, I would just go to the doctor's."[157] Mr. Whitaker, born in 1940, said of his family's doctor, "He was marvelous; he used to sit hours with me when I was a child, especially when I had whooping cough. I was very small, I was. . . . Well, the doctors said when I was born that I would never walk. So, from being a baby up to four years of age I was massaged every night with olive oil and goose grease." His grandparents did the massages.[158]

Inevitably, home care providers and physicians sometimes clashed. For example, Mrs. Washburn, born in 1900 in Preston, remembered:

If we were ill, Dr. Sellers or Dr. Hewittson would come. They never refused to come. When I had eczema very bad, it was my Aunt Mary and she said, "I wouldn't pay for the doctor, get some Zambuck [a patent remedy] as it is the finest thing out." The morning after it came up in great big scabs. So she gook me to Dr. Sellers and he played Hamlet. He said, "Have I ever asked for your money at more than sixpence a week? If you can't afford sixpence a week, give me three-pence a week. Never do anything like this again. You will have marked Emily for life." She had to make cold starch, thick, and put it on every scab and it brought them all off. When I was grown up, I went, and he said, "Well Emily, I know you have rouge on, but your skin's marvelous. You must never

money.

156. Mrs. C7L, 5, 51. See also Mr. K2P, 199.
157. Mrs. R3P, 60.
158. Mr. W7P, 44.

have scratched it." I had no marks. She didn't use quack stuff.[159]

Similarly, Miss Meade, born in 1902, said, "I remember having a very bad earache and the doctor being sent for. I remember Grandma putting a piece of onion in it and he made her take it out."[160] And Mrs. Owen, born in 1916, commented, "Doctors don't believe in rubbing, do they now, of course they have tablets, antibiotics. But we were always rubbed with goose grease, and a spoonful of it an all."[161] These accounts suggest tension between informal and formal health care authorities and techniques as well as the retrospective presumption that doctors' expertise and prescriptions were superior to informal knowledge and home and patent remedies.

To what extent did informants expect doctors to be able to cure them? Many, particularly in the older generation, had very low expectations. Comparing past with current effectiveness of professional medicine, Mrs. Oxley, born in 1902, commented: "The doctoring wasn't the same. They used to die with measles then. It's very rare that a baby dies with measles now. And, of course, they didn't have the injections that they do today for whooping cough. . . . [T]errible, they were, and they'd no injections for them, they did nothing. Old fashioned remedies, oh, they'll have it [whooping cough] until next May. And it was true, they did. I had my children with it from September till May."[162] Mrs. Marley, born in 1914, said about the medicine she bought from the GP, "It was old Dr. Thomas and he used to get it out of the tap. He had a whole row of bottles, all colors, and he'd pick the prettiest color and put just a little bit in the bottom of his bottle, and he had a water tap and then it got filled up with water, so Lord knows whatever I took."[163] Similarly, Mr. Ford, born in 1906, commented, "We couldn't afford a bottle of medicine from the doctor. Nobody had any faith in them anyway! My dad, he sometimes went to the doctor and if he got medicine he would pour it down the sink."[164] This opinion was validated by Dr. Kuppersmith, who said of his interwar practice, "Most of the medicines were of no value, none whatever. The medicines that we dispensed, they could just as well have done without. The very thought of having a bottle of medicine helped to cure them. It was psychological."[165]

Some informants also remembered questioning doctors' explanations. Mr. Danner, born in 1910, remembered a situation where "hard work and worry had me looking thin in the face and black under the eyes and Mother was worried. When I reported with a cold one day, Mother packed me off to

159. Mrs. W4P, 22.
160. Miss M4L, 12.
161. Mrs. O1B, 55.
162. Mrs. O1P transcript, no page number.
163. Mrs. M1B, 18.
164. Mr. F1P, 74. See also Mrs. M5L, 13.
165. Dr. K1P, 4.

the quack's. The family doctor was a young man. I suppose he had just read Freud, and because of this his answer to my inquiry on behalf of my mother about looking washed out, pale and thin in the face was, you have guessed it, sex," an explanation the informant found inaccurate and offensive.[166] Mr. Fleming, born in 1917, said, "Well, they didn't want doctors as much in them days as they do now, like, because they had to pay for him themselves like, you see. So, if you had no need to have the doctor, you've no need to have him and put up with fairy godmother stories, like, and all this. This is good for that and this is good for the other."[167]

However, this situation changed in the mid-twentieth century. As indicated above, younger informants were more likely as children to have regularly seen a general practitioner than older informants—and much more likely to consult physicians for their own children. This was due, in part, to a consensus that modern doctors knew more and were more effective than doctors in earlier times.[168] For example, Mrs. Young, born in 1915, said, "Medicine is much better now. In those days, the doctors only had pink water, hadn't they."[169] Rising dependence on GPs paralleled declining knowledge and use of home remedies, which were no longer associated with laudable independence but with ignorant old-fashioned behavior. When asked if she had had any "pet cures" for her children when they were young, Mrs. Christy, born in 1939, replied, "No, I don't think I did have. I think most of the cures I had were what the doctor had prescribed in the first place. You know, things like nose drops for colds, that kind of thing."[170]

Rising dependence sometimes threatened doctor-patient relationships. Mrs. Howard changed doctors in the 1970s because her GP refused a prescription she expected when her son was ill:

On the Wednesday, I said, "If you can get up, I'll drive you down to the surgery and you can get some antibiotics for that." Because he had to go back to work as soon as he could. . . . Anyway, funny thing was, I stayed outside waiting for him to come out. "Give me your prescription and I shall go and get it dispensed." And he said, "He didn't give me anything." I said, "What?" I was really against that, you know. So when I came home I wrote a letter saying that I didn't approve of them not giving him anything. You know, I explained it. But I said, "What did this doctor say?" Well, more or less he said, you've got to look after yourself, and heal yourself. I says, "How stupid!" So aired my feelings on a letter you know, and through this, we got thrown out of the surgery. . . . My

166. Mr. D2P, 42.
167. Mr. F1L, 29.
168. See, for example, Mrs. O1B, 58; Mr. N2L, 58.
169. Mrs. Y2P, 13. See also Mrs. B2P, 32.
170. Mrs. C8P, 87.

doctor came up to see me, he said he was very surprised that I should write such a letter. And do you know, it absolutely threw us at the time that doctors could set themselves up as little tin gods, as though they can't really be spoken to. You are not supposed to have an opinion. I wasn't saying anything about the doctor, just that, why couldn't he have given him some tablets, just to get him back? Because if they do give you them, you do get back to work quicker. It's unbelievable this, but after being my doctor for 25 years, and I'd never, ever aired my feelings before, and we were pretty close. He felt as he had to terminate . . . [us] on his panel because of me writing this letter. So, as a matter of fact, . . . well if that's what they think of us, who wants to be with them anyway?[171]

This account illuminates late-twentieth-century lay reliance on biomedicine, the GP's role as gatekeeper for prescription drugs, tension in the by then normative passive-patient/authoritative-physician relationship, and, ironically, lay resentment of the doctor's suggestion that the sufferer care for himself. Coming at the end of the study period, this encounter make sense only in light of the mid-century transformation of working-class health culture.

HOSPITALS

Between 1880 and 1948, the functions, structures, and importance of hospitals to study city residents in general, and working-class residents in particular, changed dramatically. In the late nineteenth century these facilities were used mainly by the badly injured, some surgical patients, paupers, and the mentally ill or handicapped, and were considered an undesirable alternative to safer, cleaner, more comfortable home care. Few middle-class people or children were hospitalized for any reason; virtually no women gave birth in hospitals. By contrast, in the mid-twentieth century, hospitalization became a routine part of life experience for members of all age groups and social classes. Institutions that had previously been run by honorary boards, matrons, general practitioners, and semitrained attendants became the professional arenas of medical specialists (referred to as "consultants"), formally qualified nurses, and technicians. Instead of a last resort when other therapeutic attempts had failed, both inpatient and outpatient hospital care became aspects of predictable, almost factory-style production of health. This change was multifaceted, and will also be addressed in other chapters of this book. This chapter will focus mainly on working-class use of, payment for, and attitudes regarding voluntary and Poor Law hospitals before 1948.

171. Mrs. H5L, 113.

In 1880 hospitalization was a minority experience in Barrow, Lancaster, and Preston, although demand for hospital facilities by local employers and physicians was growing. Indeed, it is clear that hospitals were regarded both as charitable obligations and as representations of civic responsibility and pride. Each city had a voluntary hospital that mainly served deserving poor people recommended for admission by subscribers drawn from socio-economic elites.[172] The Royal Lancaster Infirmary had been established as a dispensary for the sick poor in 1781 and merged with a House of Recovery founded in 1815; in 1880 the institution still inhabited the city-center Thurnham Street building constructed for it in 1832. A new, much larger building, heavily funded by the mill owner, James Williamson, opened in 1896.[173] Similarly, Preston's first dispensary was established in 1811, followed by a House of Recovery (mainly used as a fever hospital) in 1813. The Preston and County of Lancaster Royal Infirmary opened in 1870.[174] In 1866, responding to the large number of work injuries in its booming new factories, Barrow opened a cottage hospital with five beds. This facility, which would later be named the North Lonsdale Hospital, moved into a 25-bed facility in 1875.[175]

Poor Law institutions in each city housed paupers, many of whom were chronically ill, who relinquished their independence for the stern security offered by the workhouse.[176] Preston and Barrow had large workhouse infirmaries: Sharoe Green Hospital, which opened in Preston in 1869, and Roose Institution, which opened in Barrow in 1880. After 1929, these facilities were transferred to the control of local public health authorities, which converted them to municipal general hospitals and sought to diminish the stigma associated with them. Lancaster had a workhouse, dating back to the eighteenth century and enlarged in the 1840s and 1880s, which by the late nineteenth century contained an infectious diseases hospital and an infirmary. However, these facilities were used only by workhouse inmates and did not become a public hospital in 1929.

Outpatient treatment offered by voluntary hospitals was more popular than inpatient care. For example, in 1882 Preston's Royal Infirmary treated

172. See, for example, Steven Cherry, *Medical services and the hospitals in Britain, 1860–1939* (Cambridge: Cambridge University Press, 1996), 44–47; Hardy, *Health and medicine*, 15.

173. Blacktop, *In times of need*, 8, 17, 18, 42.

174. Wilkinson, *Preston's Royal Infirmary*, 27, 29, 35, 41.

175. J. D. Marshall, *Furness and the Industrial Revolution: An economic history of Furness (1711–1900) and the town of Barrow (1757–1897) with an epilogue* (Barrow-in-Furness: Barrow-in-Furness Library and Museum Committee, 1958), 322–23, 378.

176. See the Web site created by Peter Higgenbotham, "The Workhouse," http://users.ox.ac.uk/~peter/workhouse/index.html (accessed 12/5/05), for information about workhouse institutions in Barrow, Lancaster, and Preston. See also Ruth Hodgkinson, *The origins of the National Health Service: The medical services of the new poor law, 1834–1871* (Berkeley and Los Angeles: University of California Press, 1967), 451–574, for discussion of the workhouse infirmary's transition to the public hospital.

800 inpatients and 4,093 outpatients; in 1907 the Lancaster Royal Infirmary treated 4,002 outpatients and 625 inpatients.[177] This is not surprising, since free outpatient treatment was more affordable than consultation of a general practitioner, and sufferers could be cared for at home, beyond the reach of professional authority and institutional rules. However, comparatively low inpatient utilization also reflected the small size of local hospitals (Preston Royal Infirmary had 30 beds in 1870, when the city's population was 85,000) and the necessity for inpatients both to be unable to pay for care and to have a recommendation from a hospital patron.[178]

Another barrier to sufferers' acceptance of hospitalization was the very real threat of infection that endangered both patients and staff. For example, in Preston in 1875, "It became necessary to close the Infirmary for about eight weeks in order to disinfect thoroughly and paint the wards in an attempt to prevent the spread of erysipelas, a very acute inflammatory condition caused by a rather virulent microorganism which proved a scourge in hospitals generally."[179] Furthermore, although the Lancaster and Preston infirmaries were unusual in their willingness to admit contagious disease sufferers, mixing infectious with noninfectious patients was not a successful arrangement. For example, in 1876 the Lancaster Infirmary admitted 46 cases of smallpox, which spread to other patients, forcing evacuation of the hospital. This event motivated construction of an isolation hospital in the city in 1880. Preston's attempt to offer paying beds for nonpauper fever patients in the Harris Wards of the Royal Infirmary attracted few users, but arguably both limited provision for the needy and delayed construction of a purpose-built isolation hospital until 1907.[180]

In the late nineteenth century, because of the financial challenges besetting voluntary hospitals and the eagerness of employers to have somewhere to send accident victims (as well as, one presumes, a way to patch employees up and get them back to work as soon as possible), insurance-based worker contribution schemes were organized to pay for hospital care.[181] Barrow's scheme, composed of penny subscriptions from workmen supplemented by

177. Wilkinson, *Preston's Royal Infirmary*, 68; Blacktop, *In times of need*, 44–45.

178. Wilkinson, *Preston's Royal Infirmary*, 41; Blacktop, *In times of need*, 49. The Lancaster reference is to 1908, when the Royal Infirmary's management committee "had great anxiety in finding out if patients who used the institution were of a class for whom it was intended. . . . It was important that those not suitable, but who might reasonably be expected to pay for their own medical advice and attention, should not be brought into the institution."

179. Wilkinson, *Preston's Royal Infirmary*, 43.

180. Pickstone, *Medicine and industrial society*, 160–65, 170.

181. In *Furness and the Industrial Revolution*, 322–23, J. D. Marshall argues that a series of bad work injuries stimulated the campaign for foundation of Barrow's first cottage hospital in 1866. See the excellent collection, Roger Cooter and Bill Luckin, eds., *Accidents in History: Injuries, fatalities and social relations* (Amsterdam and Atlanta, GA: Rodopi, 1997), particularly Cooter and Luckin, "Accidents in history: An introduction" (1–16), and Cooter, "The moment of the accident: Culture, militarism and modernity in late-Victorian Britain" (107–57), for attempts to locate injuries in their social and medical contexts.

contributions from employers, helped to fund building of the North Lonsdale Hospital in 1875, as well as guaranteeing free care for workers and, eventually, their family members.[182] In Lancaster, a Hospital Saturday Fund was set up in 1879, giving workers a chance to contribute to the Infirmary and obtain care at no charge; a Workpeople's Committee was formed in 1889.[183] In 1882 the Preston Royal Infirmary established "the Workpeople's Committee and the start of weekly collections in the mills and workshops throughout Preston."[184] Worker contribution schemes, which continued up to the establishment of the National Health Service, offered free hospital attention, first to workers and later to their dependents. In addition, with other fund-raising efforts such as Hospital Saturdays or Sundays, parades, and dances, these programs fostered the transition of voluntary hospitals from charitable institutions controlled by wealthy patrons to community facilities concerning which working people had a sense of ownership and pride.[185]

Oral history informants were aware of local hospital histories. Mr. Hancock, born in Barrow in 1894, remembered: "The hospital first of all was chiefly started by railway men who took the place in Cross Street and then they went into Church Street into a larger house there and ultimately became domiciled in the present North Lonsdale Hospital which had been converted from private dwellings. Then there was the Devonshire Road Hospital for infectious diseases. There was the smallpox hospital which was never used, Rakesmoor, and, of course, there was always Roose Institution."[186] However, the oldest interviewees had little personal or family experience of hospitalization. Mrs. Ackerman, born in 1892 and one of seven siblings, said, "Our own family, I never knew any of us going into hospital, and I haven't been in my life yet, touch wood."[187] Mrs. Steele, born in 1898, recalled, "You never went to hospital unless it was for an operation or a fever."[188] Reflecting on the older generation's continued avoidance of hospitalization, Mrs. Walker, born in 1936, said, "I mean, Father was one of those and Mother was, and they have all been very healthy, till they have started creaking as they get older, you know. But then, they don't go into hospital, they doctor themselves up."[189]

In addition to preference for home-based management of ill-health, one reason for avoiding inpatient hospital care was fear. Mr. Quayle, born

182. Marshall, *Furness and the Industrial Revolution,* 378.

183. Blacktop, *In times of need,* 35, 39, 44–45.

184. Wilkinson, *Preston's Royal Infirmary,* 45.

185. Mr. Finch, born in 1900 in Barrow, said that Hospital Saturday Parades had only recently been abandoned at the time of his interview: "Indeed, they now provide extra pin money as it were for doing something which doesn't come under the authority" (Mr. F2B, 15).

186. Mr. H1B, 27.

187. Mrs. A3B, 41.

188. Mrs. S5P, 13.

189. Mrs. W6B, 82.

in 1897, remembered, "If anybody was taken to the Infirmary on account of illness, I don't know whether they did operations there or not, but if they took them to the infirmary you'd as good as said good-bye to them."[190] And Mrs. Harte, born in 1889, said she knew Nurse Whiteside who worked at the Royal Lancaster Infirmary, "the old one . . . Thurnham Street. . . . I remember once we were talking and they said that the dustbins was full of legs and arms that they'd chopped off at the Infirmary. They were trying to frighten us to death, some of them."[191] Fear deterred hospitalization, even when a physician recommended it. Mrs. Atkin, born in 1944, said: "Mum [had] an over-active thyroid gland. Now, she'd had this right from being little and if she got worked up about anything, especially my eldest brother, this lump would appear in her neck. It was very pronounced and the doctor used to say she'd to have an operation, but the thought of going in a hospital! You see, Mum had never been in, not to have us either, we were all born at home, would bring it even bigger, and so he gave her tablets."[192]

Another reason older people avoided hospitalization was the stigma of pauperization—both before and after 1929 when former workhouse institutions became public hospitals. Mr. Best, born in 1897, explained:

> Now, if I may speak about the workhouse, there was one section which was called the infirmary which is now called the hospital, so in connection with the workhouse there was the infirmary side, which had nothing to do with the fact of a person having misbehaved or fallen at the way, but just fallen on hard times. People who could not be admitted into North Lonsdale Hospital or shall I say geriatric who had to lay in until they were removed then to what was know then as Roose Infirmary. But because of the name "workhouse" this was a stigma and the people of Barrow said, "Whatever you do, don't put me in the workhouse," which was a great mistake, meaning don't let me have to go into the infirmary, . . . [a]nd even today among the older people, shall I say round the seventy mark, who can recall the workhouse days, still feel they would not like to go into Roose Hospital.[193]

Mr. Hancock, born in 1894, explained why people felt this way:

> My first impressions of the workhouse was the home of a last resort. The old workhouse in those days was inhabited by very poor people who

190. Mr. Q1B, 2.

191. Mrs. H2L, 17. Mr. Rust, born in 1890, said that before her marriage, his mother had been a nurse with Nurse Whiteside at the Thurnham Street Infirmary location. At that time, the staff consisted of a part-time physician, Dr. Dean, who also had a private practice, the Matron Mrs. Craig, Nurse Whiteside, Nurse Rimmer, and his mother, Nurse Robinson (Mr. R3L, 12).

192. Mrs. A3L, 36.

193. Mr. B1B, 6–7.

were sick in the infirmary or men who were often imbeciles, young and old men, and vagrants. . . . Their clothing was very rough worsted suiting. Women with their longish skirts, blouses—very often striped skirts, I remember. . . . The women too were young women with no homes or having left their homes. Some again I remember were imbeciles and they were a cosmopolitan crowd, really. In fact, they were people who had come down in the world.[194]

The workhouse was the place where girls who became pregnant out of wedlock, children and old people whose families could not or did not want to care for them, and drifters without homes were sent. Thus, workhouse inmates were shamed by both acceptance of charity and lack of conventional family support. This sense of shame continued after 1929. Mrs. Ackerman, born in 1904, commented: "They knew it was the end, once they got in the workhouse they knew they'd never come out again, the end of their life practically. . . . I think that fear still exists in a lot of very old people's minds because they'd rather go anywhere than go down to Roose. It's amazing, and yet it is so nice down there, it's upgraded to such an extent, but it takes a bit of convincing to some of the very very old people to tell them things are not like they used to be."[195]

Another barrier to institutional treatment was financial. Reflecting both on reasons for hospital treatment and fee-based care in the early twentieth century, Mr. Carson, born in 1902, said:

You paid so much a day in those days if you were in. There was what they called an Outpatients, anybody who'd had an accident could go and get free treatment even in those days. That was known as the Outpatients. If anyone was taken ill, appendicitis or operation, and they were in hospital for so many weeks and they used to send you a bill. They didn't force you to pay it, but they would ask you to pay something or make a donation to the hospital if you couldn't afford to pay the bill, which more or less everybody did something. . . . I was once scalded as well, but at work on m'face. All m'skin came off and m'hair. I was scalded when a steam pipe burst in m'face. . . . I spent m'twenty-first birthday in Lancaster Infirmary through that. . . . I got a bill for it. Six bob a day.[196]

Mrs. Hancock, born in 1893, remembered, "My father really was a boilermaker by trade, but a piece of steel, off the gentleman he was working

194. Mr. H1B, 8.
195. Mrs. A2B, 76. See also Mr. A2B, 76; Mr. B1B, 6–7; Mr. Q1B, 2.
196. Mr. C1L, 27. Mr. Horton, born in 1904, also got a hospital bill for treatment in 1933. He belonged to a hospital scheme, so he talked to the representative from his works committee. "He said, 'They send everybody 'em chance it's somebody who has a bit of money and they give a bit extra.' That's the way they used to do" (Mr. H3L, 59).

with, broke off and a piece went in Daddy's eye, so my dad had only one eye, but you couldn't have told because it was such a good eye. He went to Manchester for the treatment, and he was only a young man when he lost it." Her father had to pay for the treatment "because there was no National Health. In fact, in those days you didn't get compensation of no kind. There was no such thing as compensation."[197] Dr. Kuppersmith remembered hospital care in Preston between 1920 and 1948 being free, "except [for] those who went privately." He said, however, "Eventually they did start charging certain cases when the hospitals were getting in debt."[198]

Informants recalled situations where there was no charge for the hospital, but they paid a daily fee for attendance from their general practitioners.[199] They also remembered paying for private nursing home care or a bed in a hospital's private ward. Mr. Hardine, born in 1904, said:

> Now this is a thing and it come to pass that she [wife] had to go into care. She couldn't go in the Infirmary, you couldn't get in the Infirmary. Dr. Ruxton got her into this nursing home. It come out like this, my wages were about three pound something and her cost in that nursing home without extras was four and half guineas a week in them days. This was in 1930. Then you'd to pay for incidentals. She had brandy every night and stout every dinnertime because she'd lost so much blood. She was in three weeks and she couldn't be moved.
>
> *Mrs. Hardine:* He said to me once, "I'm running out of money." He asked Dr. Ruxton how much it was. He said, "Your wife shouldn't really go home, she should be in the Infirmary." I said to the doctor, "I can't afford it here any more, Doctor."
>
> *Mr. Hardine:* I'd take a bottle of stout up every night and this was Doctor's orders again. Anyway, her mother took her, and then of course what happened then, I got these bills. I got a bill from the doctor and I got a bill from the nursing home. So I went to the G.P.O. [post office savings account] and I said, "I want to draw out." He said, "Don't draw it all out, leave a quid [pound] in." I left a quid in. When I went to the doctor, I'd money then in m'pocket to pay. I said, "Your bill, Doctor." He said, "Look, would you like to have it paid monthly, give it to me monthly, it will be all right." I said, "No, I'll pay." He said, "Well, I'll knock that thirty bob off." That must have been the bit of profit to him.[200]

197. Mrs. H1B, 3.
198. Dr. K1P, 12.
199. See, for example, Mrs. W2L, 214.
200. Mr. H1L, 14. See also Mrs. O1B, 24–25. According to the on-line *OED*, a guinea was originally "An English gold coin, not coined since 1813, first struck in 1663 with the nominal value of 20s., but from 1717 until its disappearance circulating as legal tender at the rate of 21s." Currently, a guinea is "A sum of money equal to the value of this coin. In present use,

Similarly, Miss Alder, born in 1899, remembered her sister "going private" rather than waiting for a free hospital bed:

> Alice [her sister], she was full of pain and the doctor couldn't get her in hospital as there were no beds as usual. I told them they would have to do something for her. I couldn't do to see her, my mother had gone then. I worked myself up a bit and I went to the Infirmary and asked if there was anything they could do for her. I told them I couldn't do to keep watching her as she was suffering. They said it would be twelve months before there were any beds. They asked if she could afford to pay. I said she couldn't really, she just had her hard-earned savings like everybody else. We had been thrifty as we had been fetched up to be thrifty. I asked if she could go somewhere privately. In three days she was in Mount Street Hospital. We didn't choose, they chose. Doesn't that just show? It makes me feel bitter.[201]

These accounts indicate both increasing demand for hospital beds in the interwar period and the growing role of physicians (as opposed to voluntary hospital subscribers or employers) as gatekeepers for hospital and nursing home care.

Despite these examples, paying for hospitalization was rare. More commonly, informants remembered coverage through hospital schemes that were typically administered by major employers. A small weekly sum was deducted from the worker's wages; then, when a family member needed hospital treatment, the worker applied for a recommendation from the employer and received hospital admission and care free of charge. According to Mrs. Ackerman from Barrow, "Now, I was in hospital when I was eighteen and at that time I think they used to pay so much out of wages and when Dad worked it would be stopped out of his wages. I know I went into North Lonsdale Hospital with an appendix and we got a recommend into hospital. They didn't have anything to pay for me." When asked, "What were these recommends?" Mrs. Ackerman replied, "They were issued by Vickers for people who had entered the hospital scheme. I think it was two-pence a week out of the wages. He paid for years and years, and if you had anyone who needed to go into hospital you applied at Vickers and got this recommend and that was it."[202]

---

a name for the sum of £1.05 (21s). The guinea is the ordinary unit for a professional fee and for a subscription to a society or institution; the prices obtained for works of art, racehorses, and sometimes landed property, are also stated in guineas. Otherwise the word is now only occasionally used."

201. Miss A3P, 4. Mount Street Hospital was founded as St. Joseph's Institute for the Sick Poor in 1877. See David Hunt, *A history of Preston* (Preston: Carnegie Publishing, 1992), 215.

202. Mrs. A2B, 66. See also Mr. C1B, 15; Mrs. J1B, 21; Mrs. M6B, 13; Mr. P1B, 41. It is interesting that the word "recommend" was used for both insurance-based hospital admission and, as we have seen in the section on doctors above, outdoor medical relief offered by the Poor Law.

Mr. Carrington remembered a similar program in Lancaster: "The only thing was through that working at Storeys [mill] they used to make a deduction of a penny a week and that was per person and that paid into the Infirmary. You might call it voluntary because in the first place they might have called a meeting of the workers: 'Have you any objections to one penny being deducted from your wage?' Then it was automatic, that was that. . . . If you paid you did [get free treatment] and if you couldn't you couldn't."[203] Mr. Grand, born in 1904, said the Lancaster scheme initially covered only the worker. "There was a scheme brought out later which covered the wife and children, non-working children, but as soon as you became of working age and started work you had to join in your own right. It was three-pence a week. . . . If . . . you had to go into hospital for treatment your treatment was free. . . . There's a building down South Road which they're putting scaffolding up at it now, and that was where you used to go to pay your three-pence a week, because I used to go and pay my wife's and m'mother-in-law's once a quarter."[204] Mr. Eckley, born in 1895 in Preston, said, "All the people in the mill, they paid a penny or two-pence a week to the hospital, and then if you wanted to go to the Infirmary you went to the office and you got a paper. That certified that you had paid through it and they would attend to you."[205]

An important and popular aspect of hospital schemes was that they gave insured people the right to hospital care and eliminated the earlier expectation that sufferers ask permission and express gratitude for charity. Mr. Thomas, born in Preston in 1903, said: "When I started work on the railway as we have today, we had a hospital sick fund which was 3d. a week deducted from your wages. When you go in hospital, you go to your local man and ask for a certificate for the hospital. You go into hospital and when they saw that, they moved the furniture for you in hospital in those days because you were a sick man and you just walked in."[206] Hospital schemes also guaranteed members outpatient treatment. Miss Coyle, born in 1902, said her family paid into the Lancaster Royal Infirmary scheme. "I was only treated at Outpatients, but m'mother had x-rays and that was all free. Our Gladys had an operation on her knee and we didn't have to pay. I only visited Outpatients with a poisoned thumb, and that was enough for me: keep out if you can!"[207]

For many working-class families, the first encounter with hospital care came as a result of job-related injury. Indeed, as we have seen, Barrow's first hospital was founded because these injuries were so common. Informants' accounts are colored by implicit comparisons between then and now; they

203. Mr. C3L, 14. See also Mr. C1L, 74; Mr. H3L, 59; Mr. L1L, 16; Mr. M1L, 21; Mr. M3L, 38; Mr. P1L, 52; Mr. P2L, 8; Mr. T1L, 13

204. Mr. G1L, 14.

205. Mr. E1P, 45. See also Dr. K1P, 12–13; Mrs. P1P, 93; Mr. T2P, 74.

206. Mr. T2P, 74.

207. Miss C2L, 17. See also Mrs. M3P, 28.

reflect current expectation of compensation in cases of work-related health problems as well as the presumed contrast between good, modern and poor, old-fashioned hospital care. They also document the danger of work environments and everyday expectation of injury. In answer to the question, "Your father was a miner, was he?" Mr. Ford replied:

> Oh yes. He was crippled by the mines [in Cumbria]. In those days there was no compensation. I mean, today, if the same accident happened he would have been into the five-figure mark of compensation. He was doubled up; there was a fall of iron ore and he was doubled up with his head between his legs with all the weight on his back. Of course, there was no surgery in those days like there is today. They would dash to the local, well it wasn't a hospital, it was a little country place. They took the fever cases, they took anything in those days to these places. His back was broken, and one leg, and it left him a cripple for life.[208]

Mrs. Mallingham, born in 1896, said her father had several serious work accidents. In the first, when he was seventeen, he lost his hand. Later, he fell 45 feet from a crane. "There was no hope for him, and they did not bother about him at the hospital. They left him from the Tuesday, I think, to the Sunday with all his dirty working clothes on because they had no hope whatever. He was a hardy Scotsman and survived." Mr. Mallingham added, "He fell again, just before I knew you, 21 feet, but not off a crane. His trouble was he had to go to work between four and five in a morning to fire a crane and he had to have steam up . . . and he was working to nine and ten o'clock at night. . . . When he had the big fall, he split all his skull, I think he broke his leg, injured his elbow and they said it was hopeless. He only had one hand."[209] Mrs. Drake, born in 1899, worked in a munitions plant during World War I. She remembered a workmate's injury and hospitalization:

> She hadn't a hat on and of course it was a drilling machine. They're easy enough to work, them drilling machines, you just drill a hole, the hole for the screw. Anyway, she just happened to turn her head and her hair was loose and caught her hair in it. The screams, it was terrible, I remember it now. She hadn't the sense . . . she likely couldn't reach, I don't know, but one of us ran and stopped the machine and that is how they got her out. Well, it give her a shock. . . . She was taken in the ambulance, and I don't think she come back to work any more, but it was through not wearing a hat.[210]

208. Mr. F1P, 1. See also Mr. A4L, 22–23; Mr. B4B, 71–72; Mr. C1L, 27; Mrs. D1P, 20; Mrs. G1P, 76; Mrs. H1B, 3; Mr. H3L, 4; Miss H4L, 46; Mrs. N1L, 46; Mr. P4B, 17; Mr. T3P, 6; Mrs. W1B, 13; Mrs. W4P, 5.
209. Mrs. M6B, 1, 13.
210. Mrs. D1B, 39.

Mr. Danner, born in 1910, remembered having outpatient treatment when he was injured as an apprentice cabinetmaker. "I cut my hand and had to have 5 stitches. I wrapped my hand in shavings (we had no first aid kit, or even a tap, at work) and I walked about one mile to Preston Royal Infirmary." Describing the same accident later in the interview, he said, "I had four stitches put in by a young doctor and there was nothing to ease the pain. The needle hurt going in and out. I had gone to the hospital without a proper dressing on or recording the accident—something that must be done today. I still had to work with my hand bandaged. You can imagine how mucky the bandage was when I got home at night."[211]

As bad as these experiences were, hospital treatment seemed a better option than do-it-yourself first aid on the work site. Mr. Hardine, born in 1904, remembered working as a bricklayer in remote job locations:

Goggles weren't thought of in those days. The idea was that if you got something in your eye and you couldn't shift it, somebody would give you a pinch of snuff and at least you'd sneeze. So I got into that. Talking about crude methods to get things out of your eye, one of our masons got something in and it was a bit of metal as it turned out. When you're half-way between stations and you can't hop on a bus or a bike, to get down to a doctor or infirmary for some sort of attention. They laid this fellow down and poured water on it to try and irrigate it. Do you know how it was got off—one of his mates goes over to him like the kiss of life act and put his tongue in. Pulled it down and felt for it with his tongue and swished it off. It worked.[212]

As time went on, along with compensation and sick pay, working people grew to expect hospital care when they got hurt at work.

Hospital stays were longer in the early twentieth century than they would later become. For example, in 1908 the average stay at the Royal Lancaster Infirmary was 20 days, while in 1938 the average stay had declined to 16.6 days.[213] By 1960 the average stay in an acute-care bed in a British hospital was 12 days.[214] The most common hospital experience of older informants was for a contagious disease in an isolation hospital; this experience, which will be discussed at greater length in chapter 4, involved a long stay mainly to minimize exposure to infection of healthy family members, neighbors,

211. Mr. D2P, 4, 42.
212. Mr. H1L, 22. See also Mrs. S5P, 21.
213. Blacktop, *In times of need*, 44, 54.
214. Gordon Forsyth and Robert F. L. Logan, *The demand for medical care: A study of the case-load in the Barrow and Furness Group of Hospitals* (London, New York, and Toronto: Published for the Nuffield Provincial Hospital Trust by the Oxford University Press, 1960), 82.

and school- and workmates. However, other types of health problems also confined sufferers to hospital for lengthy periods. Mr. Eaton, born in Barrow in 1902, was injured as a child: "While I was at school a piano fell on me. . . . They took me home in a car, and I was that eager to get back to school and I went back again in the afternoon. It wasn't long after that, about a month, a big lump came on my stomach caused through a chill and I was in hospital for well over six month. After the operation I'd tubes in and I used to have to attend the hospital [outpatient department]. They used to do that until it dried up."[215] Mrs. Huddleston, born in Preston in 1917, remembered that her mother had a breast removed when she (the informant) was four years old. "She might have been away for six weeks as it was a longer period then with operations."[216] Mr. Rowse, born in 1903, spent four months in the Royal Lancaster Infirmary after an appendectomy when he was thirteen.[217] Mr. Rust's father was in the same hospital with bladder problems for six months during the interwar years.[218]

As a result of factors including increased hospital capacity, the trend toward doctors recommending admission for a growing number of conditions, increasingly routine recourse to surgery (including prophylactic removal of children's tonsils and adenoids), and people's rising willingness to accept inpatient care, hospitalization became more common during the interwar period. Mrs. Calvert, born in 1919, found herself running the family household at age 14:

> I had my brother at Christmas, my father at Easter, and my mother at Whitsuntide, I had all three of them in hospital that year. Our Jimmy hadn't been out so long, he had double pneumonia and then my dad had to go in and he came out on the Saturday as my mother went in the Saturday after. She was in seven weeks and she lost seven stone [98 pounds] in seven weeks. . . . We had to teach her how to walk when she come out. My dad was troubled with his chest and his lungs, that was regular for my dad. I was only 14 then and it pushed me in at the deep end and I had to bake and cook.[219]

Mr. Goodwin, born in 1945, reported having had his appendix and tonsils out in hospital as a child. "You went into hospital for all these sort of things, and you were in there for some—a week or ten days. You think it must have been months I was in there, you know, but it would only be a week or so." When asked, "How did you enjoy being in hospital," he responded, "I didn't like it because I was—well, we was always home with

215. Mr. E1B, 3. See also Mr. T1P, 36.
216. Mrs. H7P, 2.
217. Mr. R2L, 48.
218. Mr. R3L, 16.
219. Mrs. C5P, 12.

the family, and to be away from the family was something strange, you know, not something I would like."[220]

Hospitalization involved increased contact with medical specialists and trained nurses, as well as hospital rules. Some working-class informants, in accounts that had obviously been told many times, remembered consultants as heroic miracle-workers. For example, Mrs. Tinley, born in 1910, said she had injured her spine as a toddler and been given up as a hopeless case by her Barrow GP. Her mother demanded a referral to "Sir Robert Jones of Liverpool," who treated her at an orthopedic hospital in Shropshire where she was an inpatient for eighteen months, and who later described her as "one of his marvelous cures."[221] Similarly, Mrs. Washburn, born in 1900, said her brother was wounded in World War II:

> He was paralyzed all down one side. He was at Heaton Park in Manchester. . . . The doctor asked how he was situated at home, financially. My cousin told him that he only had sisters and a brother who was still in the army. The doctor said, "I can cure him, and if I don't cure him, I shall kill him." Do you know, he cured him. He was as straight as a die after he did it. . . . He [doctor] operated on his back. He [brother] was a stretcher-bearer and this bomb had gone off and Arthur had got it all at the back. The chap on the stretcher was killed and the other fellow, he wasn't so badly hurt.[222]

However, informants also found consultants intimidating. Mrs. Fleming, born in 1921, described her daughter's long battle with osteomyelitis (a bone infection), for which she was hospitalized for about five months in 1950. She said of the consultant, Mr. Kitchen, "Well, you couldn't get near him then, they were like gods. They really were."[223]

Much more frequent than patients' contact with consultants was attention from nurses—matrons, sisters (staff nurses), and probationers (trainees)—who staffed the hospitals and provided all bedside care. While the history of hospital nursing is beyond the scope of this study, many qualified nurses worked in local institutions, as well as for public health departments, schools, factories, and voluntary nursing associations.[224] All study cities had

220. Mr. G6P, 62.
221. Mrs. T3B, 1.
222. Mrs. W4P, 5.
223. Mrs. F1L, 117. Consultants' godlike characteristics had positive as well as negative attributes. Mr. Adderley, born in 1926, credited Mr. Kitchen for saving his arm after it was injured by a machine at Williamson's Mill shortly after World War II. In this case, the surgeon's heroism was expressed through both his disagreement with two other doctors about whether the arm needed amputation and his technical competence with the surgery and after-care. See Mr. A4L, 23.
224. For contrasting accounts of the history of nursing in Britain, see Dingwall et al., *Social history of nursing;* Brian Abel-Smith, *A history of the nursing profession* (London: Heinemann,

hospital-based nurse training programs.[225] Photographs and films of local hospitals invariably show uniformed nurses undertaking various tasks.[226] Thus, it is noteworthy how rarely oral history informants mentioned nurses, in contrast to their volubility about ill-health, doctors, and hospital treatment. This bears out Margarete Sandelowski's observation, "Anyone embarking on a history of nursing is soon confronted with the problem invisibles pose, that is, with how to study the relatively unseen."[227]

A possible explanation for the invisibility of nurses, compared to physicians, relates to nurses' familiarity and subordinate status. As female caregivers, they were official representations of the grannies, mothers, and neighborhood health authorities who felt brows for fever, administered remedies, and governed the environment of the sick; always there, rendering care rather than dramatic intervention, they attracted less attention than did physicians. In addition, as members of an occupation dedicated to service and obedience to doctors' orders, nurses were both skilled versions of uniformed domestic servants—also ideally invisible in the middle-class social world—and embodiments of what Barbara Melosh has called "the physician's hand."[228] Celia Davies points out that "a central issue for an understanding of gender and profession in the contemporary era turns not so much on the *exclusion* of women, but on a particular form of their *inclusion.*" She views professionalization as a historically masculine project where "ideologies of gender and gender imagery . . . explain and encapsulate the relations between the 'professional' work of men and the 'supportive' activities of women."[229] While there is some controversy about whether nursing should be considered a profession, it is clear that trained nursing was a distinct occupation with increasingly well-defined preparation, structure, hierarchy, and career options.[230] Perhaps nursing's unusual pseudo-military characteristics, which emphasized uniformed expertise, devotion

1960); Celia Davies, ed., *Rewriting nursing history;* Ann Bradshaw, *The nurse apprentice, 1860–1977* (Aldershot: Ashgate, 2001).

225. Wilkinson, *Preston's Royal Infirmary,* 46; Blacktop, *In times of need,* 51. The "Northwest Evening Mail," dated 12/5/05, contains an article and a photograph regarding nurse training at the North Lonsdale Hospital in the 1960s. See http://www.nwemail.co.uk/unknown/viewarticle. aspx?id=307663 (accessed 12/8/05).

226. See, for example, "The Royal Infirmary, Preston" (1936), film #104, North West Film Archive; "Tuberculosis Sanatorium at Ulverston" (1926), film #163, North West Film Archive; "Children's ward, North Lonsdale Hospital, 1890s," "Wattsy's Page" Web site, http://www.wattsys page.homestead.com/Nursespage.html (accessed 12/8/05).

227. Margarete Sandelowski, *Devices and desires: Gender, technology and American nursing* (Chapel Hill, NC: University of North Carolina Press, 2000), 15.

228. Barbara Melosh, *"The physician's hand": Work culture and conflict in American nursing* (Philadelphia: Temple University Press, 1982).

229. Celia Davies, "The sociology of professions and the profession of gender," *Sociology* 30:4 (1996): 663, 669.

230. In *Physician's hand,* 29, Barbara Melosh argues that nursing is not a profession. Nonetheless, much scholarship on the history of nursing focuses on its professionalization.

to authority of both nursing superiors and physicians, and submergence of individual personality traits and emotional responses, suggest one reason for nurses' comparative invisibility to patients; as virtual interchangeable parts, nurses became part of the technology of modern health care.[231] A complementary view is that as medical specialties developed and were glamorized in the mid-twentieth-century zenith of professional and institutional medicine, consultants absorbed all the light in the room. Nurses, as support staff and performers of mundane personal and maintenance tasks, were overshadowed.

Although accounts are rare, as we have seen, some informants discussed encounters with nurses. Mr. Rust remembered his father's appreciation of the work of Royal Lancaster Infirmary nurses:

> What do you think he talked about? Nobody had no idea, the conditions of how the nurses were working in those wards. . . . He was appealing for workpeople to give more than their penny a week. "These 'ere girls up at five o'clock in a morning going round giving cups of tea and one thing and another, and what was this penny a week doing towards it all?" The Chairman of the Work People's Committee came to see him in Beaumont Street thanking him for what he'd said.
>
> *Interviewer:* What year would this be?
>
> *Informant:* It would be before the Second World War, it would be in the late thirties.[232]

Like chemists, hospital nurses arguably helped to bridge the gap between traditional working-class health culture and biomedicine by interpreting doctors' orders while administering hands-on care and comfort. Unlike physicians, nurses more often came from working-class backgrounds and socialized with working people. As we have seen in chapter 2, some informal neighborhood health authorities were rumored to have been nurses before marriage.

However, nurses also helped to create and enforce increasingly rigid hospital rules that separated patients from their friends and family members. In addition, they served as uniformed representatives of medical authority and gatekeepers for access to consultants. When Mrs. Fleming's daughter was hospitalized with osteomyelitis, she could visit the four-year old only from 3:30 to 4:30 in the afternoon: "Sister Ballisteen, well she was the sister in charge of orthopedics, this sister. She would not let you see Mr. Kitchen, that was the surgeon. We asked her one day about seeing him, and all she said to us was, that she was lucky she [daughter] didn't have it

---

231. Sandelowski makes this argument in *Devices and desires.*
232. Mr. R3L, 17. This informant's father was an active trade unionist.

[osteomyelitis] over seven year old, and that if she was as old as us we'd be a cripple. And a year out of a child's life was nothing. Anyway, we demanded again, well Cliff [husband] did, and he saw him and he just more or less told him the same." This informant also said, "Old Bally [the nurse] loved to tell you bad news. Anyway, the day before the operation, she met me and told me about this, that she was going to theatre. Yes, I said, 'What chance? You know, what outcome?' She said, 'Well, you already have five more at home.'" By contrast, however, the same nurse arranged for the child to see a fireworks display and receive a doll that had been donated to the ward; the child herself asked to visit Nurse Balisteen after her discharge.[233] This account suggests that in the mid-twentieth-century hospital, nurses assumed the authority and control over the care environment and patient that wives and mothers exerted in working-class homes; however, nurses had the might of professional medicine behind them.

Mr. Monkham, who spent several months in hospital with gall bladder trouble as an eleven-year-old in 1959, described a transition in health care authority from home and neighborhood to hospital and medical staff. He recalled that his mother and Nana Riley, an elderly informal neighborhood health authority, went with him in the ambulance to the hospital and his mother signed the consent form for surgery. He felt like a celebrity because his case was discussed by several doctors. When asked, "Was there much attempt on the part of the nursing or medical staff to explain to you what was actually going on?" he said:

> Only in the simplest terms. You know, it was, "We are going to do this now," da, da. . . . It was kept very simple, but I remember wondering many many times really what it was all about, but being perhaps too young, too naïve, non-assertive to actually ask. And perhaps feeling socially intimidated in terms of, "Well, I was only a poor working-class kid," These were obviously much higher up the social scale than me, and being far too intimidated to actually assert myself. And really leaving it to my parents to a large degree, Mother taking the lead, Dad always went, but he was stood in the background and he never asked. Mum did all the talking, Mum did all the consenting, she signed the papers, not Dad.[234]

This account illustrates both growing working-class trust in and use of formal medical treatment during the mid-twentieth century and the continuation of women's role as health care decision-makers. It also suggests the relegation of neighborhood health authorities to supportive friends.

233. Mrs. F1L, 112, 113, 117.
234. Mr. M10L, 7.

CONCLUSIONS

Between 1880 and 1948, working-class residents of Barrow, Lancaster, and Preston increased their use of formal professional and institutional health care, diluting their reliance on informal neighborhood- and home care. While continuing to deal with even serious health problems at home, use homemade and patent remedies, and ask chemists and neighborhood health authorities for advice, working-class people called general practitioners and accepted hospital admission for themselves and their children more often during the interwar period than they had at the turn of the twentieth century. Indeed, the interwar years may be viewed as a watershed for the transformation of working-class health culture in the study cities—a transformation that, while not apparently inevitable at the time, was completed with the introduction of the National Health Service in 1948. This chapter has emphasized the role of neighborhood chemists in providing a bridge between traditional and official health care, the impact of insurance-based programs that reduced financial barriers to professional and institutional medicine, growing compulsion to consult the physician as gatekeeper, and rising perception of the efficacy of biomedicine in facilitating working-class use of doctors and hospitals. In chapter 4, we will turn to the relationship between public health services and working-class residents of Barrow, Lancaster, and Preston.

Chapter Four

"No fever in our house"

Contagion, Prevention, and the Working Class

In his 1975 study of the development of modern prisons, Michel Foucault observed, "The plague as a form, at once real and imaginary, of disorder had as its medical and political correlative discipline."[1] This chapter illustrates how this argument worked itself out in conceptualization and management of contagious disease in late-nineteenth- and early-twentieth-century Barrow, Lancaster, and Preston. It begins by injecting the element of social class. Although middle- and upper-class people experienced and died of diseases known to be communicable, the natural source and home of these diseases, as well as other forms of disorder, was understood to be working-class neighborhoods, dwellings, and bodies.[2] The chapter maintains that contagious diseases were both "real," in the sense that they sickened and killed many people, particularly in the early years of the study period, and "imagined," in the sense that they were constructed as threats and challenges to be overcome by national legislation and local elites. The chapter observes, on the one hand, the dynamics of official and professional power, which attempted to discipline working-class behavior and thoughts, and, on the other, traditional working-class health culture, which exercised wide-ranging discretion about ways to deal with contagious diseases and official health authorities. Although nineteenth-century political economists and evangelical philanthropists, together with an eclectic mix of turn-of-the-century social reformers, certainly favored top-down imposition of change in working-class lifestyles to improve general health, the years between approximately 1880 and 1948 witnessed both long-lasting

1. Michel Foucault, *Discipline and punish: The birth of the prison* (New York: Vintage Books, 1979), 198.
2. See, for example, Bryan S. Turner, *Medical power and social knowledge,* 2nd ed. (London and Thousand Oaks, CA: SAGE Publications, 1995); Gerry Kearns and Charles W. J. Withers, "Introduction: class, community, and the processes of urbanisation," in Gerry Kearns and Charles W. J. Withers, eds., *Urbanising Britain: Essays on class and community in the nineteenth century* (Cambridge: Cambridge University Press, 1991), 1–11.

working-class resistance to and a multifactored hegemonic process resulting in working-class acceptance of biomedical approaches to disease prevention and management.

The period also hosted development of a new professional discipline—public health or social medicine—and a series of subdisciplines related to new occupations under this umbrella. Adapting national trends to local environments, medical officers of health, health visitors, district nurses, sanitary inspectors, and others helped to invent and pilot their new occupations, disciplining themselves, each other, and the working-class people (mainly women) who composed the justification for their activities. The order they attempted to impose was moral, social, and scientific; paralleling the mortality decline, the apparent success of this attempt first justified the expansion of public health and eventually supported arguments for its irrelevance.[3]

But let us begin with local experience of contagious disease. Between April and August, 1889, successive epidemics of measles, whooping cough, and diphtheria swept through Preston. Measles killed 233 children under age ten. Diarrhea slaughtered 263, of whom 205 were infants under age one. Typhoid murdered 53 city residents. With relief, the Medical Officer of Health, Dr. H. O. Pilkington, reported that only 17 children had died of scarlet fever—less than the average of 50 in each of the previous six years.[4] The year 1889 was not unusual, nor was Preston's experience unique. For much of the nineteenth century, contagious disease was regarded as both the major threat to and the major danger posed by the English working classes.[5] While disproportionately affecting poor people, like political disorder, ailments understood to be transmitted from one person to another threatened to seep past the boundaries of working-class neighborhoods and harm the prosperous. Contagion had at least as great an impact on the public imagination as it had on individual bodies.

Furthermore, sickness and death from diseases thought to be preventable, which included an increasing number of contagious ailments, motivated leaders to address problems that damaged both industrial productivity and city reputations. Although hindsight confirms that by the end of the nineteenth century mortality from most infectious diseases had already begun the rapid decline that continued after 1900, this trend was not apparent to contemporary local governmental officials, voters, or ratepayers (property-tax payers), who had been blasted by epidemics and

---

3. See, for example, Jane Lewis, *What price community medicine: The philosophy, practice and politics of public health since 1919* (Brighton, Sussex: Wheatsheaf Books, 1986).

4. Preston MOH Report, 1889, 2–3, 19, 21.

5. See Dorothy Porter, *Health, civilization and the state: A history of public health from ancient to modern times* (London and New York: Routledge, 1999), 111–46, which provides a useful discussion of links between urbanization, social class divisions, poverty, disease, and development of state medicine in Britain.

shaken by devastating infant mortality rates that actually remained stable or rose between 1880 and 1900.[6]

While not always eager to spend the money required for major public works, local decision makers certainly viewed contagious disease as a serious problem and the new public health professionals and infrastructure as an important solution.[7] Furthermore, although mortality rates were dropping, morbidity from infection continued—particularly among the working classes—and reformers linked contagion to susceptibility fostered by factors such as dirt, heredity, crowding, ignorance, vice, and poverty. For these reasons, the sanitation projects motivated by miasma theory in the mid-1800s, the concepts and tools offered by bacteriology after about 1880, and the moral and social improvement agendas straddling the turn of the century provided powerful, and not necessarily mutually exclusive, weapons in the battle against the most dramatic killers of the industrial era.[8]

Agents of this struggle, MOsH and their growing staffs concentrated their efforts on both the environments and the individuals within which sickness bred. These efforts focused especially on the neighborhoods, dwellings, bodies, and activities of working-class people, whose rights to privacy, self-determination, and liberty were considered less important than the danger their attitudes, actions, and excreta posed to the wider community. Proliferating public health approaches including notification, surveillance, isolation, disinfection, and education (later referred to as "propaganda") were directed at both an increasing range of medically defined disorders and their human hosts.[9] It is not coincidental that the language of public

6. See, for example, Simon Szreter, "The importance of social intervention in Britain's mortality decline c. 1850–1914: A re-interpretation of the role of public health," *Social History of Medicine* 1: 11–37, regarding the nineteenth-century rise and decline of mortality from "the classic sanitation and hygiene diseases." Anthony S. Wohl, *Endangered lives: Public health in Victorian Britain* (London: J. M. Dent & Sons Ltd., 1983), remains the most thorough national study of the development, challenges, and operation of public health administration in nineteenth-century Britain. See also R. I. Woods, P. A. Watterson, and J. H. Woodward, "The causes of rapid infant mortality decline in England and Wales, 1861–1921," *Population Studies* 42:3 (1988): 343–66; Nigel Morgan, "Infant mortality, flies and horses in later-nineteenth-century towns: A case study of Preston," *Continuity and Change* 17:1 (2002): 97–132.

7. See Morgan, "Infant mortality, flies and horses," 106–11; Wohl, *Endangered lives,* 169–75.

8. Michael Worboys, *Spreading germs: disease theories and medical practice in Britain, 1865–1900* (Cambridge: Cambridge University Press, 2000), argues that, rather than being a kind of prescientific theory, "the meanings of miasmas were refined until they were subsumed within a spectrum of contagious and infectious diseases" (38). Therefore, MOsH's "inclusive" attacks on environments believed to breed disease coexisted with their later "exclusive" focus on keeping individual sufferers from endangering populations (108–50, 234–76).

9. See, for example, David Armstrong, *Political anatomy of the body: Medical knowledge in Britain in the twentieth century* (Cambridge: Cambridge University Press, 1983). In *An introduction to the social history of nursing* (London: Routledge, 1988), Robert Dingwall, Anne Marie Rafferty, and Charles Webster make the related argument that trained nurses and health visitors were agents of social control, determined to change the behavior and improve the moral and physical health of working-class people.

health suggests military strategy and law enforcement; its agents, wielding powers conferred by statute, science, social class, and (sometimes) gender, believed themselves to be engaged in a war against disease and the dirt, ignorance, and vice that fostered it. Furthermore, declining mortality rates fueled consensus that the war was being won by health professionals. This explains the apparent paradox that as the threat of contagious disease declined after 1880, the services, bureaucracy, and personnel devoted to its control grew.

At the same time, working-class families expected fatalistically and managed traditionally the vicious infections that sickened or killed one child after another and, when affecting wage earners or homemakers, threatened family viability. Like other health events, women customarily dealt with these ailments at home with support from relatives and neighbors. The oral evidence shows that working-class people understood the dangers of common contagious diseases. Many informants had children, siblings, other relatives, or neighbors who died from killers including diphtheria, scarlet fever, typhoid, whooping cough, and tuberculosis.[10] More interviewees said that they or members of their families had experienced and survived these ailments, with or without permanent damage. Informants also remembered that some diseases, particularly smallpox and tuberculosis, were feared more than others, such as mumps and chickenpox. This evidence demonstrates that both public health authorities and working-class people perceived contagious diseases as threats.

However, their respective judgments about prevention and management of these diseases were markedly different. For example, from the 1890s isolation by home quarantine or hospitalization was the approach MOsH increasingly favored to limit the spread of infection. It is clear that isolation of sufferers in working-class homes and neighborhoods was always difficult and often impractical because of space challenges, the many demands on caregivers' time and attention, and the incubation periods and durations of many communicable ailments. Measles was contagious before it was symptomatic, and typhoid could be carried for years by people without symptoms. Whooping cough usually lasted for several months, and the standard isolation period for scarlet fever in the early twentieth century was six weeks. Furthermore, isolation discouraged mutual aid services, advice, and emotional support—as we have seen, far more important to working-class families than were professional and institutional health care. In addition, the main purpose of isolation was not to cure the sufferer, but to protect the well—a goal that was understandably a higher priority for MOsH than for working-class mothers. Presuming on the basis of

10. See, for example, Mrs. B1L, 4; Miss C2L, 16; Mr. D2P, 34; Mrs. G1P, 61; Mrs. H2L, 1; Mrs. H2P, 19; Mr. M2B, 2; Mrs. M3B, 2; Mrs. M3L, 32, 34; Mrs. O1P, 3; Mrs. P1P, 14; Mrs. R1B, 19; Mr. R1L, 12, 63; Mr. T1B, 6.

long experience that children were likely to contract whatever ailment was "going around," some mothers deliberately exposed children to a mild case of measles or scarlet fever in order to "get it over with."[11] Parents also sometimes resisted enforcement of home quarantine or removal of the sufferer to isolation hospital because these measures deprived families of aid, comfort, and control. Furthermore, in diseases such as tuberculosis or venereal disease that were associated with vice or poor heredity, formal diagnosis carried a stigma that could damage family reputations. Like working-class opposition to compulsory smallpox vaccination, which was especially strong in the North of England and common among study informants, professional medical involvement in cases of contagious illness was accepted unenthusiastically and sometimes evaded or resented.[12] As we have seen, official help was often accompanied by criticism of the housekeeping, management, and child care skills of working-class wives and mothers—key elements of their identities and reputations. Thus, public health and working-class perspectives on the correct ways to deal with contagious illness differed, particularly before the interwar period. It is also clear that the contested terrain of working-class bodies, homes, and neighborhoods was not level; against the might of science, superior social status, financial resources, and enforcement powers, working-class people exercised mainly the weapons of passive resistance.

By the mid-twentieth century, consensus had developed in working-class families and neighborhoods that "germs" were responsible for many diseases and that official medicine and public health offered reliable information about prevention and the best therapies for those ailments. This consensus had complicated roots, but owed more to public health authorities, whose access to working-class homes was mandated, than to general practitioners who entered and stayed by invitation only. Health authorities had enforcement powers over matters immediately affecting working-class households, including notification of birth, death, and illness from certain diseases; isolation of sufferers and their family members (in either home quarantine or hospital); inspection of homes, yards, and (after 1907) schoolchildren; and disinfection of houses and personal property. Public health offered the first reliable tools for diagnosis (laboratory tests), prevention (vaccinations), and specific treatment (antitoxins) of contagious diseases. Furthermore, official health advice delivered in homes, clinics, schools, and public venues infiltrated the cultural space previously governed by tradition. By the interwar years, public health personnel, welcome or not, were everywhere in working-class neighborhoods, where they undermined the position of traditional neighborhood health authorities and home-based care, at the

11. See, for example, Mr. B2B, 40; Mr. F2L, 79; Mrs. H4P, 36; Mr. K2P, 83.
12. See, for example, Nadja Durbach, "'They might as well brand us': Working-class resistance to compulsory vaccination in Victorian England," *Social History of Medicine* 13:1 (2000): 45–62.

same time substituting new sources of authority and service. Enforcement partnered with hegemony to create a new working-class health culture around the same time that the National Health Service improved access to clinical medicine.

Unlike John Welshman's excellent study of public health in twentieth-century Leicester, this book does not offer a comprehensive administrative history of public health in Barrow, Lancaster, and Preston.[13] Nor will this chapter provide a systematic account of local public health responses to major contagious diseases modeled on that offered by Anne Hardy for late-nineteenth-century London.[14] Rather, in keeping with the overall theme of the book, this chapter will emphasize cultural and social issues associated with contagious diseases and the relationship between public health authorities and working-class residents in the study cities between about 1880 and 1948. Opening with an overview of local experience of infectious diseases for which public health authorities were responsible, it will consider the changing perspectives and activities of public health personnel, particularly MOsH and health visitors, and provision of sanitation, advice, and institutional (mainly hospital and sanatorium) services. It will also explore working-class experience and management of contagious diseases and perspectives regarding public health domiciliary and hospital services. Finally, it will offer conclusions about the relationship between public health and professional medicine, on the one hand, and mid-twentieth-century changes in working-class health culture, on the other.

CONTAGIOUS DISEASES IN BARROW, LANCASTER, AND PRESTON

In terms of incidence, mortality, and emotional impact, the diseases threatening public order and productivity in Victorian Britain were not equal.[15] For example, while standard histories of public health legislation and initiatives emphasize the role in catalyzing reform of the "shock disease," cholera, this ailment's demographic impact—particularly in the late nineteenth century—was minimal.[16] By contrast, Anne Hardy's research shows that in the 1860s whooping cough, measles, scarlet fever, diphtheria, smallpox, typhoid, typhus, and tuberculosis "contributed nearly 30 per cent of the

---

13. John Welshman, *Municipal medicine: Public health in twentieth-century Britain* (Oxford: Peter Lang, 2000).

14. Anne Hardy, *The epidemic streets: Infectious disease and the rise of preventive medicine, 1856–1900* (Oxford: Clarendon Press, 1993).

15. Charles Creighton, *History of epidemics in Britain* (Cambridge: Cambridge University Press, 1891).

16. See, for example, George Rosen, *A history of public health* (Baltimore and London: Johns Hopkins University Press, 1993. First published in 1958), 254; Porter, *Health, civilization and the state*, 95.

total annual deaths in England and Wales."[17] While authorities observed differences in the means of transmission of these ailments, they also observed that contagion flourished especially in the homes and neighborhoods (the "slums" or "rookeries") of poor people who themselves were perceived, in the words of Beverly Skeggs, "as dangerous, polluting, threatening, revolutionary, pathological and without respect."[18]

Medical Officers of Health spearheaded local battles against contagion.[19] Driven after the 1889 Notification of Infectious Diseases Act by locally negotiated obligations to report "notifiable" ailments and by their own training and perspectives, early MOsH in Barrow, Lancaster, and Preston focused on "zymotic" diseases, a term originating with William Farr that, from 1842, categorized such ailments according to a theory articulated by the German chemist, Justis von Liebig, in which "Disease was seen as 'a spreading internal rot, that . . . came from an external rot, and . . . could be transferred to others.'"[20] As Michael Worboys explains, this theory served the new public health authorities well, supporting both the idea that contagious diseases could originate in the environment and "the notion that zymotic diseases struck 'susceptible individuals' . . . [which] gave meaning to the social, gender, and ethnic patterns of disease incidence."[21] The multipronged strategies adopted by MOsH, which included both "sanitary science" (advocacy of clean water and sanitation projects, associated with mid-nineteenth-century approaches) and "preventive medicine" (notification, surveillance, isolation, and education, dating from the 1880s) continued to focus on eradication of "preventable" zymotic diseases, as opposed to the "constitutional," "local," and "developmental" disorders, whose origins in individual bodies and hereditary tendencies made them unpreventable.[22]

This categorization helped to define the sphere of responsibility of public health authorities and, in an atmosphere of both heightened fear of contagion—the 1871–73 smallpox epidemic surely stimulated support for

17. Anne Hardy, *The epidemic streets*, 3. For discussion of nineteenth-century cholera epidemics and their social, policy, and medical impacts, see, for example, Margaret Pelling, *Cholera, fever and English medicine, 1825–1865* (Oxford and New York: Oxford University Press, 1978), and Wohl, *Endangered lives*, 118–25. In *The people's health 1830–1910* (New York: Homes and Meier Publishers, Inc., 1979), F. B. Smith discusses the impact of a range of contagious diseases on age groups.

18. Beverley Skeggs, *Formations of class and gender: Becoming respectable* (London: SAGE Publications, 1997), 1.

19. See, for example, Pelling, *Cholera*, 101–8; Wohl, *Endangered lives*, 166–204; Hardy, *Epidemic streets*, 4–8.

20. Worboys, *Spreading germs*, 34–35. See also Pelling, *Cholera, fever and English medicine*, 113–45.

21. Worboys, *Spreading germs*, 41.

22. Worboys, *Spreading germs*, 112, discusses constitutional diseases. Barrow's MOsH categorized causes of death as "zymotic," "constitutional," "local," and "developmental" diseases, as well as "violence," in annual reports for the period 1882–1910. The term "zymotic diseases" was used in Preston MOH reports until 1925.

the 1872 and 1875 Public Health Acts—and growing anticipation of scientific victory over microbes, intensified public concern about contagious diseases. The MOsH appointed in growing numbers after 1870—in Barrow, Lancaster, and Preston as well as elsewhere—benefited from this concern since contagious diseases both justified their positions and supported arguments for expansion of public health activities.

Public understanding of contagious disease was increasingly based on epidemiology—public health officers' conceptualization, collection, analysis, and reporting of statistics regarding births, deaths, and the incidence of and mortality from notifiable diseases. In an era when science was changing rapidly and roles and responsibilities regarding local health and illness were in the process of being conceptualized, these statistics reflect medical officers' shifting perceptions about disease identification and causation; they also reflect resource issues and public health arguments. Should community efforts and funds be directed toward housing reform or isolation hospital construction? Were the annual summer epidemics of infant diarrhea caused by poor sanitation (remediable) or hot weather (beyond MOH control)? It is possible to view late-nineteenth- and early-twentieth-century English cities as laboratories where changing hypotheses about morbidity and mortality were tested. Another appropriate metaphor, however, might be the sales demonstration, where data are mustered to support a predetermined result. Regardless, public health attention focused on the incidence and prevention of zymotic diseases.

By the 1880s, when data for Barrow and Preston were first reported by MOsH, the zymotic diseases appearing as causes of death were smallpox, measles, scarlet fever (also referred to as scarletina), diphtheria, whooping cough, continued fever (including typhoid, typhus, and other unspecified fevers), and diarrhea. In 1882 zymotic diseases accounted for 221 (22.5 percent) of the 980 deaths in Barrow.[23] In 1889 these diseases were responsible for 777 (25.7 percent) of the 3,019 deaths in Preston.[24] Zymotic diseases disproportionately killed children. Of the 777 deaths from these ailments in Preston in 1889, 347 (44.6 percent) were of infants under one year old, and 681 (87.6 percent) were of children aged five and younger. Of course, zymotic diseases were not the only killers of infants and small children; in 1889, 548 Preston infants under age one and a further 116 children aged between one and five died of teething, convulsions, premature births, and debility—the so-called "developmental diseases."[25] However, as ailments deemed preventable, zymotic diseases attracted the most attention and action from late-nineteenth- and early-twentieth-century MOsH. They were joined after 1883 as a special focus of public health interest and activity

23. Barrow MOH Report, 1882, 215.
24. Preston MOH Report, 1889, 19.
25. Preston MOH Report, 1889, 19.

by tuberculosis, which, while now determined to be contagious, was never included within this category.

Although zymotic diseases were classified together, they exhibited different patterns of incidence and severity, with measles and whooping cough, for example, coming in epidemic waves every few years, while typhoid maintained a small but steady presence that declined earlier in Barrow and Lancaster than in Preston.[26] Zymotic diseases also inflicted widely differing levels of mortality. For example, in Preston diarrhea remained an important cause of infant death until the early twentieth century, killing between 103 (1903) and 343 (1893) children each year between 1889 and 1906. By contrast, during the same period diarrhea accounted for the deaths of between 9 (1902) and 61 (1906) Barrow residents. In Lancaster, this ailment caused 38 deaths in 1906, but fewer than 18 per year thereafter. Indeed, since at no point in the period under consideration did contagious diseases account for a majority of deaths in the study cities, one important question is why they attracted such a disproportionate amount of attention and resources. This question is particularly appropriate regarding Lancaster, where in 1910 zymotic diseases accounted for only 33 (5.9 percent) of 555 deaths compared to 170 (9.6 percent) of 1,758 deaths in Preston and 134 (14 percent) of 937 deaths in Barrow.

As other scholars have observed, contagious diseases had contrasting cultural meanings and powers to generate individual or collective responses that shifted over time.[27] Thus, for example, smallpox, which caused comparatively little morbidity and mortality in Barrow, Lancaster, and Preston after 1880, lingered in collective dread, stimulating maintenance of separate, rarely used smallpox hospitals in each city, detailed investigations of each case reported, and annual reference to smallpox and related issues, such as vaccination, even when no cases were notified.[28] Unlike other zymotic diseases, smallpox was rarely thought to be generated locally but was associated with external exposure—a threat to a known community from an unfamiliar other. Barrow, which attracted many sailors

26. See Anne Hardy, *Epidemic streets,* for detailed discussion of the diverse behavior of whooping cough, measles, scarlet fever, diphtheria, smallpox, typhoid, typhus, and tuberculosis, and efforts made by London's public health authorities to control their spread.

27. See, for example, David Arnold, *Colonizing the body: State medicine and epidemic disease in nineteenth-century India* (Berkeley: University of California Press, 1993); Worboys, *Spreading germs,* 236.

28. See, for example, Barrow MOH Report, 1883, 211; Barrow MOH Report, 1888, 195; Barrow MOH Report, 1897, 150, 178; Barrow MOH Report, 1927, 277; Preston MOH Report, 1915, 3; Lancaster MOH Report, 1910, 41; Lancaster MOH Report, 1916, 16. J. D. Marshall, *Furness and the Industrial Revolution: An economic history of Furness (1711–1900) and the Town of Barrow (1757–1897) with an epilogue* (Barrow-in-Furness: Barrow-in-Furness Library and Museum Committee, 1958), 373, provides an account of the 1872 smallpox epidemic in Barrow, which sickened 730 and killed 85. He attributes the severity of the outbreak to overcrowding in the rapidly growing town, and attributes to it new interest in constructing houses for workers and raising money for an isolation hospital.

and migrants, was particularly worried about this challenge, in 1883 and 1885 reporting importation of this "loathsome disease" by local people who had visited Staffordshire, Cardiff, and Yorkshire.[29] Health authorities also associated smallpox transmission with tramps moving from town to town, thereby adding to suspicion of an already stigmatized group. In 1888, of six Barrow cases, one victim was "a tramp who had been living at the lowest lodging-houses, so that it was not difficult to explain his contracting the disease." Another sufferer was the female manager of a common lodging house who came into constant "contact with the tramp class arriving from all parts."[30] Similarly, in 1890 Barrow's MOH reported one case of small-pox: "This man—a lodger—had come from Belfast within the incubation period, and although I could not learn of his having been near to any case of the disease, he no doubt brought the poison of the disease with him from Ireland or from some place on his way to our town."[31]

Preston's health authorities also associated smallpox with external sources of infection, common lodging houses, and poverty. An outbreak in 1902–3 originated with diagnosis of "a hawker who had in all probabil-ity contracted the disease during his journeys in the surrounding coun-try districts." The MOH, Dr. Pilkington, "found him amongst a number of other patients in the surgery of a Medical man doing a large working class practice, and two later cases . . . who were then present, undoubtedly contracted infection at that time." This patient "decamped" from hospital without permission. Although Pilkington "had him safely back within three hours time, he had in the meantime done his best, by visiting public houses and barbers shops, to cause as much mischief as possible. . . . The fact that he was crippled in body, and not very strong mentally, alone prevented my taking proceedings against him." Of the total of 16 cases during this outbreak, which resulted in two deaths, "12 were removed from Common Lodging Houses."[32]

In 1904 a larger epidemic sickened 99 Preston residents, of whom seven died. The outbreak began in April when "the disease was . . . imported by means of an unvaccinated tramp, who had walked from Manchester, through Bolton, and had passed the night, previous to notification of the disease, in one of the Common Lodging Houses in this town." Other victims included a "boiler maker, who had been traveling the country in search of work, [and] arrived at the residence of a relative—a Public House—com-plaining of illness" and a man who lived "in a small, ill-ventilated, and dirty house, occupied by a large family, and used for the purpose of an old clothes shop. Failing any definite history of the source of infection, it would seem not improbable that the disease had been conveyed in some

29. Barrow MOH Report, 1883, 211; Barrow MOH Report, 1885, 155.
30. Barrow MOH Report, 1888, 195. See also Barrow MOH Report, 1893, 202–3.
31. Barrow MOH Report, 1890, 185.
32. Preston MOH Report, 1903, 3–4.

cast-off clothes which had been used by, or had been in contact with a case
of smallpox, either in this or some other town." In a table allocating a number to each victim as well as noting his or her sex, age, vaccination history,
nature of the disease (e.g., variola confluent, modified, or semiconfluent),
and its outcome, Dr. Pilkington also remarked when victims had a family
relationship with another victim (18), were alcoholic (6), or mad (1). In
addition, he observed a decline in incidence of smallpox among tramps
and residents of common lodging houses, but attributed this to the "great
amount of vaccination and revaccination carried out among persons of
this class, both in the Lodging Houses and in the various Casual Wards [in
workhouses] throughout the country"; thus, not to the improvement of
transients' behavior, but to the intervention of public health officials.[33]

Mrs. Parke, born in 1898 in Lancaster, recounted a family experience of
smallpox in which the disease was imported from outside the city:

> Smallpox broke out once, and my cousin had smallpox and they sent
> her up to Littledale Hospital. An aunty of mine in Bolton had sent some
> of her cast-off clothing. . . . Well, she sent this niece of hers some of her
> cast-off clothing and they even went to Bolton to try and find out and
> trace it. They never found out how she got it. I remember them saying
> that all her hair came off. She had beautiful hair, but it all came off,
> but it all came back beautifully curly. She was a very fine smart looking
> girl. She was married and her children had to go into isolation as well,
> and, of course, they kept them for about a fortnight or three weeks,
> and then they were allowed home. But the whole family were up in
> Littledale Hospital.[34]

Mr. Eckley, born in Preston in 1895, recalled a smallpox epidemic,
probably in 1904: "There was a plague of smallpox. On Moor Park they
had to put marquees and tents up and they had to put the children in there
with smallpox. We used to go and watch, and it was funny to see the nurses
going in and out. They were dying like flies. Every Friday night we would
look in the paper and it took a great toll of children in them days did the
plague."[35] Remembering general dread of smallpox, Mr. Hunt, born in
1888 in Barrow, said, "We used to be frightened to death. Oh, somebody
has got smallpox. It was just fear really."[36]

By contrast with smallpox, measles, which was so infectious that the
study cities were loath to incur the effort and expense of making it a notifiable disease (requiring a home visit for each case) and so deadly in epidemic years that it killed 282 Preston children in 1897, 89 Barrow children

33. Preston MOH Report, 3–8.
34. Mrs. P1L, 52.
35. Mr. E1P, 1.
36. Mr. H2B, 81.

in 1889, and 57 Lancaster children in 1907, was often considered by work-ing-class informants an "ordinary childhood disease"—an inevitable, if dan-gerous, hurdle in the obstacle course of young childhood.[37] At the same time, informants remembered measles being a greater threat in the past than the present. Mrs. Oxley, born in Preston in 1902, said, "They used to die with measles then. It's very rare that a baby dies with measles now."[38] And Mr. Grove, born in 1903 in Preston, lost his first child to measles.[39]

Reflecting on these issues, Dr. Pilkington of Preston wrote to Preston's Sanitary Committee in 1889:

> It may at first sight appear strange that the death-rate should have been so much higher than in the year 1888, when the visitation of Small Pox caused such general consternation; and it may perhaps be pointed out that the measures then taken were more vigorous and effective than those adopted during the epidemics of the past year. But the circumstances connected with the outbreaks are widely different. Small Pox is a disease which, especially during an epidemic, is readily recognized, and one, of which people, as a rule, stand in such terror, that they gladly consent to the patient's removal to hospital. In Measles and Whooping Cough, the mischief of transmitting infection is already done before the nature of the disease is known, often before medical assistance is called in, and the parents almost invariably refuse to allow of the child's isolation in the hospital wards. Infantile Diarrhea again, though capable, like Typhoid Fever, of being transmitted through the patient's discharges, can hardly be classed as an infectious disease. In the one case, then, ample hospital accommodation is of the first impor-tance, and can be utilized, in the other its effect would be very limited. The large building erected in Moor Park, and intended as a convales-cent SmallPox hospital, but never actually so used, has been allowed to remain, in order that if required it could at any time be opened for the reception of patients.[40]

In 1888 smallpox had killed 31 Prestonians; in 1889 it had no local mortal-ity. However, measles, which killed two in 1888, accounted for 233 deaths in 1889, while diarrhea, which had caused 263 deaths in 1888, slaughtered 310 in 1889.[41]

The influenza epidemic of 1918–19 provides yet another contrasting

---

37. Preston MOH Report, 1897, 19; Barrow MOH Report, 1889, 210; Lancaster MOH Report, 1907, 4, 27. See, for example, Mrs. H4P, 36; Mrs. H8P, 51; Mrs. L3B, 70; Mr. L4B, 35; Mrs. F1L, 48; Mr. F1L, 27.

38. Mrs. O1P transcript, no page number.

39. Mr. G1P, 61.

40. Preston MOH Report, 1889, 7–8.

41. Preston MOH Report, 1889, 19.

Table 4.1 Mortality from Influenza in Barrow, Lancaster, and Preston, 1917–20

City	1917	1918	1919	1920
Barrow	4	214	81	14
Lancaster	5	84	32	3
Preston	31	391	166	37

Source: Annual reports of Medical Officers of Health for Barrow, Lancaster, and Preston, 1917–20.

example of public health and popular responses to contagious disease.[42] By this time, both the germ theory of disease causation and mechanisms for isolation of sufferers were well established in the study cities, and public health bureaucracies had grown dramatically. Furthermore, contagious disease had significantly diminished in both incidence and mortality. For these reasons, a more pronounced impact on both public health activities and contemporary memory might have been expected; the epidemic might have *meant* more—particularly considering the large numbers of local fatalities. (See table 4.1.) However, it is possible that routinized processes for dealing with infection and rising expectations of medical intervention increased local confidence about weathering epidemics.

Lancaster's MOH, Dr. J. D. Buchanan, reported that influenza broke out in 1918 in two waves: a mild form in June, which killed only four people, and a more severe form in October and November, when the largest number of deaths occurred. Affecting young adults most extremely, "The chief complication was a septic pneumonia which was speedily fatal even before the signs in the lungs showed much involvement of these organs." Commenting that the flu frequently caused abortion among pregnant women, Buchanan reflected both on other complications and on cooperation with local GPs in dealing with the disease: "Pneumococcic vaccine was, in the opinion of doctors who used it, the means of saving a number of lives. Relapses were frequent and recovery, where such took place, was very tardy. Many are not fully recovered. The after-effects noted are infective arthritis, neuralgias, and a condition of the lungs similar to that found in soldiers who have been gassed." Public health responses to the outbreak included school closure and the disinfection of and exclusion of children under age 14 from "Entertainment Houses," as well as distribution of "warning posters and leaflets."[43]

In Preston, Dr. Pilkington reported that the influenza epidemic had increased local mortality rates. Although he provided instructions to the

42. See, for example, Howard Phillips and David Killingray, eds., *The Spanish influenza pandemic of 1918–19: New perspectives* (London and New York: Routledge, 2003); Alice Reid, "The effects of the 1918–1919 influenza pandemic on infant and child health in Derbyshire," *Medical History* 49:1 (2005): 29–54.

43. Lancaster MOH Report, 1918, 20, 34–40.

local press for avoiding the flu, he commented, "Once started in the town the disease in a very short time became so widely spread that nothing short of absolute seclusion would ensure anything like immunity from the constant danger of infection."[44] His cursory and fatalistic comments about this epidemic contrast sharply with his much greater attention to tuberculosis and venereal disease during the same time period—perhaps a reflection of the ways mandated services and reporting influenced the documentation of morbidity and mortality and, thus, the historical record.

Few oral history informants talked about the influenza pandemic. Those who did remembered its deadliness. Mr. Horton, born in Lancaster in 1903, recalled his brother dying from flu after returning from military service in World War I. Mrs. Horton said, "They dropped like flies with flu. I remember it."[45] Mrs. Winder, born in 1910 in Lancaster, said that her father was given compassionate leave from his military unit because her mother and two siblings were so ill with flu.[46] Mr. Gridley, born in Preston in 1903, remembered: "They all had it. My father had it, my sister had it, and my brother had it. My brother was in the army then and he was in India at the time so he wouldn't have it. I think my mother had got run down with nursing. She hardly complained about not feeling well and then old Doctor Rigby came along and my father saw him and Dr. Rigby told him she was very ill. He said he thought it was pneumonia so she was probably run down with doing so much nursing and dashing about and that was that."[47] Mr. Burnett, born in 1904 in Preston, said his brother, a joiner, was kept busy making coffins during the epidemic.[48] However, considering the number of informants who were old enough to remember the outbreak, it is noteworthy how few mentioned it. Like people elsewhere, they seemed to participate in a collective amnesia about the pandemic that killed greater numbers than World War I, to which they referred far more frequently.

Returning to the issue of the contagious diseases to which public health officials devoted most attention, it is worth remembering that each zymotic disease sickened many more people than it killed. Consequently, morbidity was a bigger challenge for both health authorities and working-class families than was mortality. For example, of the 99 Prestonians who became ill with smallpox in 1904, 7 died.[49] In 1914, of 1,137 cases of scarlet fever notified in the city, only 42 died.[50] In Lancaster, diarrhea sickened 318 in 1898 and 329 in 1899 (the two years it was a notifiable disease), but killed 38 in 1906 and

44. Preston MOH Report, 1918, 7.
45. Mr. H3L, 20.
46. Mrs. W2L, 75.
47. Mr. G2P, 14.
48. Mr. B7P, 6.
49. Preston MOH Report, 1904, 7.
50. Preston MOH Report, 1914, 5.

15 in 1907.[51] In 1909, 495 cases of scarlet fever were notified in Lancaster; 14 sufferers died.[52] In Barrow in 1898, there were 58 notifications of and 7 deaths from typhoid.[53] This record suggests the burden of contagious diseases in the study cities. Because of health officials' focus on these ailments, however, it also obscures the impact of nonzymotic infections, such as bronchitis and pneumonia, which continued to be major causes of mortality into the mid-twentieth century, accounting for 178 deaths in Barrow in 1920, when the total death toll from zymotic diseases was 36; 78 deaths in Lancaster in the same year, when zymotic diseases killed 12; and 307 deaths in Preston in 1920, when 70 people died from zymotic diseases.

What did public health officials think caused zymotic diseases? This depended, to a large extent, on their ages, when they were educated, and local conditions, which varied widely. While germ theories were making headway nationally and were uncontroversially applied to some diseases including smallpox, MOsH speculated about multiple causes for many ailments, thereby justifying both inclusive sanitation measures intended to clean up domestic and working environments and exclusive approaches targeting infected individuals, including notification, inspection, isolation, and fumigation. For example, in 1889 Dr. Pilkington of Preston, who had completed his education before his appointment as MOH in 1874, wrote: "There is a tendency to report and register as diphtheria all severe cases of laryngeal inflammation attended with a membranous exudation, and so in many instances no cause for the disease could be found, except a sudden chill, or exposure to cold. On the other hand some cases, without doubt, were due to insanitary conditions, or to actual contact with some previously infected person."[54] In the same year, Barrow's MOH, Dr. John Settle, reported a single case of typhus regarding which "I could not get at any possible source of infection unless the filthy condition of house, bed and bedding could have originated the disease *de novo*."[55]

Dealing with a situation where origins of disease were uncertain and common sense suggested a range of associations, including age, sex, weather conditions, location, "rough" or "respectable" lifestyle, and filth, MOsH in Barrow, Lancaster, and Preston mapped incidence and mortality from contagious diseases by neighborhood, month, and temperature, as well as sex and age. They drew conclusions from these investigations that reflected diverse theories of disease causation. For example, during an 1899 diphtheria epidemic that made 116 Preston children ill and caused the deaths of 36, Dr. Pilkington ordered inspection of each house where

51. Lancaster MOH Report, 1907, 27, 51.
52. Lancaster MOH Report, 1910, 33, 57.
53. Barrow MOH Report, 1898, 179.
54. Preston MOH Report, 1889, 4–5.
55. Barrow MOH Report, 1889, 211. For discussion of germ theory crediting the possibility of *de novo* origins of germs, see Worboys, *Spreading germs*, 132–49.

a case had occurred. He reported: "Although as I have said, in certain instances the infection could be traced to contact with a previous case of illness, in many no definite cause could be discovered. The absence of any special insanitary condition in many of the houses affected, and the general prevalence of the disease throughout the country, would seem to point to some cause of a wide-ranging character, but as yet undiscovered."[56] By contrast, when the continuing fever rate in Hindpool, a working-class district of Barrow, dropped in 1891, the Medical Officer of Health, Dr. John Settle, concluded, "It has followed immediately upon the improvement in its drainage system. Those streets which supplied a great portion of the typhoid of former years, and which had a drain running from end to end under the basements of the houses, are now, since the removal of this drain, almost free from fever."[57] Similarly, in 1907 Lancaster's MOH, Dr. G. R. Parker, explained the low death rate in Scotforth ward and the high death rate in Bulk ward as "no doubt due to the fact that a large number of the houses [in Scotforth] are new and built on soil which is clean and healthy, not having been the site of dwellings before. Once again, I must point out with regard to Bulk Ward that only a small portion is occupied by cottages, and this is densely crowded . . . and this Ward also contains much old property." He went on to explain high infant mortality for the year: "The climatic conditions of the year 1907 were not of the best, and favored the occurrence of Pulmonary diseases, especially after an attack of measles."[58]

Dr. Pilkington believed that contagious diseases flourished because of Preston's crowded housing, unpaved yards, and unsatisfactory waste disposal services. He was especially concerned about the city's large incidence of infant diarrhea, which he blamed on, among other factors, housing in "the poorer and more crowded parts of the town, where the small space at the back of the house is in a great measure taken up by the privy and ashpit, where the yard pavement is often defective and so allows of soakage for a considerable depth below the surface, where there is no back passage to permit air and light to reach the rear of the dwelling, and where too often there is little or no attention paid to the sanitary requirements of the infant itself." In addition, like other MOsH, he linked diarrhea outbreaks with hot weather, bottle-feeding, and maternal employment that required infants to be "minded out."[59]

As indicated elsewhere, Pilkington held parents responsible for their children's health, illness, and deaths: "Better results may be expected when

56. Preston MOH Report, 1899, 6.

57. Barrow MOH Report, 1891, 207.

58. Lancaster MOH Report, 1907, 12, 21.

59. Preston MOH Report, 1893, 3; Preston MOH Report, 1898, 7; Preston MOH Report, 1899, 10–14. See also, for example, Barrow MOH Report, 1895, 186–87; Barrow MOH Report, 1899, 185.

the advance of education has taught the working classes to place a proper value upon good health, to understand that a sound untainted constitution is the best provision which their children can inherit, and to feel how much depends upon their own neglect or observance of a few simple rules of hygiene."[60] He believed that good parenting could and should overcome poor environmental conditions, while improvements in housing and sanitation could not necessarily compensate for parental ignorance and negligence.[61] In addition to parents' influence on the moral and physical factors associated with susceptibility or resistance to infection, as time passed, Pilkington and other study city medical officers focused particularly on working-class mothers' carelessness about isolating victims of contagious diseases—an observation linked to advocacy for construction and enlargement of isolation hospitals.

In the early twentieth century, in addition to the zymotic ailments, other types of contagious diseases, including puerperal fever, tuberculosis, and venereal disease, attracted the attention of policymakers and public health officials. Although mortality from tuberculosis had been declining since the 1840s, in both its pulmonary and nonpulmonary forms it remained a major cause of death in the early twentieth century, second only to heart disease in 1900 and accounting for approximately one in eight deaths in Britain between 1900 and 1910.[62] Identified as a contagious disease in 1882, TB (also referred to as "phthisis" or "consumption") generated a national campaign resulting in local education, dispensaries, home nursing, and institutional isolation. After 1911, Part 1 of the National Insurance Act guaranteed free medical and sanatorium treatment to insured workers, and empowered insurance commissioners to extend these benefits to workers' dependents.[63] In 1913 notification of tuberculosis became compulsory. As was true of the zymotic diseases, despite declining incidence of and mortality from tuberculosis, policy and institutional attention shone a spotlight on the disease resulting in increased official and lay attention and fear.

How big a problem was tuberculosis in Barrow, Lancaster, and Preston in the late nineteenth and early twentieth centuries? Between 1890 and 1900, "consumption" killed an average of 162 of Preston residents per year, 6.4 percent of an average total of 2,509 deaths. In Barrow during the same period, an average of 52 people died annually of TB—6.2 percent of an average total of 830 deaths. By 1910–20, the decade during which compulsory notification increased reporting and special local provisions were

60. Preston MOH Report 1891, 7–8. See also Preston MOH Report, 1899, 14.

61. See, for example, Preston MOH Report, 1895, 8.

62. Thomas McKeown, R.G. Record, "Reasons for the decline of mortality in England and Wales during the nineteenth century," *Population Studies* 16:2 (1962): 113; Linda Bryder, *Below the magic mountain: A social history of tuberculosis in twentieth-century Britain* (Oxford and New York: Clarendon Press, Oxford, 1988), 1; Hardy, *Epidemic streets*, 211.

63. Bryder, *Below the magic mountain*, 36.

made for the prevention, isolation, and treatment of the disease, an average 5.6 percent of all deaths in Preston, 6.1 percent of all deaths in Barrow, and 6.8 percent of all deaths in Lancaster per year were from pulmonary tuberculosis. Unlike the zymotic diseases that mainly killed children, most TB deaths were among adults between the ages of fifteen and forty.

Tuberculosis, which had been widely thought to be hereditary during the nineteenth century and continued to be associated with bad working and living conditions, ignorance, and vice, like other contagious diseases experienced both a gradual local shift in perception of causation and an ongoing multipronged attack. Preston's Dr. Pilkington's views illustrated this transition, expressing, first, belief in hereditary and environmental causes for the disease, then gradual and rather begrudging acknowledgement of contagion in a multicausal explanation for TB's high incidence among working people. In 1892 he associated lung disease with use of excessive steam and dust in the city's weaving sheds. He also blamed overcrowded, poorly ventilated bedrooms: "In many cases the window is seldom opened, the chimney, which ought to serve as a ventilating shaft, is kept hermetically closed, and no thought is taken for renewing the air, rendered foul by the previous night's occupation. In this way many cases of Pulmonary disease are engendered, especially in young children; and any hereditary taint, or predisposition to Phthisis or Scrofula, is fostered and developed."[64] The following year, he wrote, "The teaching of modern Science goes to show that the disease [TB] is one capable of being transmitted through the media of the expectoration and exhalations from the lungs from an infected to a healthy person." However, he continued to argue that traditional working-class preference for closed bedrooms encouraged spread of the disease: "In some cases this is the outcome of negligence and apathy, in others of example and inherited custom, and so from generation to generation the habit is handed down, and, with the habit, its unfortunate results."[65] Furthermore, he continued to argue for hereditary predisposition to tuberculosis, on the one hand, and the power of sanitation to prevent it, on the other.[66] In 1904, although stating that the "germs of Consumption are given off from the breath, and dried expectoration of a patient," he continued to push for environmental improvements as well as "the efforts of the people themselves, who by gradual education will learn to appreciate the dangers of ill-assorted marriages, of crowded bedrooms, of intemperance, and indeed of all those conditions which lower the vital stamina, and so prepare the body for the reception of the tubercular poison."[67] Not until after 1911, when passage of the National Health Insurance Act required provision of TB services

64. Preston MOH Report, 1892, 11.
65. Preston MOH Report, 1893, 7–10.
66. Preston MOH Report, 1898, 8; Preston MOH Report, 1902, 8. See also Barrow MOH Report, 1906, 201.
67. Preston MOH Report, 1904, 12.

by public health authorities, did Dr. Pilkington focus his comments on contagion and clinical treatment.[68]

Even after this time, traditional multicausal explanations of tuberculosis lingered in the study cities. In 1920 Dr. J. Walker, Preston's newly appointed Tuberculosis Officer, while indicating that most people contracted the disease from inhaling dried sputum or drinking infected milk, argued that resistance to TB was reduced by factors mainly affecting working-class people: pre-existing health problems, unfavorable living and working environments, poor nutrition, and heredity. "They shew the importance of the social, as well as the purely medical, aspect of the question, and also that not along one path alone is success to be sought."[69] While this explanation implied passivity and lack of agency among sufferers, it was also common to assign responsibility for preventing tuberculosis to vulnerable groups— particularly working-class families. Emphasizing both germ theory and the possibility of prevention, in 1913 Lancaster's MOH Dr. J. D. Buchanan observed of tuberculosis, "Much ignorance still exists as to the infectious nature of the disease, and much education will be required before the sufferer can be taught the advantages that will accrue to himself and his family by his following the advice and instructions given." Concerned about crowding in working-class homes, he advocated informed self-isolation as the best way to prevent transmission.[70]

Oral history informants remembered a lot of tuberculosis in their communities, which they occasionally associated with hereditary tendencies. For example, Mrs. Simpson, born in 1914 in Preston, said: "Unfortunately, in my mother's family there must have been TB. She was one of four girls and her mother died when she was 36, and that was young to die. She died of TB and my mother's two sisters died of TB, but they grew up. One went into the mill and the other one was my godmother and she did marry, but she died soon after she married. My brother died of TB when he was 22."[71] Some informants linked tuberculosis with inherited racial inferiority, and vice. Mr. King (born in 1907) and Mrs. Melling (born in 1917), both from Lancaster, said the disease ran in the families of Potters, formerly travelers, who lived in the Skerton area of the city. Mr. King said, "They're darker and they're inter-bred, you know. They used to marry into each other's family. You got a lot of TB amongst them. I know a family on Main Street that all died with TB."[72] In other accounts, such as that of Mr. Pratt, born in 1899, whose father married a woman, three of whose four children had died of TB, the implication was that living and sleeping close together may

68. Preston MOH Report, 1911, 9.
69. Preston MOH Report, 1920, 47.
70. Lancaster MOH Report, 1913, 77–79.
71. Mrs. S7P, 7.
72. Mr. K1L, 35; Mrs. M3L, 40.

have been more important than heredity.[73] Some informants recognized the link between tuberculosis and polluted milk. Mr. Tomlinson, born in 1884 in Barrow, remembered: "We'd plenty of milk to drink. It used to be grand if you were out in the country and see them milking a cow in a bit of a shed or in an open field, and they'd give you a glass of milk straight from the cow. You'd drink it all warm. It wasn't cooled, pasteurized or anything else. It was good but full of tuberculosis. A lot of people died of TB in those days."[74]

As we have seen in chapter 2, informants were most likely to ascribe cases of tuberculosis to poor working and living conditions, poverty, and hunger. However, unlike public health authorities, they were not inclined to blame the victim. For instance, Mrs. Wilson, born in 1900, said about her mother:

> I think tuberculosis was her bogey. She used to worry over my father for tuberculosis because I can hear her saying sometimes now, "Now, I've got to look after your father. If I got left with all you lot, what would become of us?" He was so thin and he looked as if a good meal would kill him. . . . Of course, that was his job, he was moulder in Vickers and it was a horrible job, very hot pouring molten metal into moulds. He'd sweat any fat off him and he used to wear what they called a "sweat rag," a piece of toweling round his neck to absorb the sweat, but his shirt and vest were wet just the same. It was good pay because it was such a rotten job, and she was always frightened that the dust would get on his chest and he'd start with tuberculosis, especially with him being so pale and thin.[75]

As this account indicates, people feared TB, which incapacitated people long before it killed them, disrupting everyday activities and livelihoods. Mr. Madison, born in 1910 in Lancaster, had tuberculosis as a nine-year-old, and spent nine months in a sanatorium in Helmsley, North Yorkshire.[76] And Mrs. Smith, born in 1895 in Barrow, remembered her brother being diagnosed with TB at age 16 and being unable to work or play soccer for six months.[77] These examples recall fortunate cases, where sufferers recovered in comparatively short periods of time. More common were memories of the hopelessness associated with a diagnosis of tuberculosis. According to Mrs. Chase, born in 1887, "If you got TB you never got better. I had a sister died at 23 with it. . . . She was in bed for nearly two years."[78] Such experi-

73. Mr. P2L, 10.
74. Mr. T1B, 6.
75. Mrs. W1B, 17.
76. Mr. M1L, 7.
77. Mrs. S2B, 27.
78. Mrs. C2B, 29.

ences account for widespread early-twentieth-century working-class efforts to prevent tuberculosis, discussed in chapter 2.

Perhaps no ailment so exemplified the link between disease and social disorder as venereal diseases. Lacking state attention after the 1886 repeal of the Contagious Diseases Acts, which had required examination by a naval or military surgeon of women believed to be "common prostitutes" and detention for up to one year in locked hospital wards of those found to be diseased, VD attracted new medical and public interest with development of an effective remedy for syphilis, Salvarsan, in 1909 and growth of the social hygiene movement, which was concerned with "racial" degeneration.[79] Concern about increased incidence of venereal diseases and their negative impact on an already health-compromised working-class population gained a national forum in 1913 with the formation of a Royal Commission, whose report helped pave the way for the 1917 Venereal Diseases Act that provided state funding for local health authorities to offer, free of charge, diagnosis, treatment, and "moral instruction."[80]

There can be no doubt that venereal diseases constituted a real health problem. However, the fact that they are mentioned in neither the annual reports of Medical Officers of Health nor the oral history evidence before 1915 is noteworthy and suggests that in Barrow, Lancaster, and Preston, as well, perhaps, as other parts of the country, the venereal disease "crisis" was to some extent constructed by national legislation and propaganda produced by voluntary organizations, such as the National Committee for Combating Venereal Disease. It is also possible that, because of its association with sexual vice, before public health attention was mandated VD had been too disreputable to mention and study city residents had received neither the education nor the treatment necessary to prevent or manage it. Regardless, suggesting the social hygienists' connection between venereal disease and racial degeneration—an arguably natural segue from his long-standing concern about the declining birthrate and the low health quality among working-class children—in association with his 1915 comments about infant mortality and stillbirth, Dr. Pilkington mentioned a "crusade" against VD "now being arranged."[81]

None of the oral history informants provided accounts of experiencing venereal disease, although since personal and family respectability hinged,

79. Lesley A. Hall, "Venereal diseases and society in Britain, from the Contagious Diseases Acts to the National Health Service," in Roger Davidson and Lesley A. Hall, eds., *Sex, sin and suffering: Venereal disease and European society since 1870* (London and New York: Routledge, 2001), 120–36; F. B. Smith, "The Contagious Diseases Acts reconsidered," *Social History of Medicine* 3:2 (1990): 197–215; Greta Jones, *Social hygiene in twentieth century Britain* (London: Croom Helm, 1986); Porter, *Health, civilization and the state*, 130–34.

80. David Evans, "Tackling the 'hideous scourge': The creation of the venereal disease treatment centres in early twentieth-century Britain," *Social History of Medicine* 5:3 (1992): 413–33.

81. Preston MOH Report, 1915, 12.

to a large degree, on sexual demeanor and reputation, this is not surprising.[82] Furthermore, male informants would have been unlikely to discuss
this type of illness experience with a woman interviewer. One informant,
Mrs. Anston, born in 1900 in Preston, told a story from the interwar years
that suggested both the shame of getting treatment for venereal disease
and her own innocence and respectability: "I went to the hospital when I
first started injections for anemia and I sat there one Tuesday and one of
the nurses came out where I usually sat and they were smiling and looking at me and one of them said, 'Come here. What are you sitting here
for?' I said, 'I always sit here.' She said, 'Well, for goodness sake, come
away! That's the VD clinic!' They used to draw the curtains round and they
hadn't."[83]

By the 1920s, when venereal diseases had joined the throng of contagious ailments for which public health authorities were responsible, it is
clear that MOsH saw VD as primarily a working-class problem and, as was
also true of other contagious diseases, one whose solution went beyond
treatment. In 1925 Preston's MOH reported 508 new cases, up from 456 in
the previous year. He wrote:

> The work of combating Venereal Disease is progressing, but the medi-
> cal side, although of vast and profound importance . . . is not of exclu-
> sive importance. There is no disease—perhaps no group of diseases—in
> which medical, social, and moral problems are so closely, so inextricably
> interwoven. No mere medical attack on Venereal Disease will ever of
> itself achieve victory. . . . There is a very close connection between the
> level of the standards of sexual morality and the conditions of housing,
> the conditions for recreation, and the conditions of life generally.[84]

This holistic perspective provided a steady undercurrent for the diverse
ways public health authorities attempted to prevent contagious diseases in
the study cities from the late nineteenth century onward.

FIGHTING DIRT AND GERMS: PUBLIC HEALTH
PROVISION IN BARROW, LANCASTER, AND PRESTON

Although major public works and services, including provision of clean
water, sewerage, and garbage collection, began before 1880 in Barrow, Lancaster, and Preston, Medical Officers of Health continued into the early

82. See, for example, Lucinda McCray Beier, "'We were green as grass': Learning about sex
and reproduction in three working-class Lancashire communities, 1900–1970," *Social History of
Medicine* 16:3: 461–80.

83. Mrs. A2P, 30.

84. Preston MOH Report, 1925, 69.

twentieth century to emphasize sanitation and domestic hygiene as the first lines of defense against contagious disease.[85] Each city presented a different challenge. Barrow, a planned new town, had modern housing, including flush toilets, and, after a rocky start, a superior sewage system (although the city's waste continued to be dumped raw into Walney Channel into the 1920s).[86] Both Lancaster and Preston had large stocks of old city-center housing with communal outdoor water supplies and dry-earth closet privies.[87] Lancaster, having suffered a mid-nineteenth-century economic slump, was slow to spend on public improvements until the town began to expand in prosperity and population after the late 1870s.[88] By contrast, in Preston, where industrial development stimulated the building of many small terraced houses between 1850 and 1880, the typical "lobby-plan" working-class dwellings lacked the large backyards and alley access that would have enabled improved lavatory and rubbish facilities and removal.[89] All of the study cities had many open "middens" located close to homes into which both human and animal waste and household rubbish was thrown. As Nigel Morgan has observed, the cities also had increasing numbers of horses, whose droppings attracted large numbers of flies that helped to spread the diarrhea and typhoid fever particularly common in Preston.[90]

In Lancaster and Preston, early MOsH set out to replace dry-earth closets with water closet (WC) lavatories. This goal had largely been achieved in Lancaster by 1900 and in Preston by 1910.[91] However, as we have seen in chapter 2, many of these WCs continued to be shared into the interwar years.[92] Many of the housing problems identified as threats to health were beyond owners' and renters' capacity to remedy. In 1914 Lancaster's MOH observed:

85. See E. C. Midwinter, *Social administration in Lancashire 1830–1860* (Manchester: Manchester University Press, 1969), for discussion of development of public water supplies in Preston and Lancaster (98–99, 111). See Morgan, "Infant mortality, flies, and horses," 108–12, for discussion of rubbish collection, privy emptying, and nuisance abatement in Preston.

86. Marshall, *Furness and the Industrial Revolution,* 407; Barrow MOH Report, 1925, 314; Elizabeth Roberts, *A woman's place: An oral history of working-class women 1890–1940* (Oxford: Blackwell, 1984), 133.

87. Michael Winstanley, "The town transformed 1815–1914," in *A History of Lancaster 1193–1993,* Andrew White, ed. (Keele, Staffordshire: Ryburn Publishing, Keele University Press, 1993), 181; Nigel Morgan, *Deadly dwellings: Housing and health in a Lancashire cotton town. Preston from 1840 to 1914* (Preston: Mullion Books, 1993).

88. Winstanley, "The town transformed," 181.

89. Morgan, "Infant mortality," 107.

90. Morgan, "Infant mortality." Morgan argues that Preston's dismal infant mortality record was principally due to the explosive growth in its number of horses. Since there is no evidence that Preston had more horses than other industrial towns or that other kinds of dirt could not have accounted for proliferating numbers of flies, I am more persuaded by Morgan's argument that Preston's housing was comparatively unhygienic.

91. Roberts, *A woman's place,* 133.

92. See, for example, Lancaster MOH Report, 1918, 13; Lancaster MOH Report, 1925, 33, 43.

The defects found to exist among the insanitary houses dealt with are those peculiar to houses erected in the middle of the last century. These are dampness and darkness, insufficient ventilation around and within the dwelling, want of facilities for the cleansing of the body and clothing owing to the absence of water-tap and slopstone, insufficient closet accommodation, and unsatisfactory means of storage for house refuse. Provision for storage of food does not seem to have received any consideration in the past, though it need not have cost much. Another defect frequently met with is the undrained cellar, which often contains matter of an offensive character. The high incidence and mortality rates of Tuberculosis are, in my opinion, not unconnected with the housing conditions that exist in certain parts of the town.[93]

One solution to inadequate or outdated housing was demolition. In 1907 Lancaster's MOH reported on replacement of "insanitary property" with "good houses." His remark, "My only regret is that I can see no prospect of low-rented houses being built, and this is a serious matter in a town like Lancaster with so many people earning small wages," indicates that this MOH, at least, understood the potentially negative impact of housing reform on low-income renters—a situation that continued into the interwar period and affected access to council housing.[94]

Another approach adopted by MOsH was to encourage renters to clean and maintain their domestic environments. In 1889 Dr. Pilkington complained, "The operative class as a rule are careless in looking after the surroundings of their dwellings. Too often they seem to look upon the house simply as a place in which to sleep and take certain of their meals."[95] In 1892 he repeated the recommendation that people whitewash the lobbies, yards, and buildings at the back of their homes. "It does good not only from its disinfecting properties, and the increased light and cheerfulness which it gives, but also from the stimulus which its use imparts to cleanliness in other directions and to the removal and destruction of those heaps of useless lumber which somehow collect at the backs of most cottage houses."[96] This type of advice was closely linked to a reform agenda that observed the origins of working-class disease in working-class culture.[97] The necessary clean-up was moral as well as functional.

At the turn of the twentieth century, public health authorities were convinced that the education of working-class homemakers and mothers was central to reduction of infant mortality and contagious diseases, and that

93. Lancaster MOH Report, 1914, 36.

94. Lancaster MOH Report, 1907, 61–62; Lancaster MOH Report, 1930, 25.

95. Preston MOH Report, 1889, 12.

96. Preston MOH Report, 1892, 9.

97. See, for example, Jones, *Social hygiene;* Jane Lewis, *The politics of motherhood: Child and maternal welfare in England, 1900–1930* (London: Croom Helm, 1980).

women who did not act on expert advice were to blame for the deaths of their children.[98] While MOsH suggested several options for educating working-class mothers, the approach most generally adopted was the appointment of health visitors which, as we have seen, was done in Preston in 1902, Lancaster in 1903, and Barrow during World War I.[99] In addition to the expectation that their advice would help to prevent infectious disease, health visitors served as inspectors of working-class homes and parenting skills and helped to enforce health policies including notification, isolation, and disinfection. More than the MOsH, health visitors conveyed official public health information and power into working-class homes.[100] They also reflected middle-class disdain for working-class customs and women, suggesting that female health visitors were no more sympathetic than male MOsH. In 1907 Lancaster's new Lady Health Visitor reported on inappropriate and unhygienic feeding practices, particularly use of the tube-style feeding bottle thought to contribute to incidence of infant diarrhea. She concluded her comments by saying, "I have . . . systematically pointed out to all careless mothers that the prevention of this epidemic lies very largely with themselves."[101]

In addition to providing advice on prevention, health visitors also visited reported cases of contagious diseases.[102] In 1912 Dr. Joseph Cates, Lancaster's MOH, described the health visitor's role in an increasingly structured system for managing these ailments:

As soon as a notification is received the Health Visitor calls at the house to obtain full particulars concerning the source of infection, the health of contacts and the sanitary conditions of the dwelling; in the case of typhoid or scarlet fever, unless there is ample provision for home treatment, the patient is removed to the Isolation Hospital. Copies of cards relating to the appropriate disease and instruction of disinfection are left at the house. The infected room or rooms are sprayed with a solution of formalin and closed for four hours, a supply of suitable disinfectant is given, and in every case the bedding and other articles are

98. See, for example, Anna Davin, "Imperialism and motherhood," *History Workshop* 5 (1978): 9–65.

99. Celia Davies, "The Health Visitor as Mother's Friend: A woman's place in public health, 1900–14," *Social History of Medicine* 1:1 (1988): 39–59; Preston MOH Report, 1902, 12; Barrow MOH Report, 1918, 249; Michael Winstanley, "The town transformed, 1815–1914," in Andrew White, ed., *A History of Lancaster 1193–1993* (Keele: Keele University Press, 1993), 181. Preston and Lancaster were early participants in this national trend, since, according to Dingwall et al., *Social history of nursing*, 185, it was only in 1904 that an Interdepartmental Committee called for "national provision of a 'health visiting' service."

100. Dingwall et al., *Social history of nursing*, 188.

101. Lancaster MOH Report, 1907, 26.

102. See, for example, Barrow MOH Report, 1933, 292; Preston MOH Report, 1904, 16–17; Preston MOH Report, 1909, 14.

removed for steam sterilization. Where the patient is nursed at home frequent visits are made to see that proper precautions are being taken, and when the illness is over disinfection is carried out.[103]

After notification of tuberculosis was mandated, this model was also followed for TB cases, indicating both the health visitor's role as an agent of the state and the emphasis placed on infected people and their families taking responsibility for limiting contagion and providing care.[104] These procedures also suggest one reason why MOsH were reluctant to make notifiable highly contagious diseases such as whooping cough or measles that could sicken thousands in an epidemic year. In 1907 Lancaster's health visitor called on 2,000 sufferers during a measles epidemic that killed 57 in six months.[105] The expectation that health visitors visit contagious disease sufferers undoubtedly inflated the number employed and increased the cost of local public health administration. Nonetheless, along with the requirement that health visitors call on new mothers, these visits, however welcome or unwelcome, accustomed working-class women to public health scrutiny of and intervention in their ways of managing the health and ill-health of their family members.

Notification was a powerful tool of late-nineteenth-century public health administration, enabling the epidemiology, isolation, and disinfection that increasingly composed its response to contagious diseases.[106] The permissive 1889 Notification of Infectious Diseases Act enabled local authorities to require either the householder or a medical attendant to report to the MOH incidence of some or all of the zymotic diseases. Made compulsory in 1899, this legislation empowered the MOH "to isolate the patient at home or remove them [sic] to an isolation hospital when he considered it necessary, and to carry out disinfection of households, clothing and bed-linen. In certain diseases, such as diphtheria or scarlet fever, the siblings of infected children could be excluded from school during the incubation period and occasionally, when an epidemic outbreak threatened, the MOH was empowered to close public establishments such as schools."[107] In Barrow, Lancaster, and Preston, although local acts required notification of some contagious diseases beginning in the 1880s, not all common or deadly infectious diseases were made notifiable, and not all notifiable dis-

103. Lancaster MOH Report, 1912, 57–58.

104. Lancaster MOH Report, 1913, 77.

105. Lancaster MOH Report, 1907, 4. It is noteworthy that regardless of whether a disease was notifiable, health visitors routinely followed up on teachers' reports of children being sent home with suspected measles or other contagious ailment.

106. See, for example, Porter, *Health, civilization, and the state*, 134–37; Worboys, *Spreading germs*, 234–40; Graham Mooney, "Public health versus private practice: The contested development of compulsory infectious disease notification in late-nineteenth-century Britain," *Bulletin of the History of Medicine* 73:2 (1999): 238–67.

107. Porter, *Health, civilization, and the state*, 135.

eases were common or deadly. Measles and whooping cough, for example, were contagious before they were symptomatic; thus, isolation, although demanded by health authorities, could not effectively limit their spread, and notification placed a heavy burden on ratepayers and public health personnel. In the study cities, measles was occasionally made notifiable, while whooping cough never was. By contrast, erysipelas, though notifiable, had little local incidence, while smallpox remained notifiable long after its regular appearance was mainly a bad memory. As in other parts of Britain, the consistently notifiable diseases in the study cities were smallpox, typhoid (or enteric) fever, scarlet fever (or scarletina), and diphtheria, joined after 1913 by tuberculosis.

Responsibility for notifying the public health authorities of suspected cases of contagious diseases fell on the sufferer or his/her parents and on general practitioners. The first challenge MOsH faced was fatalism regarding many zymotic diseases on the part of working-class adults. Warning readers about the dangers of scarlet fever and measles, Dr. Pilkington observed in 1891:

> I dwell upon these points in order that parents may first of all dismiss from their minds the idea that certain diseases are inevitably attendant upon the period of childhood, and secondly in the hope that should the children under their care contract one or other of such diseases they may be induced to bestow upon them that attentive care—not only during the actual sickness but also during the often tedious period of recovery—which so frequently determines whether the patient becomes a strong and useful adult, or a delicate and therefore more or less useless invalid.[108]

As we have seen in chapter 3, working-class people soon began to understand that failure to notify could get them into trouble. For this reason, informants remembered their families calling a doctor when the sufferer had spots or a sore throat more often than when other symptoms presented—and even remembered measles having been a notifiable disease when it probably was not.[109] However, because a notifiable disease could either present in such a mild form that it was not recognized, or be mistaken for an ailment that could be appropriately cared for without medical consultation, MOsH tried to educate the public about symptoms. For example, Lancaster's MOH reported in 1916, "Owing to cases of scarlet fever and diphtheria being 'missed' an advertisement was inserted in the local press in May, warning the public of the danger that might arise from neglect to call in a doctor or notify the Public Health Department in cases

108. Preston MOH Report, 1891, 7.
109. See, for example, Mrs. M3P, 35; Mrs. H3P, 49; Mrs. M1B, 17; Mr. T3P, 65; Mrs. A1P, 40.

of sore throat. In one house a boy died from diphtheria without a doctor having been summoned. Bacteriological examination of the larynx (post mortem) revealed the cause of death. A few days later his brother contracted the disease."[110]

Another reason cases might not be reported was the tension between GPs and MOsH, due to physicians' concern about public health's challenge to their professional authority and potential competition for patients.[111] This resulted in physicians keeping the public health department at arm's length. Lancaster's MOH reported a possibly related situation in 1920: "A boy who had been medically treated at home for a week was brought by his mother to the Health Office because, although the doctor did not think it was diphtheria, she 'had her suspicions.' Her suspicions were correct: a swab from the boy's throat was examined and found to contain diphtheria bacilli. This case demonstrates the need for the use of bacteriological aids to diagnosis, the use of which involves a little trouble but no expense to the practitioner."[112]

However, MOsH also noted parental resistance to diagnosis, notification, and isolation. In 1911 when 19 children died of scarlet fever, Dr. Pilkington observed that many cases of the disease were unrecognized or concealed: "Often medical assistance had not been called in, and it became a difficult matter to prove knowledge on the part of the parents as to the nature of the illness, otherwise a prosecution would, no doubt, have a deterrent effect upon cases, which may sometimes be due to ignorance, but which not seldom are the result of a selfish disregard on the part of one person for the comfort and welfare of others."[113] This comment suggests both the MOH's frustration and reasons parents might avoid professional attention when a child complained of a sore throat.

The push for notification partnered advocacy for isolation—a measure that had long been applied in cases of smallpox, but was demanded from the 1880s on for an increasing list of infectious diseases (both notifiable and non-notifiable). Health officials offered instructions for home isolation. For example, in 1889 Dr. Pilkington advised placement of a child suffering from smallpox, measles, scarlet fever, diphtheria, or other infectious disease in a room containing no extra furniture and "removed as far as possible from the rest of the house. The mother, or some other one person of the family, should undertake the duties of nurse and should not communicate with the rest of the household. All articles used by the patient should, before leaving the sickroom, be placed in a pail of [disin-

110. Lancaster MOH Report, 1916, 15–16. See also Preston MOH Report, 1906, 6–7.

111. See, for example, Porter, *Health, civilization, and the state,* 136; Mooney, "Public health versus private practice," 258–61.

112. Lancaster MOH Report, 1920, 23. By the 1910s all study cities were providing free laboratory testing and antitoxin for diphtheria.

113. Preston MOH Report, 1911, 6.

fectant]."[114] However, it was clear to MOsH that the cramped dwellings of the poor offered inadequate facilities for effective isolation, while the perceived unwillingness of working-class women to learn and maintain proper isolation protocols compromised the success of home quarantine.[115] Sanitary inspectors were assigned the frustrating task of making "frequent, in many instances daily, visits . . . to houses which had been notified."[116]

Enforcing home isolation posed an ongoing challenge. In 1900 Barrow's MOH reported that during an outbreak of scarlet fever, "In all cases parents were personally warned against allowing their infected children to mix with healthy children during the six weeks, but I suspect this had very little effect in most cases. Isolation would alone place an infected child in a position of safety as regards other children."[117] In 1911 Barrow's MOH similarly observed of a non-notifiable ailment that was, nonetheless, easy to diagnose: "Whooping cough appears to have been prevalent during the year. In this disease we have no means of controlling its spread, and can only appeal to the mothers or others responsible for the patient to avoid exposing the child in a public place such as tramcars and railway carriages, where there is a risk of conveying the infection to other children."[118]

Medical Officers of Health used their statutory powers to punish parents who failed to isolate children with contagious ailments. For example, in 1906 Dr. Pilkington ordered display of a placard advising isolation of children with whooping cough, which said, "Once established, the disease is readily recognized by the cough, and parents allowing a child in this condition to intermix with others are liable to a penalty not exceeding £5."[119] Public health authorities also regularly closed schools, often held responsible for transmission of an epidemic, although this approach sometimes apparently backfired, since children interacted as or more constantly on neighborhood streets than they did in classrooms. For example, regarding a diphtheria outbreak in 1911 when 139 cases were notified and 34 deaths recorded, Barrow's MOH observed: "A feature of the disease was that more notifications were received during school holidays than whilst the schools were open, indicating that other factors exist for propagating an epidemic than the much blamed schools. Probably indiscriminate visiting to and

114. Preston MOH Report, 1889, 9.
115. See, for example, Preston MOH Report, 1899, 7.
116. Preston MOH Report, 1901, 6; Preston MOH Report, 1905, 13. See also Barrow MOH Report, 1900, 193.
117. Barrow MOH Report, 1900, 193.
118. Barrow MOH Report, 1911, 221. See also Lancaster MOH Report, 1907, 43.
119. Preston MOH Report, 1906, 8. In 1913 he announced a similar fine for "willfully exposing a [scarlet fever] patient in any street, public place, shop, etc." Preston MOH Report, 1913, 6. In Barrow in 1901, the MOH reported fining one mother and trying to punish another for "gross carelessness . . . in allowing their infected children to run about and mix with healthy children." Barrow MOH Report, 1901, 193.

from infected houses has much to do with the spread of an epidemic."[120]

Public health experts realized that their capacity to enforce isolation in working-class homes and neighborhoods was severely limited. Thus, particularly after passage of the Isolation Hospitals Act in 1893, MOsH solicited support from local government for hospital isolation of certain contagious diseases—especially smallpox, typhoid fever, scarlet fever, and diphtheria. As we have seen in chapter 3, Lancaster and Preston were unusual in admitting infectious disease sufferers to their voluntary and Poor Law hospitals before the late nineteenth century. However, these facilities were unsatisfactory for a number of reasons: admission of contagious disease victims to voluntary general hospitals endangered other patients; use of Poor Law hospitals to isolate contagious disease sufferers pauperized and stigmatized nonpaupers; and the effort to attract private patients to hospitals failed because people who could pay preferred home care.[121] Furthermore, isolation hospitals constructed in the late nineteenth and early twentieth centuries were controlled by public health officials—not by Poor Law guardians or voluntary hospital boards. This created the opportunity for more effective administration of isolation, although it also exacerbated the potential for conflict between MOsH and GPs.[122] In Barrow, Lancaster, and Preston, tension was minimized by the practice of general practitioners attending patients in isolation hospitals and charging for treatment—an arrangement that worked because the isolation hospitals provided isolation and nursing care, not therapy. Mrs. Winder, born in 1910 in Lancaster, who was hospitalized with scarlet fever as a three-year-old, explained: "I think if it was same as an isolation hospital they took you in, but the doctor, our own doctor, had to go and visit me, they didn't supply a doctor, and he went during the day and any drugs that he wanted if he had to go and take them he would have wanted pay, so he told m'father that if he [father] called every evening and took down what they wanted it would save expenses."[123] This account reveals a hidden cost of ostensibly "free" isolation hospital admission.

Lancaster opted early for an isolation hospital, due to the 1876 transmission to other patients of smallpox from sufferers admitted to the voluntary Royal Infirmary.[124] The new Marsh Sanatorium "fever hospital" was built in 1880, but replaced in 1891 by the Luneside Hospital, which was used until 1934.[125] In 1899 a facility specifically intended for smallpox patients

120. Barrow MOH Report, 1911, 220.

121. John V. Pickstone, *Medicine and industrial society: A history of hospital development in Manchester and its region, 1752–1946* (Manchester: Manchester University Press, 1985), 160–65, 170; John Wilkinson, *Preston's Royal Infirmary: A history of health care in Preston 1809–1986* (Preston: Carnegie Press, 1987), 43–44.

122. Worboys, *Spreading germs*, 262.

123. See, for example, Mrs. W2L, 214.

124. Pickstone, *Medicine and industrial society*, 165.

125. Lancaster MOH Report, 1910, 65; Lancaster MOH Report, 1912, 49; Lancaster MOH Report, 1934, 28.

was built on the grounds of that hospital, but never used for that purpose. Instead, in 1904 the Littlefell Smallpox Hospital opened and offered beds for smallpox victims into the interwar period, although it was rarely occupied.[126] Despite resistance from patients and their families, between 1893 and 1907 the percentage of scarlet fever and typhoid treated in hospital rather than at home rose from 30 percent to 75 percent in Lancaster.[127] In 1915 cases of diphtheria began to be admitted to the Luneside Hospital.[128] Shortly after that time, 21 beds in an outbuilding on that institution's grounds were reserved for sufferers from acute pulmonary tuberculosis.[129] However, after a flood in 1927 that killed three TB patients, use of the hospital for this purpose was discontinued.[130]

As we have seen, Barrow established its first voluntary hospital (the North Lonsdale) after a smallpox epidemic in the period 1870–71.[131] By the early twentieth century, the city's public health authorities were administering three isolation hospitals: the Devonshire Road Hospital, constructed as a temporary facility, which was used for scarlet fever and typhoid; the rarely occupied "Raikes Moor Small Pox Hospital . . . , a corrugated iron building, giving accommodation for 16 cases"; and "Sheep Island Quarantine Hospital, . . . a building on an island in the Walney Channel, . . . provided to meet the requirements of ships arriving in the Port with cases of Plague, Cholera, or Yellow Fever on board. So far as I [the MOH] can make out only one case of suspected plague has been isolated there, and I believe the case eventually turned out to be a case of venereal bubo."[132] By 1900 Barrow's MOH, Dr. John Settle, was advocating expansion of the Devonshire Road Hospital: "There can be no question that a case of scarlatina removed from a working man's house with a large family to a well-conducted Isolation Hospital is much less likely to affect others than if left at home. From various causes, and amongst them the smallness of our hospital, we have not enforced isolation in the past, but with a sufficiency of hospital accommodation I am determined that this shall be altered in the future.[133] During a 1912 diphtheria epidemic in Barrow, the MOH, Dr. James Orr, commented that of 206 cases notified, "Most . . . should be removed to the Isolation Hospital, as efficient isolation at home is obtainable in very few houses where the cases occur. Only 33 cases were treated in the Hospital. Further Hospital accommodation will be provided in the

126. See, for example, Lancaster MOH Report, 1913, 60–61; Lancaster MOH Report, 1927, 8.

127. Lancaster MOH Report, 1907, 61.

128. Lancaster MOH Report, 1927, 37.

129. Lancaster MOH Report, 1915, 17.

130. Lancaster MOH Report, 1927, 9.

131. Marshall, *Furness and the Industrial Revolution*, 373.

132. Barrow MOH Report, 1912, 245.

133. Barrow MOH Report, 1900, 192.

near future, and the powers for removal of infectious cases will no doubt be strictly enforced."[134]

As noted in chapter 3, Preston's late-nineteenth-century attempt to accommodate sufferers from contagious diseases in its voluntary hospital was not a success.[135] More accepted and effective was the portable Ducker hospital erected to accommodate smallpox patients in 1892 on "the Corporation farm of Holme Slack" at a distance from "the public road and any dwellings."[136] Dr. Pilkington described this facility's employment during the 1894 outbreak, when 47 patients were treated there and one died. "It might be feared that the admission of paupers would prevent the building from being used by the rate-paying classes, but, with a little management, this objection can be overcome, since the Hospital Ward is a republic, in which all persons are equal, have the same rights and privileges, and must conform to the same rules"—an observation that suggests why nonpaupers might prefer home quarantine.[137]

Despite its limited success with isolation of smallpox victims, Preston was late in opening a hospital for sufferers of other contagious diseases.[138] Blocked by local government because of expense, and by local doctors on the self-serving grounds that isolation hospitals were less cost-effective than home quarantine, Preston's Deepdale isolation hospital was not constructed until 1907. Advocating this measure in every annual report beginning in 1899 on the basis of both the need for isolation to curb transmission of certain diseases and requests for inpatient care from patients and their relatives, Dr. Pilkington became increasingly frustrated, writing in 1904: "There is no doubt the spread of disease to other members of a household could have been prevented in several instances, had such accommodation been available for the first case affected. In one household, five children were consecutively attacked with scarlet fever and two deaths resulted; whereas the prompt removal of the first patient might have cut short the outbreak." Going on to discuss the need for hospitalization for typhoid fever, he wrote, "Indeed I still hope that in the course of another decade or two—perchance from an (Electric) Bath Chair, with blurred vision, and imperfect understanding—I may yet see the opening ceremony."[139] In 1908, the Isolation Hospital's first full year of occupation, Dr. Pilkington reported admitting 82 typhoid, 53 scarlet fever, and 18 diphtheria patients, of whom 20 typhoid, 1 scarlet fever, and 2 diphtheria sufferers died.[140]

Before World War II, isolation hospitals mainly admitted working-class

134. Barrow MOH Report, 1912, 242.
135. Preston MOH Report, 1900, 10.
136. Preston MOH Report, 1892, 4.
137. Preston MOH Report, 1894, 6–7.
138. Pickstone, *Medicine and industrial society*, 174.
139. Preston MOH Report, 1904, 21–22. See also Preston MOH Report, 1907, 27.
140. Preston MOH Report, 1908, 38.

children suffering from scarlet fever and diphtheria. Working-class house-holds had less capacity for isolation, and working-class parents were less able than their middle-class counterparts to mount effective opposition to hospital admission. Virtually all typhoid cases were sent to isolation hospitals. While adults were as or more likely than children to contract typhoid, that ailment had much lower and declining incidence, although it was considerably more deadly than scarlet fever and diphtheria. Thus, being an isolation hospital patient was dominantly and increasingly a childhood experience.

Hospital isolation tended to last for a long time. In 1907 Dr. Pilkington reported, "The duration of stay in hospital varied very considerably from a day or two where death followed soon upon admission to two or even three months in cases of protracted convalescence, but the average length of residence was about forty days, or nearly six weeks to each patient."[141] Hospital isolation was also quite thorough, prohibiting any face-to-face contact between patients and visitors; even parents of infants and young children had to observe their little ones through glass windows and communicate with them through hospital nurses.

It is, perhaps, not surprising that in early years, parents resisted children's admission to isolation hospital. In 1898 Barrow's MOH Dr. Settle commented, "It is impossible to get the consent of parents amongst the working classes to the removal of their children to hospital."[142] In 1909 Dr. Pilkington commented about Preston attitudes, "There is a not unnatural dislike on the part of parents to permit the removal of very young children to hospital, but invariably even the very youngest soon settle down to their new surroundings, enjoy the company of the other children, and benefit by the more careful nursing, better food, and purer air than, in the case of the great majority, they would enjoy in their own homes."[143] In 1910 Pilkington referred to the effort to make Deepdale Hospital as attractive as possible, "since there is less reluctance on the part of relatives to allow patients—especially children—to enter an institution of a bright, cheerful, and ornamental character. It also does much to remove the prejudice and opposition generally shown against the erection of an Isolation Hospital in any neighborhood."[144] In 1912 he suggested further advantages of hospitalization, for the first time arguing that patients had a better chance of survival there than sufferers cared for at home because of "gratuitous medical treatment and skilled nursing to all classes. . . . Another advantage, though one perhaps not so plainly apparent, is that those nursed in hospital are less likely to be affected with any of the complications which so frequently follow upon attacks of infectious disease." Addressing disadvantages of home quarantine, he argued that hospitalization "removes from

141. Preston MOH Report, 1907, 28.
142. Barrow MOH Report, 1898, 178.
143. Preston MOH Report, 1909, 22.
144. Preston MOH Report, 1910, 24.

the household the source of infection which might prevent the bread win-
ners from following their employment, and it does away with the danger
of spreading infection that must be associated with a case of fever nursed
under the ordinary conditions of a common home."[145]

In 1910 Lancaster's MOH reported that 71 percent of notified cases
of typhoid and scarlet fever were admitted to the Luneside Hospital: "I
am glad to say that we have now no difficulty in persuading parents to
send their children to our Sanatorium. They have seen for themselves the
advantages of institutional treatment, and are no longer afraid of it, as was
at one time the case. It is now thirty-five years since the establishment of a
Sanatorium in Lancaster for the treatment of Scarlet and Enteric Fevers,
and I well remember how difficult it was in the earlier days to induce parents to send their children there."[146] While this example may overstate
parental willingness to have children admitted to the hospital, it suggests a
trend that became more pronounced during the interwar period, indicating rising acceptance of professional medical treatment in general. By 1929
Lancaster's MOH reported that 145 (74.3 percent) of 195 notified cases
of scarlet fever were removed to the isolation hospital, despite the health
authority's preference for keeping sufferers in homes where isolation was
possible: "Whereas, at one time, parents had to be coaxed to allow a child
to go to hospital, they now ask for removal, even though there are adequate
facilities for isolation and nursing at home."[147] In 1931 the MOH reported
denial of parents' request for an isolation hospital bed for a scarlet fever
sufferer, "because it was a mild case, the child an only child, and the house
had three bedrooms."[148] It is noteworthy that acceptance of and demand
for hospitalization rose at the same time as mortality from scarlet fever,
typhoid, and diphtheria declined. Perhaps study city residents identified
a cause-effect relationship between hospitalization for contagious diseases
and their decline in mortality. However, medical officers also noted increasing mildness of the scarlet fever affecting their communities in this period,
while typhoid declined in incidence as sanitation advanced and diphtheria
mortality dropped as antitoxin was routinely used in the study cities.[149]

145. Preston MOH Report, 1912, 28.
146. Lancaster MOH Report, 1910, 66. The MOH dates the establishment of Lancaster's
isolation hospital five years earlier than my source, John Pickstone, *Medicine and industrial society*,
165, which indicates that the Marsh Sanatorium opened in 1880.
147. Lancaster MOH Report, 1929, 26.
148. Lancaster MOH Report, 1931, 25. See also Lancaster MOH Report, 1927, 37.
149. Diphtheria antitoxin was developed in 1891 and began to be widely employed after
Émile Roux (1853–1933) presented a paper on its use at the Eighth International Congress of
Hygiene and Demography at Budapest in September 1894. See Rosen, *History of public health*,
305–6. However, while Medical Officers of Health urged its early use in cases where diphtheria
was suspected, and advised that it be provided at no cost, they observed that local GPs sometimes
delayed its administration—perhaps an example of friction between MOsH and GPs, who
objected to any infringement of their rights to determine appropriate treatment. See, for
example, Barrow MOH Report, 1911, 220; Lancaster MOH Report, 1907, 39; Lancaster MOH

Part of the trend toward institutionalization of isolation and care, the first local mention of sanatorium provision for tuberculosis sufferers occurred in the1898 report of Dr. Settle, MOH for Barrow.[150] In 1905 Preston's Dr. Pilkington expressed both operational and moral reservations about construction of TB sanatoria.[151] Believing it impossible to offer sanatorium beds to all TB sufferers, and opposing rewarding with luxury accommodation the undeserving patient whose disease was his or her own fault, Pilkington also argued that institutional care might even be counterproductive in the attack on this ailment, which required a holistic approach rather than a quick fix.[152] The contrast between this medical officer's position on isolation hospitals for other contagious diseases and his thoughts about TB sanatoria is noteworthy, suggesting he believed that sick children, removed from the care of their working-class parents, might be redeemed, while adult tuberculosis sufferers were unworthy of public investment and could be saved only by their own moral transformation and hard work.

As we have seen, Pilkington was conservative about tuberculosis in general, continuing to associate the disease with heredity and vice after the tubercle bacillus was identified, and resisting institutional isolation as pubic health consensus moved toward this solution. By contrast, in 1913 Dr. Buchanan, MOH of Lancaster, displayed both bacteriological and environmental orientations in his thoughts on this matter: "Certainly, in a great many cases where, owing to housing and economic conditions, patients can neither get suitable and sufficient food, nor proper sleeping accommodation, removal to sanatorium for a longer or shorter period would be of undoubted advantage. There are, however, cases in which the home can be made a 'Sanatorium,' to the benefit of the patient and without any risk to the rest of the household." However, Buchanan commented that many houses offered inadequate accommodation, so that patients shared the only available beds and bedrooms were overcrowded. "Of 64 cases, 30, or less than half, had a separate bedroom. Seven had a separate bed, but shared the room with one or more others; no less than 21 shared the bed with another, and in six cases there were two others in the bed with the patient."[153] Indeed, the new understanding of TB as a communicable disease lent strength to previous concerns about overcrowding and helped fuel advocacy for housing reform at local as well as national levels. More immediately, after passage of National Health Insurance it stimulated arrangement for local beds for TB treatment, somewhat earlier in Barrow

Report, 1912, 61; Lancaster MOH Report, 1920, 23. Comparative continuation of fatalities from this disease in Preston, coupled with the MOH's silence about supply and administration of antitoxin, suggests that routine administration of antitoxin came somewhat later in that city.

150. Barrow MOH Report, 1898, 179.
151. Preston MOH Report, 1905, 18.
152. Preston MOH Report, 1916, 9; Preston MOH Report, 1917, 8.
153. Lancaster MOH Report, 1913, 78–79.

(1913) and Lancaster (1915) than in Preston (1920), although disagreement continued about whether sanatorium beds were more necessary for sufferers with advanced cases (the approach taken in Lancaster) or for patients in early stages of the disease where an arrest was possible (the protocol in Preston).[154]

Experts agreed that sanatorium admission helped to reduce the spread of disease by increasing professional control over patients' behavior. In a revealing 1916 statement, Lancaster's MOH observed, "The County Council [–funded] beds at the Isolation Hospital are helping considerably in the prevention of the spread of infection, but powers are required to enable us to prevent careless patients from leaving the Institution and returning to homes where there are not the requisite facilities for isolation."[155] It is worthy of remark that sending patients to remote rural sanatoria at considerable distance from their home communities, such as the High Carley facility in Ulverston (the destination of many Lancashire patients during the interwar years), may have strengthened professional control over inmates' behavior and contacts, and decreased the likelihood that "careless patients" would leave too soon and infect other people. Sanatorium care, which often lasted for years, emphasized fresh air, bed rest, outdoor exercise usually involving "graduated labor," and large quantities of food. By the 1930s, surgical therapy involving pneumothorax (the artificial collapse of an infected lung) became increasingly common in British sanatoria. However, not until streptomycin was introduced in the late 1940s was there a truly effective treatment for tuberculosis.[156]

Sanatorium admission was a minority experience for TB victims in Barrow, Lancaster, and Preston. Many more attended dispensaries, which from 1913 offered diagnostic testing, notified cases, provided home visiting and nursing services, and supplied limited types of treatment and supplies. For example, in 1918, when only 30 sanatorium beds at diverse locations were available to Preston sufferers, the city's dispensary "treated 469 insured persons and 452 non-insured patients, most of whom were children."[157] Together with venereal disease clinics and school medical services, tuberculosis dispensaries added treatment to the surveillance, reporting, and isolation responsibilities of public health authorities.[158] In theory a strong link between public health, clinical medicine, and tubercular patients, in practice dispensary services were met with resistance by both sufferers and general practitioners, according to MOsH.[159]

154. Lancaster MOH Report, 1920, 26; Preston MOH Report, 1916, 9.

155. Lancaster MOH Report, 1916, 17.

156. Bryder, *Below the magic mountain.*

157. Preston MOH Report, 1918, 2.

158. See, for example, Lancaster MOH Report, 1926, 34; Armstrong, *Political anatomy of the body,* 10–12.

159. Preston MOH Report, 1920, 52.

Another institutional approach to tuberculosis control was the open-air school movement, designed to prevent the disease developing and spreading among children. Supported by local authorities beginning in the interwar period, these schools offered delicate children outdoor exercise and an enhanced diet, while also removing them from crowded classrooms where they might contract or spread infection.[160] Preston's Tuberculosis Officer began advocating local establishment of an open-air school in 1916; such a facility was opened in 1919, admitting "pre-tubercular children and very early non-infectious cases of tuberculosis. Meals are given at the school and periods of rest are arranged for the children."[161] Barrow opened an open-air school on Roa Island in 1928.[162]

While antituberculosis initiatives emphasized isolation and prevention, local anti–venereal disease efforts focused on diagnosis and treatment. By 1917 Preston's Dr. Pilkington was working with local people to determine how to carry out the requirements of the Venereal Disease Regulations of 1916 to arrange for laboratory testing and treatment of VD sufferers. Although, in keeping with recommendations of the 1913 Royal Commission on Venereal Disease, Pilkington presumed "that the Royal Infirmary should be the treatment centre for the town and district," he encountered resistance from the voluntary hospital, similar to that displayed in other parts of the country.[163] However, the opposition to providing outpatient services was overcome, and thereafter, VD patients from Preston and the surrounding area (including Lancaster until 1946) received treatment from the Preston Royal Infirmary.[164] In Barrow, the venereal disease clinic was first established in the North Lonsdale Hospital, then moved to the Devonshire Road Infectious Diseases Hospital in 1943.[165] Public health authorities also provided Salvarsan substitutes to general practitioners.[166] In addition to treatment of adults, newborns were increasingly checked and treated for *ophthalmia neonatorum*.[167] For example, reporting on 11 Lancaster cases in 1918, the MOH commented, "This disease which is the chief cause of blindness is the result of Venereal disease in the mothers."[168] However, despite the availability of services, because of the continuing stigma of venereal diseases, it was difficult for health officials to successfully deal with these ail-

160. Bryder, *Below the magic mountain*, 148–51.

161. Preston MOH Report, 1916, 10; Preston MOH Report, 1919, 34.

162. Barrow MOH Report, 1928, 38.

163. Preston MOH Report, 1917, 12. Evans, "Tackling the 'hideous scourge,'" 424–25.

164. Preston MOH Report, 1917, 12. Lancaster MOH Report, 1918, 44; Lancaster MOH Report, 1946, 13.

165. Barrow MOH Report, 1925, 327; Barrow MOH Report, 1947, 29.

166. See, for example, Preston MOH Report, 1920, 63.

167. Some towns began notifying *ophthalmia neonatorum* from 1909, and the Local Government Board made its notification compulsory in 1914. Personal communication from Graham Mooney, 5/19/06.

168. Lancaster MOH Report, 1918, 44.

ments. For example, in 1919 the MOH commented that almost no women attended for treatment; also, that it was difficult to get patients to complete courses of treatment.[169]

Linked to the establishment of local VD clinics were educational efforts, including lectures, pamphlets, posters, and films.[170] Preston was in the vanguard of towns using the new media, film, for this purpose.[171] In Lancaster in 1920, "Propaganda work, begun in the previous year by a local committee, was continued during the spring when meetings for men and women were held, and later addresses were given by County Council lecturers to mothers and school teachers."[172] In 1921, however, the MOH commented, "Three lectures were given in connection with the campaign of the County Council against these [venereal] diseases. The meetings were badly attended."[173]

Several informants remembered educational programs about venereal diseases. Men learned about these ailments when they joined the military.[174] Mrs. Peterson, born in 1899, said that during World War I, she went to a lecture at a cinema that "was showing people what they were like when they had got this disease. It showed a walled place in Italy where they kept them and they wouldn't let them out. It showed cripples and all sorts. I thought it was terrible!"[175] Mr. Danner, born in 1910, said that at about age 15, he saw the film "Dangers of Ignorance": "I saw all the genital organs that I had till then only guessed about, and the effect of V.D. and the like. The picture was based on man meeting girl, the latter a daughter of shame. After all this, I was sure one could live a decent life, and, in my case, I could not let such good sisters down."[176]

Health education was an important prevention technique used by twentieth-century public health authorities. However, it would be remiss to ignore perhaps the oldest and most effective prevention technique available to them—smallpox vaccination. Compulsory after 1853, vaccination was nonetheless resisted—particularly by working-class people who objected to governmental interference with their liberties, parental rights, and bodies.[177] Medical Officers of Health perceived vaccination as both an

169. Preston MOH Report, 1919, 38.

170. See, for example, Preston MOH Report, 1918, 13.

171. Preston MOH Report, 1920, 63. See also Preston MOH Report, 1926, 75; Preston MOH Report, 1941, 33; Timothy Martyn Boon, "Films and the Contestation of Public Health in Interwar Britain," unpublished PhD dissertation, London University, 1999; Hall, "Venereal diseases and society," 129.

172. Lancaster MOH Report, 1920, 27.

173. Lancaster MOH Report, 1921, 19.

174. See, for example, Mr. N3L, 62.

175. Mrs. P1P, 43.

176. Mr. D2P, 39.

177. See, for example, Nadja Durbach, "'They might as well brand us': Working-class resistance to compulsory vaccination in Victorian England," *Social History of Medicine* 13:1 (2000):

important weapon against a nasty, highly contagious disease and the reason for decline in smallpox's incidence, virulence, and deadliness. Thus, at the turn of the century they were outraged by mounting resistance to the procedure that resulted in the 1907 "conscientious objector" legislation, which made it possible for parents to refuse to have their children vaccinated without threat of prosecution.[178] When outbreaks occurred, the unvaccinated were most likely to contract, spread, and die from smallpox—a pattern Dr. Pilkington blamed on "the unsatisfactory manner in which the Vaccination Act has of late years and in many places been carried out."[179] In 1911, commenting on the three cases of smallpox occurring that year, he reflected on "exemption from vaccination, which has not for some years been so frequently sought, and so easily obtained," creating a large number of people susceptible to the disease.[180] In 1920 Lancaster's MOH called for restoration of compulsory vaccination for smallpox, arguing, "The public safety should take precedence of the liberty of the individual." In the city that year, of 963 babies born, 670 were vaccinated, 64 died, 142 (15 percent) were exempted, 2 proved insusceptible, and 84 were unaccounted for.[181]

In light of continued objection to smallpox vaccination, lack of popular resistance to the use of antitoxins in the early twentieth century and diphtheria immunization in the interwar period is noteworthy.[182] Serum treatment for diphtheria was in general use in the study cities from about 1906.[183] In 1911 Barrow's MOH reported: "During the year the Sanitary Authority resolved to supply anti-diphthertic serum free for the poorer inhabitants, and this has been largely taken advantage of. Comparatively large doses of the serum have been encouraged, and your Medical Officer's experience is that large, and in some cases what appears to be heroic doses have been the means of saving life, and in at least two cases have saved the patient from tracheotomy."[184] It is clear that general practitioners required some guidance in the use of this new intervention, which MOsH recommended be applied at the first suspicion of diphtheria.[185] As late as 1929,

45–62; Durbach, *Bodily matters: The anti-vaccination movement in England, 1853–1907* (Durham: Duke University Press, 2005).

178. Preston MOH Report, 1896, 5; Barrow MOH Report, 1898, 178.

179. Preston MOH Report, 1903, 6. See also Preston MOH Report, 1909, where Dr. Pilkington deplored the "reactive stance which leaves too many unvaccinated until an epidemic arrives" (4).

180. Preston MOH Report, 1911, 4.

181. Lancaster MOH Report, 1920, 25.

182. See, for example, Preston MOH Report, 1910, 5.

183. See, for example, Barrow MOH Report, 1906, 200.

184. Barrow MOH Report, 1911, 220. See also Ann Hardy, "Tracheotomy versus intubation: Surgical intervention in diphtheria in Europe and the United States, 1825–1930," *Bulletin of the History of Medicine* 66 (1992): 536–59.

185. See, for example, Lancaster MOH Report, 1912, 61.

Lancaster's MOH reported, "There is still a tendency on the part of some practitioners to withhold antitoxin, which is supplied free by the corporation, until the diagnosis is bacteriologically confirmed."[186] This comment links serum treatment to bacteriological testing—another resource managed by the public health service (often at isolation hospitals) and, thus, arguably an additional component in the turf contest with GPs.

By the 1920s, techniques had been developed making possible large-scale immunization for diphtheria.[187] However, public health authorities in Barrow, Lancaster, and Preston did not proactively advocate or use this tool before the mid-1930s, perhaps because hospital isolation for this disease was by then routine. It is possible that parents actually led the way in demanding immunization for their children, which was administered differently in the three study communities. For example, in Lancaster in 1932, when a diphtheria epidemic sickened 70 and killed 6, the MOH observed, "An increasing number of parents have had their children artificially immunized against diphtheria. This preventive method continues to be practiced at one of our residential institutions [an orphanage], ensuring complete immunity from the disease. The Isolation Hospital staff is now also immunized, and measures are being taken to extend the practice amongst the general child population of the area."[188] Stimulated by an epidemic, Barrow officials immunized 805 children in 1935. In the same year Preston became the earliest of the study cities to begin routine immunization of schoolchildren. However, in 1945 that city's MOH reported that because some parents resisted the procedure, only 37.5 percent of preschoolers and 77 percent of schoolchildren had been immunized.[189] Not until after World War II began did Lancaster health authorities offer diphtheria immunization to all school children.[190]

A final weapon in public health officials' arsenal in the war against contagious disease was disinfection of victims' possessions and homes after recovery or death. Beginning in the 1880s, this technique was used for an expanding range of ailments, eventually (during the interwar years) including cancer, and applied to spaces such as bedrooms, homes, and school classrooms, and materials including bed linens, clothing, toys, and library books. It is clear that MOsH believed that germs could be transferred from person to person through contact with contaminated surfaces and materials; it is also apparent that MOsH believed disinfection was an effective way to limit spread of contagion. In 1883 Barrow's MOH credited disinfection and limewashing the home of a smallpox victim for preventing an epidemic; similarly, in 1891 the dwellings of five continued fever suffer-

---

186. Lancaster MOH Report, 1929, 27.
187. Rosen, *History of public health*, 312–13.
188. Lancaster MOH Report, 1932, 28. See also Lancaster MOH Report, 1934, 27.
189. Preston MOH Report, 1935, 68; Preston MOH Report, 1945, 34.
190. See, for example, Lancaster MOH Report, 1941, 3; Preston MOH Report, 1945, 34.

ers were "cleansed and disinfected; beds and bedding were destroyed or disinfected, and a serious outbreak of this terrible disease was averted at this point."[191] In 1897 Dr. Pilkington reported that 587 Preston houses were fumigated.[192]

By the early twentieth century, disinfection had become part of a systematic response to contagious disease, consuming significant time and resources.[193] In 1912 Barrow's MOH reported that 504 people suffered from notifiable diseases. Of these, 82 were hospitalized, 432 cases were notified to the Education Authority, and the borough librarian was informed of 361 whose books were collected and disinfected before being issued to other patrons. A total of 357 homes were disinfected.[194] In 1915 Lancaster's MOH reported that "3,835 articles (bedding, clothing, etc.), were disinfected in addition to 260 articles of clothing for the rural district. 215 houses and 39 library books were also disinfected."[195]

Various methods of disinfection were used. In 1907 Lancaster's MOH reported disinfection of houses with "formic Aldehyde, Perchloride of Mercury, Sulfur Dioxide," and of clothing and bedding, with "super-heated steam."[196] Mr. Grove, born in 1903 in Preston, remembered:

> They had the Town Doctor and he used to come to the house and they would say as we had had scarlet fever and this house had to be stoved. They would ask where the child was, and they would say in such a bedroom. I remember it was a three-bedroomed house and they came and they did all three bedrooms. They left the rest of the house. It was like sulfur in a round tin and they put one in each bedroom and they lit it. They sealed all the bedroom doors and windows up with sticky brown paper. They would do that in the morning and then at night they would come and take this brown paper off and open the doors and windows.[197]

Lancaster's MOH reported in 1912, "The infected room or rooms are sprayed with a solution of formalin and closed for four hours, a supply of suitable disinfectant is given, and in every case the bedding and other articles are removed for steam sterilization."[198] Formalin spray was still being used in the interwar period; steam disinfection of bedding, clothes, and

---

191. Barrow MOH Report, 1883, 211; Barrow MOH Report, 1891, 207.
192. Preston MOH Report, 1897, 13.
193. See, for example, Preston MOH Report, 1905, 13, 19; Preston MOH Report, 1909, 10: This report also refers to disinfection of schools.
194. Barrow MOH Report, 1912, 293.
195. Lancaster MOH Report, 1915, 17.
196. Lancaster MOH Report, 1907, table LX, no page number given.
197. Mr. G1P, 11. See also Mrs. W2L, 188.
198. Lancaster MOH Report, 1912, 57–58.

books was done at the isolation hospital.[199] It is worth mention that in the mid-twentieth century public health authorities also undertook responsibility for disinfecting furniture infested, or suspected of being infested, with bedbugs and other vermin—particularly during transfer from private to council house property. In this case, HCN gas was applied to furniture in moving vans.[200]

There was some resistance to disinfection. For example, in 1910 Lancaster's Lady Health Visitor commented:

> The Scarlet Fever epidemic of the two previous years diminished in frequency of attacks on the latter part of 1909, but has also continued all through 1910, and each month has furnished its quota of cases, although the total number is much diminished. I am still convinced that these epidemics might be much lessened both in duration and extent if it were possible to secure the more cordial cooperation of parents in the disinfection of articles of clothing, etc., which may possibly have been in contact with the sick person. At present we are able to disinfect the beds and bedding, the walls of the room, and, in fact everything in the sick room. I think, however, that benefit would result if the whole house could be disinfected, and especially the better clothing, which is put away in drawers or other receptacles all the week.[201]

Oral history informants suggest why some people resisted disinfection. Mr. Southwort, born in 1915 in Preston, remembered that after home quarantine for scarlet fever, "It was a process my mother called 'stoving,' everything that I had used or touched had to be burnt. All my clothes and all my toys, anything that I had used at all was destroyed. Some chaps came from somewhere and there were some ghastly smells. I think they called it 'stoving' of the room took place."[202] For already poor households, demolition of still-useful possessions must have seemed terribly wasteful, and the expense of replacing them a financial burden. However, regardless of the unpleasantness of the process, like other public health interventions, disinfection was mandated and enforced.

WORKING-CLASS EXPECTATIONS, EXPERIENCES, AND MANAGEMENT OF CONTAGIOUS DISEASES

The memories that oral history informants contributed to this study span multiple transitions in expectations and experiences of contagious diseases.

---

199. Lancaster MOH Report, 1927, 39; Lancaster MOH Report, 1932, 32.

200. Lancaster MOH Report, 1941; Lancaster MOH Report, 1942; Preston Borough Council, "Preston Slum Clearance" (1938), North West Film Archive, Film No. 518.

201. Lancaster MOH Report, 1910, 35.

202. Mr. S4P, 4. See also Mr. A2B, 73; Mrs. C8P, 148.

The oldest interviewees recalled a cultural environment where these ailments were expected, dreaded, sometimes deadly, and invariably managed at home by mothers or wives and experienced older female relatives and neighbors; professional interventions, such as vaccination or doctors' visits, were rare and often viewed with suspicion. Somewhat younger respondents' memories suggested the new resources and powers of social medicine, where the main alternative to home care for still-vicious communicable diseases (increasingly associated with childhood) was isolation hospital or sanatorium, while the attentions of medical and public health professionals often continued to be avoided or resented. Still younger informants' accounts indicated transitions in perceptions of both contagious diseases, generally thought to be minor (if inevitable) hurdles in the obstacle course of childhood, and professional attention, newly considered part of a natural order of things and welcomed as working-class women entered adulthood without traditional knowledge, skills, and confidence in their competence to treat and nurse serious illness. The youngest informants revealed both virtually complete dependence on biomedical management (including immunization, diagnosis, and treatment) of communicable diseases and the sense that public health and medicine had disarmed these ailments as health challenges.

The boundaries between these sets of experiences and expectations are porous and difficult to date precisely; informants' childhood memories both differed from and informed their experience of contagious diseases in their adult households. Furthermore, as we have seen, younger informants from very traditional families remembered traditional home-based management of communicable ailments long after their age contemporaries from self-consciously "modern" families recalled relying on professional advice and care for most health challenges. Nonetheless, since working-class contagion and culture were the primary targets for public health services and most scholarship on this topic is based on professional sources and perspectives, it is important to explore working-class experience of both communicable diseases and the growing range of official interventions intended to prevent or contain those diseases.

Oral history informants' memories of contagious disease were often linked to the early deaths of siblings or neighbors. When asked during her first interview whether she had brothers and sisters, Mrs. Harte, born in 1889 in Lancaster, said that of her mother's eleven children, three died:

Then we buried Maggie May. She was born on Saint Margaret Mary's birthday. Miss Dillon was an old woman that went round such as m'mother, and they'd do it for nowt in those days. She was the loveliest little thing that ever walked and she started with diphtheria and I've heard m'mother say that she rolled from the top of the bed to the bottom to get her breath. There was no immunization, no nothing. The poor little thing died. Then there was John died and he died with

consumption of the bowels I believe, and there was no cure then. There was a Polly died, I believe, but I'm not sure about Polly.[203]

This account indicates the horror of the communicable diseases that attacked young children, the expectation that victims suffer and die at home, and support offered by neighborhood health authorities such as Miss Dillon (who prepared the baby for burial). Another informant, Miss Coyle, born in Lancaster in 1903, remembered the random quality of mortality from contagious disease. One of four children, her infant sister died at "six weeks old—twins. They had whooping cough when they were a fortnight old. Our Edward [brother] had it and I had it. She was the finest baby, and yet our Gladys [the other twin] lived through it."[204] Mrs. Howe, born in 1898 in Preston, remembered, "A neighbor of ours, Mr. Ratcliffe, they lived round the corner, and he had two dead in the house at once with diphtheria, Nellie and John Ratcliffe. . . . [T]hey lived on Fishwick Parade. They were both in their coffins at the same time."[205]

Working-class people feared contagious diseases. Mr. Tomlinson, born in 1884 in Barrow, said, "Diphtheria was the killer with children. If children got diphtheria their throat fastened up. . . . [M]y sister's child died of diphtheria. I'd be about twenty-four and this little girl would be about four or five or six."[206] According to Mr. Middleton, born in 1898, "I'll tell you what was a common thing, TB. You were meeting young people all the time. If you just happen to look in the Barrow News between 1900 and 1914 and you see it all over, so-and-so twenty-three, full of babies and children. Nearly everybody lost somebody with it. TB has gone . . . compared with what it used to be."[207] Mr. Danner, born in 1910 in Preston, remembered, "Mother had fear of us getting TB which was common, and infectious diseases. I got lectured about risk of VD as I got older, and associating with people who were not nice. . . . Consumption was a real killer and diphtheria and whooping cough used to be killers too. I have heard children whooping their hearts out."[208]

Despite their dread of contagious diseases, however, working-class people were fatalistic about these ailments. Mrs. Havelock, born in Preston in 1903, said, "I'm not what you call a religious woman, but I do try to live a Christian life and I thought, if my baby is going to get whooping cough, she'll get it anyway. It was more or less faith that I relied on and she never got it. She did get scarlet fever and measles and that's about all she had

203. Mrs. H2L, 1.
204. Mrs. C2L, 4, 16.
205. Mrs. H2P, 19.
206. Mr. T1B, 6. See also Mrs. B1L, 4.
207. Mr. M2B, 21.
208. Mr. D2P, 17, 29. See also Mrs. M10B, 48.

of baby ailments."[209] Mrs. Hill, also born in 1903 in Preston, said that children who got diphtheria usually died. She observed, "There was a time of measles and chickenpox and things like that, so you kept your child in unless you spread it all round. Once they had it, that were it. There was never doctors or anything like that."[210]

This comment shows that despite increasing institutionalization of certain infectious-disease victims, most sufferers were cared for at home by mothers and their relatives and friends. Mrs. Drake, born in 1899, remembered:

> Honestly, do you know all the schools in Barrow closed for fever and in them days there was such a lot of scarlet fever that all the schools were closed and the fever hospitals full and you'd to do the best you could at home. Our mother went in and out and they used to help one another in them days because of big families. Some of them had about twenty-one children. Our mother used to go and we never ailed a thing, we never got fever and we never got anything that was going. We had measles once and I don't know how the dickens I got measles. But fever and other things that were going we never caught, and our mother used to go and look after them all.[211]

This account emphasizes both dependence on mutual aid and a common, almost mythical belief in mothers' expertise and power; beneath the surface, however, lurks perception of a real enemy always ready to attack. Contagious disease strained meager household resources. Support from relatives and friends was particularly useful during a period when professional advice and help were not routinely sought. Mr. Hardine, born in Lancaster in 1904, said of the neighbors, "They were very good indeed. They'd even sit up all night and they was always ready to help people out with garments if there was a lot of sickness and a lot of bed-wetting. There was always somebody turning up with something, 'Well, you can burn this afterwards.'"[212] This observation suggests awareness of the danger of contaminated clothing and bed linen; it may also indicate experience of officially mandated disinfection procedures that put family possessions at risk.

In addition to eliciting mutual aid, communicable ailments called on traditional knowledge and remedies. Mrs. Peel, born in 1921 in Barrow, remembered having "mumps, chickenpox and measles and tonsillitis, but my mother used to always get us well. . . . We got our throats rubbed with camphorated oil and the warm sock round our throats, when we had chick-

209. Mrs. H4P, 36.
210. Mrs. H8P, 51.
211. Mrs. D1B, 19.
212. Mr. H4L, 25.

enpox and measles she used to burn sulfur on a shovel." When asked, "What was that supposed to be good for?" Mrs. Peel responded:

> To kill the germs and to make it easier for the breathing, pull the blinds down if we had measles so that we didn't get the light in our eyes. And on the whole she used to nurse us through; I've had goose grease on my throat, that was supposed to be good; I've had sulfur blown down my throat for a bad throat—that's powdered sulfur and they put it in a white clay pipe and blow it down. . . . Liquorice sticks and cod-liver oil and malt and Scott's Emulsion. . . . I mean, mothers know if it's mumps, chickenpox or measles, you know, it's just a natural instinct, isn't it?[213]

Despite some positive outcomes, however, home care did not always turn out well. Mrs. Musgrove, born in 1886 in Barrow, said, "You see, you had to do all your own nursing yourself, and then there was the little girl [sister] that died of Scarlet Fever. There were four down with it at once, and mother had them all to nurse at home, and one died."[214]

Home care was a challenge even when the sufferers survived—particularly since some ailments lasted a very long time. Mrs. Oxley, born in Preston in 1902, remembered:

> I had three boys with the whooping cough all at once, it was a terrible thing, they nearly choked. One of the boys, he was the worst of the lot, and he would start at night after you had put them upstairs to bed. When they started coughing you used to have to dive upstairs with a cloth or something and there was nothing done about it much then. And I had a sister lived with me, an elder sister who never married, and they used to give you all kinds of recipes, old ladies, you know. One was to scoop the middle out of a turnip and put sugar in and to sort of drink the liquid from it. . . . And they used to take babies out with whooping cough and hold them, there used to be wagons go out full of tar and they used to hold them over, and they said that did them good, didn't they?
>
> *Mr. Oxley:* My sister did that, she took them and there was a place at Longridge which they call Tootal Height and they used to say if you took them on Tootal Height it would blow it away. We got our children taken there in a car, an open Sunbeam car it was, thinking it would move it, but it didn't. It has its time, they always say if you got whooping cough, it would last until May.[215]

---

213. Mrs. P6B, 117–19. See also Mr. R3L, 13, 31; Mrs. S3B, 72; Mrs. W4L, 33.
214. Mrs. M3B, 16.
215. Mrs. O1P, 3. See also Mrs. F1L, 48; Mrs. H2P, 19; Mrs. P1P, 37; Mrs. R1B, 18–19.

This story emphasizes the difficulty of dealing with an ailment for which there is still no effective biomedical treatment (although there is a vaccine), the importance of mutual aid, and the use of traditional remedies. It underscores the fatalism with which people met contagious disease: "If you got whooping cough, it would last until May." In addition, it suggests several reasons a working-class parent might take a child with whooping cough out of its home—an action that, as we have seen, attracted the ire of MOsH: the parent might reasonably do this to try a traditional treatment (exposure to tar fumes or the breeze on Tootal Height) for the suffering child. However, it was also unfeasible for a responsible low-income mother to arrange for (and pay) a child-minder or to leave a young child alone at home every time she had to go out for a period that could last as long as six months. Medical Officers' disapproval of hearing children with whooping cough out in public arguably reflects their gendered distance from primary responsibility for child care and their own middle-class experience of households supported by domestic servants.[216]

Whooping cough was not a notifiable disease in Barrow, Lancaster, and Preston. Thus, although MOsH recommended isolation, they did not enforce home quarantine or recommend admission to isolation hospital for this ailment. However, when they were not sent to hospital, victims of notifiable diseases—scarlet fever and diphtheria, in particular—were isolated at home. Mr. Ackerman, born in 1904, remembered both administration of antitoxin and the isolation and disinfection procedures required by Barrow health authorities in the early twentieth century:

> I can always remember my sister having diphtheria at home. . . . It was serious. What always sticks in my mind was the way in which they injected . . . her with something into her stomach and I remember mother and dad had to hold her while they put the injection into her tummy. . . . She was isolated in the little back bedroom and after it was all over they came and fumigated the place . . . [t]he local authority. This was an absolute essential if it's a notifiable disease.
>
> *Interviewer:* What did they do to it?
>
> *Informant:* Sealed all the doors and windows up and set one of these things alight in the room and let it burn itself out.[217]

Mr. Southwort, born in Preston in 1915, recalled his own experience with quarantine for scarlet fever:

> This was typical of my mother's utter devotion and dedication to me as a child and which probably accounts for my later shortcomings. It

216. See, for example, Barrow MOH Report, 1911, 221; Lancaster MOH Report, 1907, 43.
217. Mr. A2B, 72–73.

was unheard of for anything other than that you went to an isolation hospital, but my mother managed to prevail upon the doctor and the health authority that because I was the only one, she was prepared to take extreme precautions with regard to infection and I was immured in the bedroom for a couple of months and no one was allowed in the room except my mother. I remember the blankets and things soaked in disinfectant, hanging outside the door. It was a most peculiar period. I saw nobody but my mother and the doctor for many weeks. She moved heaven and earth to allow them to let her nurse me at home.[218]

In this case of a small family and comparatively well-educated mother, the mother became a trained nurse, carrying out the instructions of public health authorities and her general practitioner. Home quarantine also required that other family members stay home from school or work. Mrs. Peel, born in 1921, remembered that her father, who worked for the Barrow Post Office "on the engineering side," had to stay off work when she and her brother had "any of those contagious diseases."[219]

Once sanatoria were available, many tuberculosis sufferers were institutionalized for isolation and treatment; more, however, were cared for at home. Mrs. Smith, born in 1895 in Barrow, the third of ten children, recalled:

We weren't an ailing family. Alec [younger brother] was the only one. At sixteen he played football for Ulverston Town and he got a germ. I came in from work and he was in bed. He had started serving his time at the yard as a fitter and he was in bed and we sent for the doctor. I always used to feed the baby, help m'mother to put the dinners out, and the doctor came. I went to the door and let him in and took him upstairs and then went to see to the dinners while m'mother went. When the doctor came downstairs I can remember it as though it was yesterday, he just looked at m'mother and said, "I'm afraid I've very bad news for you. I don't think the boy will last six months." He'd got tuberculosis and he wouldn't go into the homes [sanatoria]. He was off work for six months and my mother fed him on eggs and sherry, egg flip and it took a lot of hard work to do it. He used to take cod liver oil and malt and he stayed off work six months and the doctor used to come visiting him. Two more boys started with it at the same time and they went to a sanatorium and they both died and he didn't. My mother used to feed him up and he was off six months and should have stayed off longer, but he said, "I'm going back to work, if I've got to die, I'll die at work." He went back to work and he used to have cod

218. Mr. S4P, 4. See also Mrs. A4L, 77; Mrs. B2P, 34; Mr. I2L, 40.
219. Mrs. P6B, 118.

liver oil and malt all the time from the doctor and medicine and he lived until he was sixty-eight.[220]

As this account suggests, sometimes the symptoms of a serious contagious ailment motivated people who normally managed illness without professional help to call the doctor. Mrs. Ralston, born in 1889 in Barrow, remembered a friend's child dying of diphtheria:

> They thought that he'd got a sore throat and giving him cough stuff, perhaps rubbing his throat, putting flannel round his throat. My husband went round—they lived in Farm Street then, and we lived in Dundee Street—to see Jackie. . . . He went round to see this lad, and when he came back he said, "Do you know, I didn't like the looks of that little lad." He was in bed and he'd heard George's voice and called him. He said to Tom, the boy's father, "I think you ought to have the doctor to that child, his breathing isn't right." The result was Tom had gone for the doctor, and the doctor had come, and whatever he'd said to Tom, Tom had broken down and he said that he was very sorry, but he was in an advanced stage of diphtheria and he died that night. They took him up to Devonshire Road [isolation hospital]. That was just after the First World War.[221]

Similarly, as we have seen in chapter 3, suspicion of notifiable disease stimulated consultation of medical professionals. Mr. Carson, born in 1902 in Lancaster, remembered: "I know a man who worked with me, and he was walking about with scarlet fever for a fortnight. He was skinning and I said, 'What the hell is the matter with you? You'd better got to the doctor's.' He went straight from work there and then to Dr. Stout. 'Get yourself home man and get off to bed and stop there for fourteen days and I'll come and see you. Let no one into the room, not your two children, only your wife to bring your dinner up and attend to you.'"[222] These experiences did not necessarily increase people's faith in professional medicine. Mr. Ritter, born in 1894 in Lancaster, remembered, "I'd a sister that died at four year old, diphtheria, no cure for it. She just choked, fetched the doctor and she died while he was there."[223] They did, perhaps, bear out physicians' complaints that people often waited too long to call them.[224]

In 1934 Mr. and Mrs. Grove's first baby, David, died of the measles in their Preston home. Mrs. Grove's account suggests both that at this time it was still usual and expected—even by medical professionals—for seriously

220. Mrs. S2B, 27.
221. Mrs. R1B, 19.
222. Mr. C1L, 29.
223. Mr. R1L, 63.
224. See, for example, Preston MOH Report, 1913, 25.

ill infants to be cared for at home and that mothers sometimes lacked the knowledge, experience, and support to manage this responsibility confidently:

At 18 months, on a Wednesday, he [David] had a running cold and my mother said that he did look poorly so I sent for the doctor. He said it was the measles and told me not to move him out of the room. When the doctor come in, he got behind the door and shut it so that no cold air could come in and then when he saw him he said that it had turned to double pneumonia. It still didn't worry me because I didn't know so much about it. I was 24 when David was born. He told me not to lift him up or anything and to just give him barley water if he cried. I always thought I did well, but I think I made the barley water too thick and it wasn't as thirst quenching as it should have been. This was on the Friday and he came Friday night and I had him on my knee and he was so forlorn. He told me to just let him lay and not to pick him up. I stopped up Friday night and the doctor told me he would send the district Nurse and she came Saturday morning. On the Friday night I did pick him up because he just couldn't cry. I realized as I got older that he must wasn't quenching his thirst. I thought I was giving him strength. The nurse came and we had made cotton laps and they were about this big and I had made him a little cotton waistcoat, just sewed it together with some tapes down. I had something on for the chest because he couldn't cough and he could hardly breathe. This nurse came and she took everything off, his vest and his pajamas and she asked for another pajama coat and she put his arms through. That night, he was up on his knees and he couldn't make a sound. I kept putting him down and covering him up and then he would be up again and all his back was burning. I think it was too drastic a treatment. Out of all that warmth into the cold. We had no heat in the house, only the fire, so the air went cold. I don't think it did him any good and she came again on the Sunday morning. They came again on the Saturday night putting kaolin poultices on back and front. One came on Sunday morning and I made her a cup of tea and I told her how he had been in the night. Then he started making such a noise. She asked how long he had been like that. I said I didn't know. She told me to go down and open the front window and she told me to go and ring the doctor. When I came back he was dying. It must have been to get us out of the way. I never had such a shock in all my life. It learned me a lesson not to smother them. He would have been 44 now, but he was a fine little boy. He was such a sturdy little boy. He was going to walk in the Whitsuntide processions that weekend. I asked the doctor if he thought he would be fit to walk and he said no. He died the week after and it was a shock. It is funny, you take a first baby on, and you come home with it and in them days

they kept you 14 days in bed, you never washed them, changed them, you never got a bath till the last day. On the last day they showed you how to bath the baby, but they did it.[225]

This story, which illustrates transition from lay to professional management of serious illness, indicates that support from the informant's mother, the general practitioner, and—perhaps most important—the district nurse, was available and welcomed. It also suggests that this young mother believed that professional and hospital care during childbirth and lying-in, still unusual in the early 1930s, may have undermined her ability to look after her baby competently. Regardless, there is the general sense that there was little anyone could do to save the infant and that Mrs. Grove blamed herself and grieved for her firstborn until her own old age. Mr. Grove commented about David, "Now, during the week he got measles about Tuesday or Wednesday, he come out in the spots. By Friday it was bronchial pneumonia and the doctor sent a nurse. He died on the Sunday morning. He died so quick. In them days measles was a more serious illness than what it is now."[226]

While home care for contagious diseases remained usual, oral history accounts clearly illustrate the trends toward increased powers of public health authorities and institutionalization for a growing range of ailments. Many interviewees remembered admission to isolation hospitals. Mr. Carson contracted scarlet fever in 1911 and was sent to the Luneside Hospital in Lancaster:

The doctor used to condemn you to hospital and this man used to come from the hospital with a blanket, go upstairs and put you in it, carry you down or walk you down, into the van. Nobody had to speak to you. You only had your eyes over the top and you were like a prisoner. You were put in this van, which had a bit of a couch in it. There was just some ventilation holes that you could just peep through. You were having a ride for nowt. You got there and you walked down the corridor—it was quite a long drive from the hospital to the gates. You'd to show a ticket to get in from there, the outside gate, up to the Matron's Office, reception office, and then you went down a long corridor and then you walked outside the wards. The patients were inside and you each had a window. It didn't open, but you could talk through the window because you were isolated or else it would be infectious. You could infect or contaminate or they could catch scarlet fever off you, even off your breath or touching anything.[227]

225. Mr. G1P, 61.
226. Mr. G1P, 5.
227. Mr. C1L, 29. See also, Mr. F1L, 27–28; Mrs. H3L, 62; Mr. P1L, 51.

This account emphasizes the patient's perception of the similarity of isolation hospital to prison and both the enforced nature of hospitalization and its purpose: to minimize the transmission of infection. It also links the family's GP with public health regulations and processes.

Mr. Grove described his family's experience with contagious disease and isolation hospitalization at about the same time: "In 1914, my mother and father had a very bad spell. I had a sister that had meningitis; she was in the Infirmary for six months. I had a sister died with diphtheria and I went in hospital with scarlet fever. I had another sister in after I came out. I came out six weeks later. I had been home about a month and my sister was taken in. For six months my mother and father said they never had their clothes off as they were up night and day." He was taken to the hospital in a horse-drawn ambulance:

> It was a horse-cab. I always remember, my mother went with me and it was a water-bed. I didn't know there was such a thing. With being on the horse and on cobbles in the streets, there was no springs on carts hardly. When you went in, you could have had scarlet fever for a week. It made no difference to them, they treated you the same. You went for three days and you were only on slops and they kept you laid down. They gradually built you up but all the time you were in hospital, you were hungry. When the meal come, you would have eaten anything. Even at tea-time or at breakfast, all you would get was bread and butter. You used to count how many pieces of bread you got as you were that hungry. Parents weren't allowed in. Later on they could come and look through the window.
>
> *Interviewer:* How did you actually spend your time for six weeks, it must have seemed to be forever?
>
> *Informant:* It was. You didn't know what the days were. . . . My mother come for me and I had never been out for six weeks. She said, "Have we to get a cab?" I asked if we could walk it as I was that pleased to be out. When I come to the sidewalk, I couldn't lift one leg on to it. . . . [The hospital was in] Deepdale Road. Blackpool Road wasn't made in them days and you went up a long drive to it. It was a long way from anywhere. Wednesdays and Saturdays your mother used to bring you oranges and eggs or something like that. . . . Well, I was in hospital for six weeks and all your skin comes off with scarlet fever. They used to take you to the bathroom with this old-fashioned bath. You would sit on the surround and your feet would be in the boiling water. The nurse would do the bottom of your feet with pumice-stone. You nearly went up in the air because the water was boiling hot.[228]

Mr. Hunter, born in 1928 in Preston, had a similar experience a gen-

228. Mr. G1P, 11–13.

eration later that is noteworthy because of increased medical and surgical intervention:

> I came home from school on the Tuesday, I thought I had a cold, and then I went into school on the Wednesday morning, I was really poorly and I could hardly swallow. And a gentleman next door whose family we were friendly with, said you had better call the doctor, I think he's got diphtheria. He came and I was rushed into hospital. And I was in there for three months. . . . Well, the first thing they did when I got there was to stick a needle about that long into me. . . . They gave me an injection of serum. And I wasn't all that bad. Some had been in about five months, six months you know. For eight weeks I had to lie entirely flat, and then you started to get pillows, you know, and then to crown things, I had to have my tonsils out there. And that was the most gruesome thing in my life, of course these days you never see the operating theatre. But then I was wheeled along on a trolley and they had a little cubicle at the end, and they brought the previous person out you know. Arrrrgh . . . and I was wheeling on and put on the table and there was a bucket alongside, and the surgeon just put a mask over and I was given ether. . . . That's the only time I've had morphine. Of course, I was obviously weak, and I heard him say, you know, give him so much morphine to keep down the pain. And after about two days I had jelly, you know. But I enjoyed being in hospital, because oranges were short and chocolate, and the hospitals always got the first choice on those, you see. This is 1941–42, but that was the only time I was actually off school, and that was eight years.[229]

After 1913, it became usual for residents of Barrow, Lancaster, and Preston diagnosed with tuberculosis to be sent to sanatoria. Mr. Madison, born in 1910 in Lancaster, remembered having had this disease as a child:

> I'd be about eight or nine years of age and I went to Helmsley. I stayed there for about nine months and the treatment in those days was isolated huts on the moors among the bracken for isolated cases and in the main hospital itself the windows were never shut and in the winter it was nothing to have about that much snow on your bed. That was the treatment to get rid of TB in those days. After about nine month I come home. I was born of small parents but when I left school I think I was about four stone, anybody could pick me up in one hand when I started work at fourteen.[230]

Mrs. Jenkins, born in 1932, contracted tuberculosis as age 17 and spent

---

229. Mr. H3P, 10–11. See also Mr. M13B, 57; Mr. R3B, 51.
230. Mr. M1L, 7. See also Mr. P6B's account of the sanatorium at High Carly, 31.

two years in a sanatorium in North Wales. Her account also reflects mid-century development of more aggressive therapy options:

> I didn't have any treatment apart from PAS streptomycin which I didn't like, they were going to operate, but they wrote to my firm and said if she can stay a bit longer, I think this was after six months, we've no need to operate. Well it ended up nearly two years. . . . No, it was medicine, horrible medicine, they were both on the trying out then, and the horrible thing about there, I loved it because it was in the country, it was by the sea which I loved, but you'd get to know people and I was there nearly two years and a lot of people died, usually the older ones, and it was all old people and teenagers, funnily enough.[231]

Family members as well as the ailing experienced isolation hospitalization. In the 1920s, Mrs. Peterson's husband was an outdoor laborer; she had temporarily given up her job as a weaver to stay at home with their four young children. The family lived in a very small house in Preston. Mrs. Peterson remembered one of her infant twins coming down with whooping cough:

> David caught it and then the little one [John] and he didn't come round after it. I had to keep them separate and I had little John at this end of the bed and David in the pram at that side to keep him away. I had them like that for a day or two and then they sent our George home from nursery school with measles. I don't like telling you this, but I must as I'll never talk about it again. It were a real tragedy. The Welfare come to see about him and I told them that it was George that had the measles. She asked if I had any other infection and I told her that the twins had whooping cough. All at once George said, "Mum, I do feel tired!" I told him to turn round to the wall and he might be better on the other side, and all sick came up. I no sooner get him cleaned and the little one at the top was sick and then the other one was sick with the whooping cough. I thought, I hope he doesn't get the whooping cough on top of the measles. I cleaned these babies up. . . . They sent somebody to take John away and then they come for David after that because of this whooping cough. They asked if there was anybody else. I told them that one had measles. They said they would have to take him as well. When my husband came home he went mad.
> *Interviewer:* Where did they take them to?
> *Informant:* Isolation Hospital. . . . When he [husband] come home at night, this was after John had died, like. I said that they had taken our George because he had asked where he was. I said that because he

231. Mrs. J1B, 5. See also Mr. C1B, 23.

had been infected they had to take them both. He said that I had no business letting them. You can't go against them people, can you? I were demented. I didn't know what I were doing. They took George as well and he did fight. I was too upset to really console him. I was sorry after. I just said, "You'll not be long, love. You will soon come back!" He were fighting in this blanket saying that he wasn't going to go.[232]

This terrible story about infant death, home nursing, public health ("the Welfare") domiciliary services, and hospital admission reveals the informant's powerlessness in the face of disease, official authority, and even her husband's questions and son's resistance to being removed from home. Her additional memories of George's and David's hospitalization, David's slow recovery, and her frustrating efforts to get follow-up care from general practitioners and hospitals indicated both her desperation to get professional help for her children and her disappointment with that help when it was provided.[233]

Hospitalization itself could be dangerous. Mrs. Winder, born in Lancaster in 1910, described losing her sight in one eye: "I went into the isolation hospital with scarlet fever and they got a disease in there at the time, a germ, a boy and I got this germ. The boy died and it caused me to have some throat infection that ate the back of m'eye away, and that's what caused it. . . . They wouldn't let them keep you home in them days."[234] When her daughter contracted scarlet fever during the early 1940s, Mrs. Winder resisted having her hospitalized. Such experiences no doubt reinforced traditional working-class belief, briefly discussed in chapter 3, that hospitals were dangerous places. In addition to the risk to patients, there was suspicion that isolation hospitals could spread infection to nearby neighborhoods. Miss Coyle, born in 1902, spent three months in Lancaster's Luneside Hospital:

I hadn't been up a week when they sent me home. A lady across the road was a Sister down there and she gave me a bath one Friday morning and said, "When do you think you're going home, Hilda?" I said, "Me go home? I don't think I'm ever going to get out of here." She said, "You never know." Instead of sending me back in to the ward, she sent me into another room to put m'own clothes on and then m'mother came for me. She walked me all the way round Freeman's Wood and instead of coming down on Canon Hill and down Wheatfield Street, she fetched me all round the ruddy Pointer. I said to m'dad, "Do you know m' mother walked me all that way through Freeman's Wood this

232. Mrs. P1P, 14.
233. Mrs. P1P, 15–16, 71.
234. Mrs. W2L, 213.

morning." She said, "Well, I thought if there was any germs on you, I'd blow them away."[235]

Mr. Hunt, born in Barrow in 1888, described related dread of ambulances: "There used to be an isolation hospital, which is now the Devonshire Road Hospital, and that was the fever hospital. Then, of course, there was a horse-drawn van. A brownish van, and you used to hold your breath as kids when it passed for fear you got something off it."[236] Expressing a similar feeling, Mr. Simpkins, born in Lancaster in 1932, expressed sentiments about the isolation hospital that had changed little in two generations:

> The things that stand out in my memory are the illnesses that were taking place at that time, because I can remember we used to dread seeing the . . . blue ambulance come on the [Lancaster Council housing] estate. Because diphtheria was widespread and we used to have a nasty little habit of spitting into the gutter and saying, "No fever in our house." . . . People died from diphtheria in those days, you know, and the isolation hospital. . . . You see, and they were not going to go in that blue ambulance, no way, you know, you was never going to come back.[237]

With the introduction of antibiotics and a proliferating range of immunizations in the mid-twentieth century, use of isolation hospitals declined in Barrow, Lancaster, and Preston, and the types of cases sent to them changed. Dr. Armstrong, who began practicing in Lancaster in 1948, remembered:

> The things that previously had perhaps been put into isolation hospitals, like scarlet fever, sometimes they were still admitted and you swabbed their throat and after penicillin for forty-eight hours and they were negative you used to get rid of them. Until it became a thing you just didn't put into isolation hospital. Measles, whooping cough, you still had youngsters with measles and whooping cough, but you wouldn't keep them very long. So the isolation in respect of you call the minor infectious things were out, and the locums I did I don't know if I perhaps had a bit of luck. I didn't have any cases of encephalitis. . . . We never had any polio.[238]

Isolation hospitals were intended to keep disease from spreading from the ailing to the well. An earlier prevention approach, vaccination for smallpox, was required between 1853 and 1907, when the "conscientious objector" legislation provided a legal loophole for parents who did not

235. Mrs. C2L, 4.
236. Mr. H2B, 81.
237. Mr. S7L, 8, 77. See also Mr. B10P, 3.
238. Dr. A5L, 9.

want to have their children immunized. Very few informants had personal or family experience with smallpox, which, as we have seen, had almost disappeared from Barrow, Lancaster, and Preston by the early twentieth century. Nonetheless, vaccination continued to be urged by public health and medical authorities until the 1980s, when smallpox officially became a dead disease. Some informants' families had their children vaccinated as a matter of routine. Mrs. Masterson, born in 1913 in Preston, remembered: "The first thing that they did was, the child was registered and the next thing was it would have to be christened very early and then it was the vaccination. They really insisted in those days. Everyone had vaccinations, some had four. Then it gradually went down to three and then two and then one. But everyone was vaccinated against smallpox because there was quite a lot of that in those days. It is dying out now."[239] Some, particularly younger, parents agreed with official arguments in favor of vaccination. Mrs. Rowlandson, born in 1945, said: "Yes, my mum always agreed on that. In fact, there was arguments over that, my dad you know, didn't bother about things like that. But my mum said, no, it's a good thing. You see, with her being a nurse during the war and that, she agreed with every-thing like that. . . . Even though . . . she wasn't politically minded, but she knew, she had very good views on things, you know what I mean. . . . But she always agreed with immunization, you know, especially with my sister having poliomyelitis when she was little. You know, and she got my sister back to normal."[240] However, objection to smallpox vaccination was also common among informants throughout the study period.[241]

In some cases, parents resisted the interference with their control over their infants' bodies. Mrs. Howe, born in 1898, said: "Our Tom wasn't vacci-nated or our Belle hadn't been vaccinated, only me, my dad didn't believe in it. We had an old man, Dr. Dunn, and he was the Vaccination Officer and he come walking in and he said he had come to vaccinate the baby. My dad said, 'You haven't, you know.' We had a doctor then and his name was Archibald Ramsey and he gave him a paper. I don't know how he worded it in but in them days they could put men in jail for not being vaccinated, but now they have the choice."[242] Mrs. Havelock, born in 1903, objected to vaccination on cosmetic grounds: "I did not see eye to eye with it at the time, and my baby wasn't inoculated at all. She has no marks. I said, 'Do you want to leave her with four big round marks like I have?'"[243]

Other parents thought vaccination was dangerous. Mrs. Washburn, born in 1900, said, "When I was vaccinated I had eczema. That was why I

239. Mrs. M1P, 49.
240. Mrs. R1P, 56.
241. See Durbach, *Bodily matters,* to consider informants' twentieth-century resistance in the context of the nineteenth-century antivaccination movement.
242. Mrs. H2P, 19. See also Mrs. T4B, 75.
243. Mrs. H4P, 36.

didn't have Brenda done. You used to have to have a paper signed by the magistrate. To this day Helen has eczema and I always say that is through vaccination."[244] Mr. Glover, born in 1913, recalled that his older brother had died at the age of 12 months: "I have heard Mother speak about this, and I was born five years later, but she blamed it on vaccinations. That was one of the reasons I've never been vaccinated for anything. He died a week or so after he had been vaccinated."[245] Mr. Grove, born in 1903, explained:

> I had an aunt and she had bad ears and they blamed it on the vaccination. It had upset her in a lot of ways as she was a bit backward. There was a book published about vaccination and there was a bit of a scandal. They said if anybody had had cowpox and got smallpox, it was never as bad. So they took from a cow that had cowpox and that's what they do. Now, they didn't bother about any other diseases that cow had, so you could be saddled with some other disease. So we never had it done and they never took any harm. We had one son . . . and he was born in 1941 and we thought it might be a smallpox epidemic, so we thought we would have him done. We had him done and he went green. Whatever the poor lad had had at that time, it was wrong.[246]

Mrs. Center, born in 1942 in Lancaster, also objected to vaccination on theoretical grounds: "I suppose we were a bit old-fashioned in that way, and I always thought, well, if they inject the germ into Phil and he's a bit prone to these ailments, is it going to do him more harm than good? So no, they were never done for anything."[247] Similarly, Mrs. Swallow, born in Lancaster in 1948, said her mother didn't believe in immunizations. "I don't think she understood it, to be truthful, and I think she thought that they were putting something in your body that shouldn't be there anyway, so no, there was never anything like that."[248] Mrs. Sykes, born in 1927 in Barrow, said her mother thought smallpox vaccination was "a messy thing and she wouldn't let us have that," although she was immunized against at least one other disease (probably diphtheria).[249] Despite widespread resistance to immunizations, however, many informants remembered them being administered without parental permission, either at school, by employers, in the military, or by local health authorities during an epidemic.[250]

244. Mrs. W4P, 18.
245. Mr. G3P, 1.
246. Mr. G1P, 90.
247. Mrs. C8L, 18.
248. Mrs. S6L, 24.
249. Mrs. S3B, 74.
250. See, for example, Mrs. B2P, 33; Mr. B4P, 34; Mr. F1L, 32; Mrs. F1L, 62; Mr. G1P, 89; Mr. N2L, 54, Mrs. S6L, 24; Mr. W7P, 45.

Informants' relationships with and attitudes toward public health staff were colored by awareness of public health's surveillance and enforcement functions. Thus, informants' memories of public health activities often reveal resentment or shame. This was particularly true of attitudes toward health visitors who were thought, particularly by older informants, to be judgmental, interfering, and nosy. This perception suggests both the centrality of housework and child care to working-class women's identities and reputations discussed in chapter 2, and the related insult that health visitors' criticism of their competence conveyed. Almost all informants recalled having health visitors inspect their hair at school, looking for head lice and nits. Many commented on being visited after a baby was born or by the health visitor from their children's school. Mrs. Nance, born in Lancaster in 1899, who did not voice an opinion about health visitors, nonetheless remembered feeling that her home and housekeeping skills were being inspected: "Every time the school visitor came, Miss Thompson, I always had the chairs on the table. Everything into the center, cleaning. I said to her one day, 'I always seem to be untidy when you come.' She said, 'You're always cleaning, and that is what we like.'"[251] Similarly, Mrs. Dent, born in 1908 in Preston, remembered the health visitor finding her home "spotlessly clean. She couldn't find any complaints."[252] Mr. Grove said, "Yes. I can remember the Health. . . . Going through your hair and one thing and another, it used to be done at school and then the health visitor for some reason occasionally used to come home. Yes, I don't think any of us looked forward to it, but . . . ."[253] Mrs. Hunter, born in 1931 in Preston, said that her mother did not attend public health clinics and, "When somebody came round, she used to tell the tale, when somebody came round no matter who it would be, she resented it. She resented it very much."[254]

Despite—or, perhaps, explaining—widespread resentment of health visitors, there is evidence that working-class housekeeping routines were influenced by perception of links between dirt and disease.[255] Mrs. Chase, born in Barrow in 1887, observed, "You used to disinfect your drains. They were very particular about their drains in those days. They were poor, but they were clean. The drains you could have eaten your meals from them, but today they wouldn't think of cleaning them."[256] Similarly, Mrs. Black, born in 1916 in Preston, said, "We only had a cold water tap. We had stone sinks and they were only about so deep. Nearly every day you put a bit of chlorous down the hole to make it clean."[257] Mr. Grand, born in 1904 in

---

251. Mrs. N1L, 52.
252. Mrs. D1P, 21. See also Mrs. C7L, 34.
253. Mr. G1P, 48.
254. Mrs. H3P, 49. See also Mrs. H4P, 6.
255. See, for example, Elizabeth Roberts, *A woman's place*, 131–35.
256. Mrs. C2B, 30. See also Mrs. H2L, 18.
257. Mrs. B2P, 15. See also Mrs. D1B, 29.

Lancaster, remembered hygiene-related challenges, ideas, and routines in
his childhood home:

> It was a tiled floor and they used to have a pegged rug which m'mother
> and father made on the hearth. Everywhere else was red tiles. I was the
> eldest and during the war when m'mother was out so busy scrubbing
> for other people, that was my job every Saturday morning to scrub those
> tiles. I used to use an awful soap by the name of Mauler soap and it was
> made by somebody in Kendall, I think. . . . It was horrid smelling stuff
> was this soap, but it was supposed to be high disinfectant. Most of these
> houses had cockroaches and silver fish and it was m'mother's idea that
> it would keep them down. I can't say we had a lot of cockroaches, but
> we had some of those silver fish things. . . . [S]he always had the inevi-
> table fly catcher up, sticky thing. . . . There were no fridges and we used
> to have a three-sided box that stood on the back kitchen shelf with a
> hinged door with a wire mesh at the front. That was the place in which
> you kept things if you didn't want flies to get at, uncooked meat or
> cooked meat that was left if you were fortunate enough to have it.
>
> *Interviewer:* Did you have a midden at the back?
>
> *Informant:* Yes. That was hand-emptied and the men had a basket
> what they called a swill. It was all shovelled into this basket and then car-
> ried from the midden to the dust cart and emptied in. The dust cart was
> an open cart and not like the closed in things we have today. . . . This
> was another thing, and some people were careless and left midden
> doors open and dogs and cats got in. They must have carried disease
> about scratching amongst the filth. I think in those days anyone who
> did care about hygiene would burn a lot of rubbish which was far easier
> than it is today with modern heating.[258]

Mrs. Masterson, born in Preston in 1913, similarly remembered:

> It [soda] was put down the toilet and they were outside toilets. It was
> used down the sink, they used to be stone sinks. Then the washing
> soda was used for almost everything. They used to scrub the floors and
> the wooden staircase because there would be no carpets on them. The
> wood was white with scrubbing and the gable top was snow white. Even
> the seat outside in the toilet, the long wooden seat, was all scrubbed
> really white. They used a lot of soda on the floors and everything. Even
> washing up they would use it. Of course, it was cheap, you could get a
> bag for a penny.[259]

258. Mr. G1L, 23. See also Mr. M1L, 51, 82; Mrs. M3L, 35.
259. Mrs. M1P, 62.

These examples demonstrate both the enormous challenges facing working-class housewives and the Herculean efforts they made to keep their rented dwellings clean; no wonder they resented the critical and patronizing attitudes of health visitors. However, interwar housing reform and postwar prosperity reduced both working-class housekeeping challenges. At the same time, with the post-1948 shift of public health focus from prevention of contagious disease and infant mortality to dealing with mental health, geriatric, and "problem families" issues, the role and demeanor of health visitors toward working-class women may have changed.[260]

Informants' attitudes toward health visitors altered somewhat after World War II, suggesting broader changes in working-class health culture. Mrs. Jenkins, born in 1932 in Barrow, observed a generational shift in acceptance of official health advice that occurred in the years after World War II. She took advice from health visitors herself, but reported that her mother-in-law, who was also raising a baby at the time, "wouldn't allow her [the health visitor] in the house. Said she was an interfering busybody or similar. But young people . . . I mean, I went regular to the clinic, my mother-in-law didn't, so you know."[261] Similarly, Mrs. Burrell, born in 1931 in Barrow, said she was more likely to take advice from the health visitor than from her own mother "because I thought the health visitor was the one to ask if I had any problems." It is noteworthy that, while this informant's mother had not allowed her to be vaccinated for smallpox, Mrs. Burrell had her own children immunized against "everything," reflecting her own acceptance of biomedicine and public health services.[262]

As their dependence on professional medicine grew, working-class people sometimes encountered friction between general practitioners and public health workers—a situation in which they tended to regard "their" doctor as their advocate. For example, Mrs. Chase, born in 1887, remembered her sister being kept home from school with "a weakness in her chest, in a lung. You could nearly see through her, she was nearly transparent, she never put any weight on no matter what she ate." The health visitor came around: "and mother said, 'Don't you lay a finger on her because she's under our own doctor and he'll tell you when she's got to come to school.'"[263] Along similar lines, Mr. Southwort, born in 1915, said: "I remember a medical inspection at school and a consequent note home to my parents to say that I needed my tonsils out. Mother wasn't for having that and trotted me along to Dr. Mooney who inspected my tonsils and said, 'Nonsense, it's a modern fad.' All these young doctors had nothing better to do than to take everybody's tonsils out. So I trotted back to school with a notice from my family doctor that in his opinion I did not

260. See, for example, Welshman, *Municipal medicine,* 241–49.
261. Mrs. J1B, 64. See also Mrs. L3L, 53; Mrs. W4L, 40; Mrs. Y1L, 52; Mrs. G5P, 45.
262. Mrs. B2B, 50–51.
263. Mrs. C2B, 18.

need my tonsils out and that was the end of that."[264] Mrs. Thornbarrow, born in 1948, remembered her parents objecting to smallpox vaccination: "When my sister was born, I think, there was some scare on about smallpox and they wanted her to get out of it. And apparently there was this sort of embarrassing thing when my dad had to get one of the doctors to sign a form to say, you know, that she didn't have to have this. And he was very embarrassed about it, because about the one doctor in Barrow who would do it, apparently his daughter had died after having this injection herself. So he knew he was a sure touch to get out of it, but he was embarrassed to have to do this."[265] Working-class perception of the GP's authority and status compared to that of public health workers indicated an important social reality that transcended the statutory power of health officials. It also became increasingly accurate after 1948, when the decline in incidence and mortality of contagious diseases paralleled both the establishment of the National Health Service and the growth in perceived effectiveness of clinical medicine.

CONCLUSIONS: CONTAGIOUS DISEASE, PUBLIC HEALTH, AND WORKING-CLASS CULTURE

After the Second World War, some of the deadly contagious diseases of the early twentieth century, including smallpox, typhoid, scarlet fever, and diphtheria, had virtually disappeared from Barrow, Lancaster, and Preston, while other former killers, including measles and whooping cough, had become minor "childhood diseases." Tuberculosis, scarlet fever, and venereal diseases could be cured by antibiotics; children were routinely immunized against a lengthening list of ailments including smallpox, diphtheria, whooping cough, tetanus, and polio. Public health services and requirements were embedded in working-class life; school inspections, workplace TB testing, and health visiting after childbirth were universal and unremarked rituals. At the same time, institutional and home isolation, once almost universal experiences, quickly faded from memory. In both professional and popular perception, modern medicine had beaten infection. This presumed victory was an important element in the transformation of working-class health culture. Mr. Madison, born in 1910 in Lancaster, made a comment about working-class people that was both formulaic and self-congratulatory: "They're more clued up on germs and things today than what they was then. They were ignorant about a lot of things."[266] This observation shows both the influence of biomedical ideas and profession-

264. Mr. S4P, 38.
265. Mrs. T4B, 75.
266. Mr. M1L, 82.

als, and the repudiation of traditional ways and people.

I have intended in this chapter to argue neither that contagious diseases were not "real" problems between 1880 and 1948 nor that public health policies and interventions were not generally effective—although both statements are debatable. I do maintain, however, that health authorities constructed contagious diseases as problems and benefited from strengthening popular belief in their expertise and support for the range of solutions they championed. Indeed, the biomedical account of its victory over contagion has become such a dominant cornerstone of standard modern history that it is easy to forget that there are other perspectives from which to view this process and other possible ways to tell this story. I think it is likely that working-class people did not traditionally classify diseases, as public health and medical authorities did, into contagious or not-contagious categories that required quite different types of decision making and management. Rather, they saw ill-health generally in terms of sickness (in the Parsonian sense of reduced ability to function in society) as a change from normal functionality (or "health").[267] Sick people, whatever their diagnoses, were cared for at home with mutual aid and occasional professional medical support; while certain contagious diseases (smallpox, later tuberculosis) were especially feared, the clear obligation to provide traditional care was far stronger than the new, alien notion of isolation. Furthermore, official criticism of working-class behavior as the cause of or vehicle for contagious disease was rejected by people who both maintained high standards for housekeeping and child care and did the very best they could with bad housing and meager resources.

However, by the mid-twentieth century the combination of enforcement of public health policies, pervasiveness of public health information and personnel, and perceived effectiveness of public health interventions changed the ways working-class people thought about and dealt with contagious diseases. After this time, these ailments were considered to be both less threatening than they had been in the past and more strictly the responsibility of professional rather than lay people. Thus, both contagious diseases and working-class health culture had been brought within the sphere of biomedical and governmental control; disorder, manifested in both infection and the traditional working-class behaviors that caused and managed it, had been disciplined.

267. See discussion in Turner, *Medical power and social knowledge*, 37–54.

Chapter Five

&

"They never told us anything"

Sex and Family Limitation

This chapter explores the related issues of working-class respectability, sex, family planning, and birth control in Barrow, Lancaster, and Preston during the years between about 1880 and 1970—a period that witnessed enormous changes in the ways Western societies dealt with sexuality and reproduction. Played out on the fields of belief, science, economics, policy, and culture, these transformations have attracted the interest of scholars from many disciplines. Most historical studies of sex take a macro view, considering large geographical areas and diverse populations.[1] While there are notable exceptions to this observation, there is little research that focuses on the working-class populations of specific English communities.[2] This focus is important because, as we have seen, the working class was considered to be both Britain's primary resource for economic and military power and the main threat to national health and stability. Working-class reproduction was central to a formidable range of theories, policies, and regulations.[3] Eugenicists warned of overbreeding and imperi-

1. See, for example, Michel Foucault, *The history of sexuality* (New York: Vintage, 1978); Jeffrey Weeks, *Sex, politics and society: The regulation of sexuality since 1800* (London and New York: Longman, 1981); Lesley A. Hall, *Sex, gender and social change in Britain since 1880* (New York: St. Martin's Press, 2000); Roy Porter and Lesley Hall, *The facts of life: The creation of sexual knowledge in Britain, 1650–1950* (New Haven, CT: Yale University Pres, 1995); Steve Humphries, *A Secret world of sex, forbidden fruit: The British experience 1900–1950* (London: Sidgwick and Jackson, 1988).

2. See, for example, Ellen Ross, *Love and toil: Motherhood in outcast London, 1870–1918* (Oxford: Oxford University Press, 1993); Maureen Sutton, *"We didn't know aught": A study of sexuality, superstition and death in women's lives in Lincolnshire during the 1930s, '40s, and '50s* (Stamford, UK: Paul Watkinds, 1992); Kate Fisher, "'She was quite satisfied with the arrangements I made': Gender and birth control in Britain 1920–1950," *Past and Present* 169 (2000): 161–93.

3. See, for example, Jane Lewis, *The politics of motherhood: Child and maternal welfare in England, 1900–1930* (London: Croom Helm, 1980); Joanna Bourke, *Working-class cultures in Britain, 1890–1960: Gender, class and ethnicity* (London and New York: Routledge, 1994); Anthony S. Wohl, *Endangered lives: Public health in Victorian Britain* (Cambridge, MA: Harvard

alists worried about declining birthrates among the laboring classes. Public health analysts explored the relationship between working-class women, child-rearing practices, and infant mortality. Proponents of birth control linked infant and maternal sickness and death with frequent pregnancies. Abortion foes and advocates discussed the dangers of illegal practices that were, nonetheless, routine in traditional working-class communities.[4] Scholarship about these concerns tends to focus on policy or demographic issues and either broad social change or the motivations and activities of influential individuals and groups. This chapter approaches the issues of working-class sex culture from a different perspective.

Like management of contagious diseases, experts' concerns about and attempts to influence working-class sexual behavior were both influenced by national trends and intensely local. Medical Officers of Health and their staff members provided services such as health education for mothers and girls, antenatal care, and family planning assistance, according to their own opinions and perceptions of community cultures. Similarly, general practitioners offered or withheld birth control advice and supported or distanced themselves from the sexually erring, such as women pregnant out of wedlock or venereal disease sufferers. Furthermore, working-class sexual behavior—particularly attempts to limit family size—varied from place to place.[5] Local circumstances, including religious beliefs, fluctuations in employment, the extent to which mothers and children contributed to family finances, and tolerance of matters including premarital pregnancy and abortion affected both working-class sexual behavior and availability of information and assistance from informal health authorities.

While authorities were mainly concerned with aggregate end results—birthrates, infant and maternal mortality, illegitimacy, the health and size of school children—all of these matters were associated with working-class sexuality. These officially conceptualized issues related, in turn, to the intensely private, culturally dictated realities of working-class sexual knowledge, attitudes, and behavior. As was true of contagious diseases, working-

University Press, 1983).

4. See, for example, Richard Allen Soloway, *Birth control and the population question in England, 1877–1930* (Chapel Hill and London: University of North Carolina Press, 1982); Audrey Leathard, *The fight for family planning: The development of family planning services in Britain 1921–74* (London and Basingstoke: Macmillan, 1980); Jane Lewis, *The politics of motherhood;* Wally Seccombe, *Weathering the storm: Working-class families from the Industrial Revolution to the fertility decline* (London and New York: Verso, 1993); Diana Gittins, *Fair sex: Family size and structure in Britain, 1900–39* (New York: St. Martin's Press, 1982); Barbara Brookes, *Abortion in England, 1900–1967* (New York: Croom Helm, 1988); John Keown, *Abortion, doctors and the law: Some aspects of the legal regulation of abortion in England from 1803 to 1982* (Cambridge: Cambridge University Press, 1988); James Thomas and A. Susan Williams, "Women and abortion in 1930s Britain: A survey and its data," *Social History of Medicine* 11 (1998): 283–309.

5. Diana Gittins, *Fair sex: Family size and structure in Britain, 1900–39* (New York: St. Martin's Press, 1982), 63, indicates that working-class family size declined in Lancashire earlier than in other parts of the country.

class people had different priorities for their sexuality than did the experts who theorized and attempted to regulate it. Working-class people were most concerned with highly gendered personal and family needs and associated community dynamics. This chapter begins by considering the ways working-class residents of Barrow, Lancaster, and Preston learned about bodies, sex, reproduction, and birth control. It documents experiences, actions, and cultural contexts regarding matters including menstruation, premarital sex, abortion, and contraception. It considers the relationship between sexuality, reproduction, and respectability in working-class communities. Finally, it observes changes that occurred regarding these matters during the study period. Because of the paucity of local evidence, it does not address issues associated with homosexuality.[6]

The chapter argues that before the interwar years, parental silence about sexual matters was traditional and normative, stemming from the desire to protect family reputations. Women's reputations were especially related to their sexual knowledge, communication, and behavior. Premarital ignorance of sexual matters, extramarital chastity, and appropriate sexual demeanor within marriage were important elements of their respectability, which was, as we have seen, the key to the mutual aid networks that were particularly important to working-class women before World War II. Attempts (or lack thereof) to plan family size were associated both with access to birth control information and resources and with working-class culture, which, for many reasons, tolerated larger numbers of children earlier than it did later in the study period. This chapter argues that attitudes and communication about sex changed dramatically between the generations born before and after about 1930, reflecting both the medicalization of sex, family limitation, and reproduction and changes in the composition of and need for respectability in working-class neighborhoods. It explores shifting attitudes about family size and parent-child relationships and observes a transition of authority regarding appropriate knowledge and behavior from working-class to professional hands.

WORKING-CLASS SEX: HOW DO WE KNOW?

Michel Foucault observed what might be called the myth of nineteenth-century middle-class silence about sex—a myth belied by the proliferation of discourse and regulation regarding sexual matters.[7] His analysis also works for the late-nineteenth- and early-twentieth-century Lancashire working class, where normative reticence between parents and children about

---

6. See, for example, Lesley A. Hall, *Sex, gender, and social change in Britain since 1880* (New York: St. Martin's Press, 2000), for an excellent national overview of these matters.

7. Foucault, *The history of sexuality*. See also useful discussion of both Foucault's ideas and normative British reticence about sex in Hall, *Sex, gender, and social change,* 4–7.

sex coexisted with traditional whispering within age- and sex-segregated groups and, also, with increasing communication from experts and the mass media. It is possible that inhibitions regarding intergenerational talk about sex and reproduction grew in the late nineteenth and early twentieth centuries, becoming part of the increased decorum that some scholars identify with the development of a distinctive working-class culture.[8] Since working-class people left few records documenting any part of their experience, their silence about this forbidden topic is hardly surprising.[9]

Nonetheless, this project's interviews contain informants' memories about sex and reproduction—particularly delicate issues for elderly working-class Lancashire people. In addition to revealing reticence, self-defense, and a desire to maintain respectability before the interviewer, the interviews elicited a wealth of information about these matters—sometimes explicitly solicited, but more often volunteered as part of a broader conversation. Accounts regarding some subjects—menarche and first pregnancy, for example—were repeated so often and in such similar language that there is little doubt that they represent common experiences. Repeated accounts regarding other subjects—most notably, complete ignorance about the mechanics of sexual intercourse before marriage—are belied by events including premarital pregnancy.[10] Especially sensitive topics, such as awareness of abortion and abortionists, sometimes elicited inconsistent information, with informants at first denying all knowledge, then later being more forthcoming.[11] Interpretation of interviews was further complicated by use of code language or euphemisms and influence of changing cultural norms on what informants said and how they said it. With these reservations in mind, however, the following discussion arguably reflects working-class experience more accurately than do accounts based solely on experts' observations. The oral evidence indicates that residents of Barrow, Lancaster, and Preston learned about sex and reproduction in much the same ways. Furthermore, comparison with information from other regions suggests that there was, indeed, a British working-class sexual culture that transcended local and regional boundaries.[12]

8. Weeks, *Sex, politics and society,* 73–74. See also Trevor Griffiths, *The Lancashire working classes, c. 1880–1930* (Oxford: Clarendon Press, 2001), 2–3.

9. The best-known exception to this rule is Robert Roberts, *The classic slum* (Harmondsworth: Penguin, 1973), which, as part of a larger discussion of neighborhood and family life, provides some information about sex and reproduction.

10. This is not to say that young women who had intercourse before marriage knew it could cause pregnancy. Regarding this matter, my evidence is consistent with that of other researchers—see, for example, Steve Humphries, *A secret world of sex,* 75. It is also noteworthy, as Fisher points out, that women sometimes hid the extent of their actual knowledge about sex and contraception to preserve their self-identity and reputations. See "'She was quite satisfied with the arrangements I made,'" 173.

11. See, for example, Mrs. D3P, 16, 26–27, 30.

12. For oral history information from London, Lincolnshire, Oxford, and Wales, see Ross, *Love and toil;* Sutton, *"'We didn't know aught'";* Fisher, "'She was quite satisfied with the

"HOW DID YOU LEARN THE FACTS OF LIFE?"

This question elicited information about menstruation, sex, pregnancy, birth, deviance, venereal diseases, and sex communication. It is note-worthy that informants' experiences cannot be neatly pigeonholed into discrete time frames. As is true of other aspects of working-class health culture, older people from socially aspiring families remember consciously "modern" approaches to sexual matters, while younger informants from more traditional families maintained "old-fashioned" ideas about sex and reproduction well into the 1950s and '60s.[13] Furthermore, informants from "rough" families were sometimes more tolerant of matters such as premari-tal pregnancy and marital infidelity than informants from "respectable" families. However, similar repeated accounts indicate both typicality and changes that occurred during the period under consideration.

Many interviewees responded to the question, "How did you learn the facts of life?" with accounts of talk (or, more usually, absence of talk) about sex within their families of birth. Almost everyone born before 1930, and many born before 1950, said that sex was never discussed between parents and children.[14] Mr. Brown, born in 1896 in Preston, said, "They [parents] never told us anything and you never read anything much and therefore you were ignorant in a lot of things."[15] According to some interviewees, sex was one of several inappropriate topics for family conversation. Mr. Peel, born in 1909 in Barrow, said, "It wasn't discussed; there was no politics, sex, other people's business discussed round the table. Because the father was there, and just a look and that would be it."[16] Others indicated that there was something especially disgusting or taboo about sex as a conversation topic. Mrs. Dent, born in Preston in 1908, commented that her mother "wouldn't discuss anything nasty with me."[17] Mr. Danner, born in Preston in 1910, said sex was a "dirty thing to talk about," while Mr. Boswell, born in Barrow in 1920, when asked whether his parents or school provided any sex education, answered, "None whatsoever, no. No, nothing at all like that, no. I've just told you they wouldn't even let you draw a toilet. It was the thing

---

arrangements I made.'" In *A secret world of sex* (36–38), Humphries observed more sexual experimentation and freedom from adult supervision among working-class children than was revealed in my interviews.

13. This observation supports Simon Szreter's observation of a wide range of fertility and nuptial practices in twentieth-century English working-class communities. See *Fertility, class and gender in Britain, 1860–1940* (Cambridge: Cambridge University Press, 1996), 387.

14. Other types of working-class parent-child communication are beyond the scope of this book. However, oral history evidence suggests that intimate parent-child conversations were more common among the smaller families of the mid- and late twentieth century. More usual in the first half of the century were households where children were "seen and not heard" and where "They [parents] never told us anything" about anything personal—including sex.

15. Mr. B8P, 5.

16. Mr. P6B, 51. See also Mrs. L3B, 68; Mrs. W1P, 37.

17. Mrs. D1P, 53.

that you never got taught anything, just found your way round that."[18]

Several informants' parents thought sex was not a proper thing for *children* to know about. Mrs. Masterson, born in 1913 in Preston, said, "If the parents were speaking about anything to do with anything at all like that [sex], it was all taboo; the children weren't allowed to listen. You were brought up innocent on matters. There was no bad-mindedness."[19] Mrs. Wilson, born in Barrow in 1900, one of ten children, reported that her mother never told the children when she was pregnant. "When she got up, I remember saying to her, 'Oh mother, you must have been poorly.' She looked at me. I said, 'Well, you've gone so thin.' Well, I didn't know it was the baby. . . . She said, 'You know far too much, get yourself out.'"[20] Adults would go to great lengths to prevent children being exposed to information about sex and reproduction. Mr. Glover, born in 1913 in Preston, remembers his mother telling him that when she was pregnant with his brother, his grandfather refused to let her into the family home, saying, "'Don't come in here in that condition,' because they had a younger family. She hadn't to let them see her."[21]

Despite normative silence, parents might talk to adolescents about sex when a teen's innocence or reputation was perceived to be at specific risk. Mrs. Drake, born in 1899 in Barrow, as a teenager took a live-in domestic service job. She said, "I knew nothing about sex, but my mother warned me before I went." The same mother was otherwise so reticent about these matters that she instructed the informant's older sister to talk to her about menstruation.[22] Mr. Parke, born in 1894 in Lancaster, remembered, "All my father ever told me was, 'You're going out to work now and you'll be mixing with boys and girls. Now, remember, always treat women as you'd like other men to treat your sister,' and I always did."[23] Mrs. Dent, born in 1908 in Preston, remembered an odd lesson in sexual etiquette: "My mother told me about a young woman and she went with this young fellow on the park and he tried it on with her. It upset her that much, she arranged to meet him again. This time she took a razor with her and she cuts it. . . . [Y]ou know what I'm talking about, don't you? His 'tea-pot.' She cut it and she nearly cut it off. She said that would teach him, as he asked for it. It nearly killed him." This woman's mother was determined to protect her daughter from premarital sex, as we have seen in chapter 3, getting the family doctor to exempt her from school once she started menstruating as a way of keeping her away from boys.[24]

18. Mr. D2P, 29; Mr. B4B, 37. See also, for example, Mrs. H5L, 54.

19. Mrs. M1P, 57. See also Mrs. M1B, 40; Mrs. A3B, 3; Mrs. M1P, 14; Mr. B8P, 5.

20. Mrs. W1B, 77. In *Love and toil*, 100, Ross provides a similar account. See also Mr. M1B, 40; Mr. G3P, 28; and Mrs. B11P, 49.

21. Mr. G3P, 28. See also Mrs. B1P, 45.

22. Mrs. D1B, 30.

23. Mr. P1L, 95.

24. Mrs. D1P, 59–60.

Adults mainly talked about sex within same-sex peer groups. Reflecting the difference between current and past norms, Mr. Best, born in 1897, said when describing the father's exclusion from a home confinement, "That was the whole point in those days; it was all a lady's life and a man's life."[25] Mrs. Masterson, born in 1913 in Preston, remembered, "In those days, things were kept very quiet and if you went in a house and they were speaking about someone, say their periods . . . you were told to go outside and play. You weren't allowed to listen to anything. You could always tell if there was anything going on because everything was so secretive."[26] Boys and girls also talked about sex with other young people of the same sex.[27] Mr. Danner, born in 1910, remembered a friend telling him the "facts of life" as he understood them: "'The father f—s the mother and in 11 months she has a baby, it comes out of her belly.' This had to be fully described to me because I did not believe it and I did not know what was meant by 'f—'. . . . Well into my teens I looked upon sex as something awful and taking advantage of females."[28] Mrs. Turnbull, born in 1932, said, "You just found out from, you know, people, kids, talk at school, a bit like that. . . . Even when I got married, I was green, honestly green as anything. . . . Now they have it all at schools, don't they?"[29]

Teenagers' conversations about sex often happened at work.[30] Indeed, for many children, the first job coincided with puberty; many started work at age 12 or 13, some "half-timing," alternating "a week of morning work and afternoon school with a week of afternoon work and morning school."[31] Mrs. Huddleston, born in 1916, said her parents did not tell her about the facts of life. "I can't understand why. Was it embarrassment, or did they think we weren't old enough? . . . There was no mention about babies, you had to gather from your friends, and then you didn't always hear it in a good light. . . . Because you heard it in the mill when you were 14, 15, or 16. It was a thing not to talk about."[32] Mrs. Arnold, born in 1910, speculated that these workplace conversations occurred "because you got among older girls and you got among girls who weren't your neighbors and they may have been a bit different, a bit freer, I think you grew up more at

25. Mr. B1B, 24.

26. Mrs. M1P, 14. See also Mrs. O1B, 28.

27. Mr. C8P, 113. See also Mr. F1P, 34.

28. Mr. D2P, 37.

29. Mrs. T2L, 39. See also Mr. M10L (born 1948), 64, 86.

30. In *A secret world of sex*, 61–62, Humphries makes a similar observation, although he emphasizes humiliating workplace initiation rituals not mentioned by my informants. In *A woman's place*, Roberts comments, "There is little evidence that women discussed sexual topics in the mill" (102). Although I did not find a large amount of information on this topic in the oral history transcripts, I found enough to suggest my alternative interpretation.

31. Roberts, *A woman's place*, 35. School attendance was compulsory until age 10, beginning in 1876. School-leaving age rose to 11 in 1893, 14 in 1899, 15 in 1947, and 16 in 1972.

32. Mrs. H7P, 24. See also Mrs. O1B, 28; Mrs. J1B, 51.

work than anywhere."[33] This comment suggests that a girl's reputation was most important and most at risk in the multigenerational neighborhood where both social life and mutual aid took place.[34] At work, she was free to explore a somewhat wider sphere of information, demeanor, and even personal identity.

Several informants said they learned about sex through experimentation with partners. Sometimes the experience was negative. Mr. Danner, born in 1910 in Preston, told a story about meeting a girl his friend had stood up. Mr. Danner walked home with her, took her into an empty house, kissed her, and "felt in her blouse. At once I was ashamed of myself. I was also aware that this person could be in trouble and I could be accused. I could not deny that I had not been in the house with her. I at once asked her to go home. I told her I was annoyed with myself and I would not, of course, see her again. I went home very distressed." He converted to the Baptist church because of his shame and guilt, although he eventually had a happy marriage and became a father.[35] More usual than Mr. Danner's experience, however, was pleasurable experimentation either preceding or in early marriage. Mrs. Jenkins, born in Barrow in 1932, met her future husband when she was 15 and remained a virgin until they were engaged. She became pregnant at 19. She said, "I think it was general, that . . . I think you found out more from each other, nobody ever told you anything."[36] Some informants defended traditional silence about sex, arguing that educating young people about this matter stimulated them to experiment. Mrs. Washburn, born in 1900, compared lack of communication about sex during her youth with the situation in the 1970s, when she was interviewed: "You just found out yourself and it was far better. Some of these kids are being taught so much that they try out what it is and what happens, they get the Pill. They are just bringing up a world of horrible prostitutes and the mothers don't know whether they are on the Pill or not."[37]

It is clear that cultural boundaries for conversations about sex limited and represented individual and family respectability. Children who "knew too much" reflected badly on parents' (particularly mothers') child-rearing standards and personal reputations. Women who talked about sex with men risked being thought "loose," while men who talked about sex in mixed company were considered rude. In crowded working-class dwellings and neighborhoods, conversational barriers regarding sexual matters arguably created both a measure of safety and privacy. However, the same constructed

33. Mrs. A1P, 28. The oral evidence indicates that not all informants talked about sex at work. Commenting about birth control information, Mrs. B1P said, "No, you hadn't time to talk in the mill, no you didn't seem to talk about it" (51).

34. See Roberts, *A woman's place*, 187–201.

35. Mr. D2P, 44.

36. Mrs. J1B, 75. See also Mrs. O1B, 25.

37. Mrs. W4P, 43. See also Mrs. F1L, 30.

sexual innocence that elderly informants remembered proudly as a badge of personal and family honor also fostered real ignorance that caused fear and shame. Furthermore, norms governing talk about sexual matters undergirded the mechanism of social control in working-class neighborhoods.[38] Being labeled a "slag" both punished women and their family members and marginalized them from social and mutual aid networks.

MENARCHE

Among the most stigmatized and secret sex-related experiences in working-class life before the mid-twentieth century was menstruation. Female informants almost invariably responded to the question, "How did you learn the facts of life?" with an account of their first menstrual period—traumatic because they had not been told that menstruation was universal, normal, and healthy.[39] Mrs. Black, born in 1916 in Preston, said, "In them days you never knew what sex was about. I was unwell when I went to school at 11 years old and it come on me all at once and I didn't know anything about it. My mother hadn't told me. It was private was that."[40] This account links menstruation with sex and being "unwell"; it also suggests that menstruation was so private it could not be discussed. Yet, of course, every woman informant had talked about her first period with someone. Mrs. Owen, born in 1916 in Barrow, remembered, "When I first started my periods, I was sleeping with my Aunty May, and I came to the toilet and I was crying and she asked me what was the matter, and I told her I was bleeding, and it was her that told me all about it. And of course she was very vexed with my mum because she hadn't prepared us."[41] It was, indeed, usual for girls to learn about menstruation from a close female relative or a sister. Mrs. Addison, born in Barrow in 1892, recalled, "We didn't know anything. They never told us anything. At certain ages, we'd to tell our sisters. . . . I'd to tell you and you had to tell her. . . . That is how we found out, we were as innocent as the grave."[42] Reticence and embarrassment about menstruation continued in some families after World War II.[43] Above all, and at the root

---

38. Melanie Tebbutt, *A social history of 'gossip' in working-class neighborhoods, 1880–1960* (Aldershot, Hants, Scolar Press: Brookfield, VT: Ashgate Publishing Co., 1995).

39. Roberts discusses menstruation in *A woman's place*, 16–18.

40. Mrs. B2P, 29. See also Mrs. P2P, 22.

41. Mrs. O1B, 27. See also Mrs. H7P, 24. This experience was usual among all social classes in the early twentieth century, according to Carol Dyhouse's *Girls growing up in late Victorian and Edwardian England* (London: Routledge and Kegan Paul, 1981), 20–21, and it remained common, according to Sophie Laws, *Issues of blood*, and Julie-Marie Strange, "The assault on ignorance: Teaching menstrual etiquette in England, c. 1920s to 1960s," *Social History of Medicine* 14: 2 (2001): 247–65.

42. Mrs. A3B, 15. See also Mrs. H4P, 17.

43. See, for example, Mrs. T2L (born 1932), 38. Mrs. G5P (born 1958), 32.

of efforts to conceal evidence of menstruation, was the importance of keeping it hidden from males.[44] So strong was the code of secrecy surrounding this matter that, according to Mrs. Masterson, born in 1913, many girls "were afraid to tell their parents even when they had started their periods. They were afraid to tell them, yet it was a natural thing."[45]

Once daughters began to menstruate, mothers wanted them to know how to manage and conceal the menstrual flow, deal with associated health hazards, and protect themselves from pregnancy. Older informants remembered dealing with periods before disposable pads became affordable (around 1940). Mrs. Howe, born in 1898, remembered, "Then when you were poorly there were no sanitary towels or anything like that. You had to have bits of rag and put your pins in and pin it and all that business."[46] Mrs. Addison, born in 1892, said, "Mother used to have a bag, there used to be brass bedsteads and mother had a school bag and we had to put them in there. Then when we come home we used to have to wash them ourselves. They weren't what they buy today, they were bits of calico and mother used to put a little bit of tape there and bit of tape there and we used to have a tape on."[47] Mrs. Needham, born in 1919, started menstruating at age 16. "And when I told her [Mother] . . . she said, 'You use one of those [homemade pads], and you make that do once a day, and put it in that bucket of water at night, with that lid on. . . . You've got six. And you have to make them do.' And she used to boil them in a bowl."[48] Informants grew up worried about staining their clothes and placing additional strain on their mother's laundry responsibilities. Mrs. Havelock, born in 1903 in Preston, remembered that she was only allowed to wear one pair of underpants per week: "You were allowed a change once a week and she [mother] could tell if you touched a piece." When the interviewer asked, "And this was on the rack in the kitchen, was it?" she said, "Yes. All the washing that she had done, and it was beautiful. If you took anything off, she would miss it. You never thought to say, 'Well, mum, I'm losing,' or anything like that. It was always a camouflaged fact, but you knew what she was talking about."[49]

Some women remembered managing without a pad. Mrs. Maxwell, born in 1898, reported, "We probably would have two or three pairs of knickers on, especially when we were unwell and that sort of thing. That was horrible work. . . . You hadn't to tell anybody else or you hadn't to let anybody else see anything. Everything was kept out of the road. There was a special bucket with a lid to put them in."[50] Mrs. Havelock, born in 1903,

44. Mrs. S4L, 68.
45. Mrs. M1P, 34. See also Mrs. H6L, 63.
46. Mrs. H2P, 17. See also Mrs. A3B, 15; Mrs. B2P, 3; Mrs. H2L, 25.
47. Mrs. A3B, 15.
48. Mrs. N3L, 44.
49. Mrs. H4P, 17.
50. Mrs. M3P, 45.

said, "I am more ashamed to have to admit it of my mother because I loved her and we were so ignorant. The point was that when you started to menstruate you were just given a pair of navy-blue knickers so that it didn't show through."[51] Elizabeth Roberts recounts the memory of an elderly woman whose mother told her "that as a young mill girl she wore no protection at all when menstruating, she simply hoped that her several layers of petticoats and skirts would both absorb the flow and hide it from the outside world."[52]

Although disposable sanitary napkins were patented in 1892, and the oldest informant to use them was Mrs. Peterson, born in Preston in 1899, few other informants reported buying them until after World War II.[53] Younger interviewees document this transition, which was accompanied by somewhat better intergenerational communication and greater assertiveness and economic independence of adolescent girls. Mrs. Owen, born in 1916, said her Aunty May, who told her about menstruation, "did give me a sanitary towel, but Mum used to make them at first, and then we started buying our own. They were sixpence a packet, I always remember."[54] She was an early consumer of this product. More typical was Mrs. Jenkins, born in 1932 in Barrow, who asked, "Did I tell you about when I started my periods? . . . My Mam just threw me a piece of old cloth and said, 'Oh, you'll get that every month.'" However, after that first period, her mother bought her disposable sanitary towels.[55] Fifteen years younger, Mrs. Lonsdale from Lancaster remembered:

When we moved from junior school up to senior school, parents were told you know, "You are going to have to tell your daughters." I mean, I knew about it because a couple of the girls had already started menstruating. But she [mother] was right nervous about it, she sort of threw me this book, this leaflet thing, and you know, "Read that." At the time she wasn't using disposable sanitary towels, she was using sort of like bits of sheet, I think, that you used to cut up and you used to wash them, and you used them again, you know. To save money, I suppose. And she said, you know, "This is what I use." And I turned round and I said, 'I'm not using one of them,' you know. So then when I started my periods she started buying, you know. Dr. Whites, yes. . . . I could speak to my [older] sister better than I could my mum, yes.[56]

51. Mrs. H4P, 16.

52. Roberts, *A woman's place*, 18.

53. Mrs. P1P, 42. John Benson, *The rise of consumer society in Britain 1880–1980* (London and New York: Longman, 1994), 73.

54. Mrs. O1B, 28.

55. Mrs. J1B, 50.

56. Mrs. L3L, 37.

Older informants remembered vague warnings about health hazards associated with menstruation. When Mrs. Dent, born in 1908, began menstruating, "She [mother] would tell me not to touch anything cold and not to sit on anything cold."[57] Several informants were warned not to bathe or wash their hair while they were menstruating.[58] Mrs. Fleming, born in 1921, said that when her eldest daughter "started her periods, she went through to have a bath. And my mother said, 'Do you know where she is going?' I said, 'She is going for a bath.' 'She is going for a bath and you know what's to do with her?' Well, that was taboo in. . . . They always thought it went to your head. . . . Well, there was all sorts of daft things, yes. They even thought, not specifically her [mother], but all these old wives' tales, that if you touched meat you sent it bad, you know."[59]

Such ideas harkened back to both humeral ideas about health maintenance and traditional notions about the destructive powers of menstrual blood.[60] They faded with the medicalization of menstruation. Mrs. Ruthven, born in 1936 in Barrow, remembered a generational gap in the way her older female relatives and her mother felt about menstruation. She had her first period at age 11 while on a visit to relatives in Ireland:

This was very, very traumatic, because my aunt, who had never been married, simply panicked, and instead of going out and buying sanitary towels like my mother would have done, which she did in fact later. My aunt and my Irish relations, who were also really quite puritanical, chopped up large bits of sheets and made these kind of nappy things with pins and I wasn't really allowed to wash my hair or paddle in the sea. It was all really going back several generations. . . . In a way it was rather more threatening by not being explained, it was these kind of things you weren't to do. As I say, when I got home and told my mother, she was very angry and pooh-poohed them, and said it was ridiculous and of course you could paddle your feet and of course you can wash your hair, and you must have a bath, because of course bathing wasn't allowed either by Aunty. And again my mother being very modern and up-to-date and sensible.[61]

To young girls themselves, more important than what might be considered theoretical traditional health hazards of menstruation was the real discom-

57. Mrs. D1P, 32.

58. See, for example, Mrs. B2P, 3; Mrs. H4P, 17; Mrs. P1L, 95.

59. Mrs. F1L, 84.

60. Humerol theory held that women's physiology made them spiritually, intellectually, and physically inferior; many traditional societies believe menstruating women endanger men, crops, food, and drink. See, for example, Lucinda McCray Beier, *Sufferers and healers: The experience of illness in seventeenth-century England* (London, 1987), 213–1; P. Crawford, "Attitudes to menstruation in seventeenth-century England,' *Past and Present* 91 (1981): 59, 61.

61. Mrs. R4B, 43–44.

fort of menstrual cramps, which presented a challenge in a gendered culture where shame generated silent endurance. Mrs. Young, born in 1915 in Preston, remembered:

> And my mother—that was something that you suffered. She used to say to me, "Straighten your shoulders up, the boys are laughing at you." And I thought, why are they laughing at me? Why do we have to suffer? What do boys have? And she said, "Oh, they have their problems." And I said, "Well, what problems do they have?" And she said, "I'll tell you some other time." And I've never found out what problems they have to this day. Because I suffered, I used to go on my knees with pain and no, no way would she get the doctor. She'd get Indian Brandy for me, and, you know, stiff upper lip sort of thing.

Mrs. Young said that the (male) mill manager was sympathetic and offered to let her go home, but her mother worked in the same mill and wouldn't let her leave. At age 19 she went to the doctor on her own and got a "big bottle of black medicine." Her mother was disgusted, saying, "'How dare you go to the doctor without me?' A girl, going to see a male doctor without a woman being with her: it was sinful. 'Don't you ever do that again!' and she poured all the medicine down the sink."[62] The irony is that, of course, men were quite aware of menstrual cramps.[63] It is arguable that the mystery surrounding menstruation made men both more tolerant of menstrually related incapacity than they might have been of other health problems, and less likely to ask about them.

Of course, until the mid-twentieth century, menstruation was regarded as evidence of female inferiority, as well as a handicap that "naturally" limited women's equal participation in employment and education.[64] Thus, it is perhaps not surprising that Mrs. Ralston, born in 1889 in Barrow, remembered, "I left school when I was twelve, and the reason why, I started with menstruation, and I used to be very ill. The doctor gave Mother a note, 'Keep her at home because she is no sooner there than she's off.'"[65] However, by the mid-twentieth century the growing consensus that menstruation was healthy, even when it caused discomfort, reduced the identification of periods with illness and handicap. In contrast to older informants' experience, Mrs. Lonsdale, born in 1947, remembered, "The only time I sort of

62. Mrs. Y2P, 14. Mrs. M3P (born 1898) had terrible menstrual cramps as a young girl. She stayed home from work and took Indian Brandy and Turkey Rhubarb, obtained from the chemist (15).

63. See, for example, Mr. C1P, 78.

64. Julie-Marie Strange, "The assault on Ignorance"; Elaine and English Showalter, "Victorian women and Menstruation," in Marsha Vicinus, ed., *Suffer and be still: Women in the Victorian age* (Bloomington and London: Indiana University Press, 1972), 38–44.

65. Mrs. R1B, 5.

felt ill was when I had period pains. And I just used to have a day off school and lay on the floor with a hot water bottle, you know." When asked, "Was that quite acceptable, did other girls of the time do that?" she said, "Yes. Some of them." She never saw a doctor for her cramps because her mother believed "it was just part of growing up."[66]

Above all else, after menarche, mothers wanted to protect daughters from the shame of premarital pregnancy. Since maintaining a girl's innocence about sex was also important, mothers' instructions were somewhat confusing. Mrs. Peel, born in 1921 in Barrow, said, "When I came to be eleven year old, I had to ask my mother what was the matter with me. And then she explained, and I was told never to let a man touch me. She didn't say why I hadn't to, 'Don't let a man touch you, or else you'll have a baby.'"[67] Similarly, some mothers also used surveillance. Mrs. Needham, born in 1919, said of her mother, "Untrusting, she was untrusting. She didn't trust anybody. Especially her own family. . . . For instance, I once missed my periods for about five months and my mother marched me all the way up to the Pointer and in that doctors' surgery. . . . But Dr. Mathers examined me and he said, 'She's virgo intact, she's got anemia.'" The same mother was equally suspicious of her sons. "If they went out, she would examine their clothes when they had gone to bed [to] see if they had been with a girl."[68] Mrs. Emery, born in 1937, remembered that her mother "used to have a calendar up on the wall. And she used to know when your periods started, and if you didn't start, she used to say, 'You should have started.'"[69] Ironically, Mrs. Needham had a baby out of wedlock when she was 20, and Mrs. Emery was pregnant before she got married.

WHERE DO BABIES COME FROM?

A visible representation of sexual activity, pregnancy was traditionally considered private, even shameful, and certainly not to be discussed with children. Thus, older informants remembered complete childhood ignorance of this matter, saying they believed new babies were found under gooseberry bushes or brought in the doctor's black bag.[70] Mothers routinely concealed a pregnancy from their other children. Indeed, parental reticence about this matter was associated with virtue. Mrs. Scales, born in 1896, said about her mother, "No, she was most strict over anything like that [menstruation]. Strict over everything. She was a good mother. . . . We were never

66. Mrs. L3L, 65–66.
67. Mrs. P6B, 9. See also Mrs. B2P, 3; Mrs. K2P, 163.
68. Mrs. N3L, 12–13.
69. Mrs. E2P, 32.
70. Mrs. N1L, 69; Mr. T5B, 81.

told anything like that [where babies come from]."[71] Mr. Barrington, born in 1927 in Preston, responded to the question, "Do you remember family gossip about people having to get married and so on?" by saying, "I don't. Of course, it might have gone on and I wouldn't understand what it was all about as they might have talked about it when the children weren't there. I think that links up with the respectability and conservatism to some extent."[72]

Nevertheless, teenagers became aware of the shame premarital pregnancy could inflict. Normative reticence about the links between specific types of sexual activity and pregnancy probably increased the vulnerability of adolescents and families to an experience, which, however disgraceful, regularly occurred. Mrs. Jelks, born in 1911 in Preston, said of her mother, "She had four girls and she would be frightened of one of them going wrong. They would, these mothers, it was so dreadful if anything went wrong." When asked, "Did you know any girl who had to get married?" she responded, "We never spoke of them but afterwards I have thought of different women who had a little boy or a little girl and my mother never told us about them. You never spoke about anything like that."[73] Mrs. McGowan, born in 1885 in Lancaster, remembered both ignorance about sex and understanding how bad getting "in trouble" was: "Sex was merely if you were masculine or feminine. The word didn't mean anything else to us, but you would hear of a girl being in trouble. Any girl that was in trouble, out, she was turned out of the house and we as youngsters never thought, 'Where is she going?' Quite a few of them were found in the river. But I think the older ones thought it was right, if they disgraced themselves, they should be sent away."[74] Women who had babies out of wedlock suffered community disapproval and shame.[75] Mrs. Crest was born in 1897 to an unmarried woman; her father was married, "And he didn't tell her. She was 36 when she had me, and I believe she tried to commit suicide. . . . She was one of those good girls who never went out and she had to stay at home and look after 10 children."[76] Mrs. Nance, born in 1899 in Lancaster, had a sister who drowned herself in the River Lune when she became pregnant.[77]

Parents' attitudes toward potential or actual pregnancy demonstrated their own respectability. Informants remembered being threatened with

71. Mrs. S4L, 68.

72. Mr. B9P, 28.

73. Mrs. J1P, 15.

74. Mrs. M6L, 9. See also Mrs. B2P, 1; Mrs. C5P, 29; Mrs. H1P, 3; Mrs. O1P, 40; Mrs. N1L, 69; Mr. D2P, 47.

75. See, for example, Mr. D2P, 47; Mrs. B2P, 11.

76. Mrs. C3P, 1, 25. Also quoted in Roberts, *A woman's place*, 77–78.

77. Mrs. N1L, 16.

whipping, expulsion from home, or commitment to the workhouse.[78] Suggesting that the dread of premarital pregnancy had contributed to local folklore, Mrs. Havelock, born in 1903, told a story about the Preston Banister Doll—a pregnant girl whose father "bound her with chains" and beat her to death.[79] These were not always idle threats. Mrs. Dorrington, born in 1905, said that when her mother became pregnant before marriage, she was horsewhipped by her strict Methodist father.[80] Mrs. Meadows, born in 1904, remembered:

> It is quite a well-known fact that quite a lot of girls did get whipped. I know a woman not so far from us, and she wouldn't have her girl in the house when she found out she was pregnant. The boy wanted to marry her, but because the boy was a Catholic and the girl wasn't, the mother wouldn't hear tell of it. Nowadays they wouldn't bother. She did really flog that girl, she threw her out, wouldn't allow her to be in the house. . . . [S]ome kind neighbor took her in for the night and somebody that worked near her found her a room somewhere. That was the only thing they could do.[81]

Mrs. Needham, born in 1919, was sent to the Lancaster workhouse by her mother when she became pregnant in 1939.[82] Mr. Best, born in 1897, worked in Barrow's Roose Institution (workhouse) as a baker. He remembered pregnant girls being sent there by their families:

> On the female side of the position, it was in the old days when a young lady fell by the way, the parents immediately said, "Well, if you're going to be like that, don't darken my doorstep again. There's only one place for you. You'll have to go to the workhouse." The ladies came in and they came into the workhouse and did domestic work, cleaning up and washing and they did that until such time as the baby was due and then they were moved into another section to have the baby. Whilst they were with the baby and providing they were feeding the baby they stayed there looking after the babies in the nursery. They came back again, if they had nowhere to go, back into the workhouse to do ordinary domestic work.[83]

Finally, as an illustration of the observation that "working-class solidarity did not always mean mutual support and help," Elizabeth Roberts pro-

78. See, for example, Mrs. A1P, 28; Mrs. W1L, 22; Mrs. H7P, 26; Mr. D3P, 30; Mrs. O1B, 29.
79. Mrs. H4P, 16.
80. Mrs. D3P, 18.
81. In transcript of Mrs. D3P, 30.
82. Mrs. N3L, 65.
83. Mr. B1B, 3.

vided a Preston account of an early-twentieth-century pregnant bride being stoned on her way to her wedding.[84]

Although informants agreed that extramarital pregnancy was a burden and a shame that fell most heavily upon the woman, men could also be disgraced by it; Mr. King, born in 1907, said, "[Mother] didn't bother who I married so long as I didn't bring any trouble home, get any girl into trouble, and that was the one thing she was bothered about."[85] And men sometimes paid a price for sexual misconduct; Mr. Parke, born in 1894, had two brothers who "got girls in trouble and they cleared off to Canada. That was a thing in those days that if you got a girl into trouble and you couldn't marry her, off you went."[86]

However, there is evidence of both a divergence between the threat and the reality, and variations in attitudes and behavior in different circumstances, times, and places. When faced with an actual pregnancy, some families minimized the shame by either bringing up the child as its mother's sibling, or sending it to live with relatives. Mrs. Hill, born in 1903, remembered:

> It was a great tragedy for a girl to come to trouble. She came home with it and that's what happened and she was looked down on for a long time after. In many ways it was covered up to the child who its mother was. We know of an instance today in this street that we didn't know about at the time. This lady, we don't know her now but we knew her mother and we thought that mother had only had one daughter which she lost tragically when she was 22, but she had another daughter and we thought it was her sister. The mother brought the child up to call her "Mum" and her own mother treated her as a sister. There were quite a few scandals in that way.[87]

Some informants mentioned mitigating factors, such as war or economic depression, that made extramarital pregnancy more likely by delaying or preventing marriages.[88] In addition, like other types of adversity, pregnancy out of wedlock sometimes elicited goodwill and support from the neighbors. Mrs. Preston, born in 1907 into a "rough" Preston family, responded to the question, "Do you remember many girls having babies when they weren't married?" as follows:

> Oh yes, it was quite common. It's more common today, but they get rid of them. It's been like that since the beginning of time.

84. Roberts, *A woman's place*, 78.
85. Mr. K1L, 35.
86. Mr. P1L, 44.
87. Mrs. H8P, 42. See also Mrs. A1P, 28, and Mr. P1L, 95, who said that it was usual for grandmothers to bring up illegitimate children.
88. See, for example, Mrs. P1P, 81.

Interviewer: But the neighbors would rally round?

Informant: And help. There would be one or two hoity-toity that were never away from church that would never do a good turn for anyone, but the majority, it's like in adversity when we have a war, everybody comes to be human. If somebody has a fire, they will help and they will give furniture. Well, people were like that nearly all the time, weren't they? They were so poor and so proud and so ashamed of being poor.

Interviewer: But why would the girls not get married then, have you any idea?

Informant: The men want their fun and games and don't want to settle down or they hadn't the money. Money was the big problem, they couldn't afford to get married. A lot of them would probably have liked to get married.

Interviewer: So who would look after the babies, can you remember?

Informant: The grandmas had to do it. Then there were baby-minders up and down the streets that took these poor kids in and they [the mothers] had to go to work.[89]

Despite general agreement that the community frowned on premarital pregnancy, the disgrace was minimized if the couple married.[90] Mrs. Hampton, born in 1911, had a sister who "come to have to be married, and there was no hysterics about it."[91] Mrs. Metcalfe, born in 1917, said, "I've seven brothers, and there wasn't one had to be married. I don't know whether dad told them about it. . . . There would have been no flying their kites and then changing their minds. They would have had to marry the girl. If she'd been good enough to do that with, she would be good enough to marry."[92] Mrs. Maxwell, born in 1898, whose mother came from a rural village and had herself been pregnant before marriage, suggested that premarital pregnancy was more usual and tolerated in the country than in her Preston neighborhood.[93] And Miss Thompson, born in 1912, speculated that mores may have become more restrictive in the early twentieth century than they had been in her parents' generation: "They didn't think nothing about it because they had nearly always had somebody in their own family that way, way back. Even in my mother's day, she can remember people coming with a baby and they weren't married, but it always seemed to be hushed up and brought up as one of their own sisters and brothers. The parents thought it was going to spoil the girl's chance of getting married."[94]

89. Mrs. P2P, 21.

90. See, for example, Roberts, *A woman's place,* 73–80, and Bourke, *Working-class cultures,* 31.

91. Mrs. H1P, 3. See also Mrs. B1L, 24.

92. Mrs. M3L, 17.

93. Mrs. M3P, 54. Roberts discusses high rates of illegitimacy in mid-nineteenth-century Cumberland and Westmorland in *A woman's place,* 76.

94. Miss T4P, 46.

Annual reports of the Medical Officers of Health indicate that study city experience of and MOH attitudes toward illegitimate births differed considerably. While all cities recorded higher numbers and rates of these births during the world wars, Preston's numbers and ratios of illegitimate to legitimate births tended to be higher than the corresponding figures for Barrow and Lancaster.[95] Regardless of both this trend and Dr. Pilkington's consistent willingness to judge Preston mothers (particularly among the working class) harshly, only in Barrow did public health officials focus on this issue, between 1889 and World War I regularly linking illegitimacy with high rates of infant mortality on the grounds that the mothers had to work, place babies with child-minders, and were more likely to neglect or even kill their babies. In 1895 Dr. Settle commented: "Proportion of deaths to births in illegitimate children, 46.1%. Proportion of deaths in wedlock-born children, 26.7%. The reason of this higher mortality in illegitimate born children is not far to seek, the mother unmarried, without a house of her own, and compelled to work for her own living, is unable to suckle her infant. It is, therefore, left to be tended by strangers, who give the child what may be going, or frequently sour milk from a commonly unclean bottle."[96] In 1898 he broadened the argument, observing, "From this it may be inferred that the child born out of wedlock has only about half the chance of attaining five years of age as compared with its brother born in wedlock. In a previous report I have concisely cited three factors bearing upon the fatality of illegitimate children, viz. Ignorance, Accident, and Design."[97] In 1907 he linked illegitimacy to national birth rates, attitudes, and policies, writing, "There is no reason for thinking that children born illegitimate are less vigorous than children born otherwise, so that there less chance of life must be due to less care and more unnatural conditions. They seldom get the mother's milk or the mother or father's care. In France, where children are scarcer than with us, the State is a good foster-mother."[98] In 1908 he developed this pronatalist imperialist argument further: "They [illegitimate children] make good soldiers for France, and they would make good soldiers and sailors for us, and for imperial and other useful purposes they are quite worth keeping alive. They die from neglect, necessary neglect,

---

95. Available figures indicate that in Barrow between 1889 and 1960, numbers of illegitimate births ranged from a low of 35 in 1906 to a high of 83 in 1917. (Figures for illegitimate births are not available for Barrow for the period 1937–45, with the exception of 1944, when 56 illegitimate babies were born.) Corresponding figures for Lancaster reveal a low of 28 in 1910 and a high of 82 in 1918 for the period 1906–60. (Figures for illegitimate births were not reported in Lancaster for 1942 and 1943.) In Preston, illegitimate births spiked at 185 in 1918 (10.3 percent of total births) and 231 in 1945 (11.8 percent of total births); however, illegitimate births normally hovered between 4 and 6 percent of total births between 1893 and 1950, and rose sharply to between 8 percent and 13 percent of total births during the 1960s.

96. Barrow MOH Report, 1895, 187.

97. Barrow MOH Report, 1898, 174.

98. Barrow MOH Report, 1907, 193.

not from any innate weakness. A little milk, keeping warm, and cleanliness is all they want."[99]

As the oral evidence indicates, the main public provision for unwed mothers before the mid-twentieth century in Barrow, Lancaster, and Preston was the workhouse. In 1930 Preston's MOH reported: "There is no provision for unmarried mothers other than that provided by the Public Assistance Committee. Illegitimate infants and homeless infants are maintained in the children's nursery in the Preston Institution up to the age of three years, and over that age, Roman Catholic children are maintained at the St. Vincent's Orphanage for Boys and the Moorfield Convent for Girls. Protestant Boys and Girls are maintained at the Cottage Homes, Brockholes View."[100] In 1944, reflecting easing social norms as well as broadening public responsibility for social welfare, Preston's City Council arranged for hostel accommodation and financial support for unwed pregnant women and follow-up social work supervision of these mothers and their children.[101] Similarly, in 1932 Lancaster's MOH wrote, "There is no special institution [for unwed mothers and their children] in the area, but during the year a House of Help for women and girls was established at 7, Queen Street, Lancaster, its main purpose being 'to provide a *temporary* refuge while the necessary enquiries are being made, and until some plan opens up for their future.'"[102] Barrow's MOH reflected comparable changes in local attitudes and support provision.[103] While it is clear that the public stance toward extramarital pregnancy and out-of-wedlock births shifted during the period under consideration, MOH reports support the conclusion that the best alternative for an unwed pregnant working-class girl was marriage.

Regardless of attempts to protect their innocence, by the time they reached mid-adolescence oral history informants understood that pregnancy resulted from sexual contact. However, despite the ubiquity of home delivery, they knew little about pregnancy and birth. Mrs. Carter, born in 1919, remembered, "When I got to about 16, I used to think, babies, where do they come from? I used to think that my mother must have been cut on her stomach six times because she had six children. I thought she must have six scars on her stomach."[104] Even after they became pregnant, many first-time mothers knew little about the mechanics of birth. Mrs. Turnbull, born in 1932, commented, "When I went in labor, I didn't know how it was going to come out. . . . I had pains and that, but I just didn't know

99. Barrow MOH Report, 1908, 245.
100. Preston MOH Report, 1930, 16.
101. Preston MOH Report, 1944, 43.
102. Lancaster MOH Report, 1932, 12.
103. Barrow MOH Report, 1943, 6.
104. Mrs. C5P, 30. See also Mrs. S4L, 68, and Bourke, *Working-class cultures in Britain*, 32.

what they were going to do to me."[105] Mrs. Barlow, born in 1928, had a mother who was "fairly down-to-earth. I can't remember her sitting down and telling me about the facts of life and looking back, I think, you know, what I did know was fairly negligible, but I did, I can remember her telling me that her younger sister, when her younger sister had her first baby she thought it was going to come out through her navel, and she was the youngest of quite a big family, and . . . had seen quite a number of nephews and nieces . . . so obviously, my mother had told me otherwise."[106] For this mother, saving her daughter from the trauma of ignorance was more important than defending her innocence.

DIRTY SEX: CRIME AND DISEASE

The code of silence that was intended to protect children's bodies from early sexual activity and their minds from moral pollution did nothing to protect them from molestation—and even put abused children at a further disadvantage because the shame of dirty sex stained the victim as well as the perpetrator.[107] Mrs. Ralston, born in Barrow in 1889, was molested by a cab driver. She told her mother, who sent her to bed, "as if we'd done something. We were wrong in going there, we shouldn't have been there."[108] Mrs. Jenkins, born in 1932, said: "I could tell you terrible stories, usually about old men exposing themselves. I mean, over the years; the rag and bone man, for instance, 'Come and feel this for a penny,' and things like this. . . . This was in Hindpool [poor working-class area], and you know, I don't think anybody even told their mothers. You couldn't talk to your mothers then. I mean, if anything happened to my family, they could come and tell me, but then you sort of kept it secret."[109]

Mrs. Melling, born in 1917 in Lancaster, was molested by a stranger as a little girl:

> When I was a little girl, I came back home at seven and not being used to brothers and then being used to six men, I was down at the bottom of the street playing with some girls and a man enticed me away and I went with him. There was a lady at one of the houses at the bottom of Lune Street looking through her window at Johnny's Field. You know where

105. Mrs. T2L, 83. See also Mrs. D3P, 16, 26.
106. Mrs. B3B, 22.
107. In *Child sexual abuse in Victorian England* (London and New York: Routledge, 2000), Louise Jackson argues that attribution of "fallen" moral status to the working-class female victim of sexual abuse stemmed from "a discourse of Christian moral economy, promoted by the middle classes" (6). The oral history evidence projects similar working-class attitudes.
108. Mrs. R1B, 30.
109. Mrs. J1B, 71–72. See also Mrs. E2P, 31.

Our Lady's school is, there is still a footpath at the bottom of the street and we used to call it the lane. He took me down there, and I went with him, but this lady saw me out of the bedroom window. She came running up to m'dad and said, "Have you got your little girl at home, Mr. T.?" He said, "Yes." She said, "I've seen a chap taking her down that lane." He [the molester] put me down on the floor, down the side of the lane, and laid on me, and I could see them all running down near the railway side. I could see all my brothers running by shouting for me. I don't know what happened, whether I nipped or what, but he rolled off and I run out and shouted, "Daddy!" That was the only time that he [father] smacked me, and he really smacked me, and then after he was sorry because I didn't know. . . . Then he [the molester] pretended to be drunk, and then after I heard our lads had given him a real good thumping. It wasn't so much sending him up to the police.[110]

Even worse than molestation by strangers was sexual abuse within families—a disgrace that retained its horror throughout the period under consideration and shamed the innocent along with the guilty. Mrs. Rowlandson, born in 1945, remembered: "One of my best friends at school, her father had interfered with her when she was at school with me. And she kind of told us, but . . . we couldn't do anything about it, and eventually he did get put in prison. Now, my mum found out about that, and she said, I hadn't to speak to that girl again. . . . She said, like, 'That girl, that's a very dirty family and you'll have nothing at all to do with them.'"[111] Mrs. Britton, born in 1936, remembered a man being imprisoned for abusing two of his daughters. "And his wife had come from Spain . . . and she went back to Spain with the children. . . . I mean, her life was shattered."[112]

Prostitution was discussed with greater equanimity, sometimes in association with public houses.[113] Mr. Metcalfe, born in 1906, remembered prostitution "for coppers" in some rough Lancaster pubs and common lodging houses. These women were "nearly all amateurs, not professionals. There was one there, Lady Alvin, who used to get drunk, but not prostitution as you know it today."[114] However, informants also recalled prostitution being denoted by certain types of speech, dress, and other behaviors. Mrs. Peterson, born in 1899, who lived in a rough Preston neighborhood, said that in the past "they were bad women that lived around here. You would be passing and you would see two women and they had shawls on and you could tell. We used to have to go through Shepherd Street sometimes and you would see these women with shawls on going at it and shouting. When

110. Mrs. M3L, 13.
111. Mrs. R1P, 59.
112. Mrs. B4L, 89.
113. See, for example, Mrs. A3L, 51; Mr. S1B, 13.
114. Mr. M3L, 24.

you were near them I've heard them say, 'There's a child coming!' and if they were swearing they would stop. They wouldn't swear in front of you. They were bad women in some ways, but they had hearts of gold."[115] Mrs. Dent, born in 1908, learned from a hospital nurse that prostitutes got venereal diseases and procured abortions from "quacks."[116] It is noteworthy that even among very poor informants who remembered women doing many kinds of home-based work to make ends meet, casual prostitution was not mentioned as an option for boosting family incomes.

HOUSING AND THE THREAT OF INCEST

In addition to denying children information about sex, working-class parents prevented girls and boys from seeing each others' bodies and, where possible, sharing bedrooms. This effort suggested concern about incest, often associated with crowded working-class dwellings, also expressed by late-nineteenth-century social reformers and policymakers.[117] Despite their general reticence about sexual matters, study city Medical Officers of Health registered awareness of problems that might be caused by cramped housing, in veiled language linking incest with other health issues. For example, in 1895 Dr. Pilkington of Preston described good working-class families as follows:

> There are numbers of households—many in which the family is a large one, and the weekly income by no means in proportion—which show undoubted signs of thrift and good management. Where the living room is clean and tidy, where the food is kept from contact with dirty matter, where the sleeping accommodation is arranged and looked after with a view to the health and morality of those using it, and where the back-yard—however small it may be—is kept for the purpose for which it was originally intended.[118]

While Pilkington called for working-class self-discipline and propriety, in 1918 Lancaster's MOH, Dr. Buchanan, called for public "provision of healthy homes for the working classes and eradicate the squalid and insanitary dwellings . . . highly favorable to the increased prevalence of tuberculosis and to the physical, intellectual, and moral degradation of those who dwell in them."[119] Regardless of the policy approach, working-class people were aware of the threat overcrowding posed to family morality and reputations.

115. Mrs. P1P, 7.
116. Mrs. D1P, 53.
117. See Weeks, *Sex, politics and society*, 31, and Humphries, *A secret world of sex*, 42.
118. Preston MOH Report, 1895, 8.
119. Lancaster MOH Report, 1918, 5.

Older oral history informants tended to come from large families and to live in small terraced houses where it was unusual for there to be more than three bedrooms and rare for a child to have a bed to him- or herself; people did not commonly sleep downstairs. Often in connection with parental strictness regarding other sexual behavior, informants spoke with pride about their parents' success in keeping boys and girls from seeing each other naked or sleeping in the same room. Mrs. Sykes, born in Barrow in 1895, said, "They moved up there with ten children and m'grandma, thirteen of us. Yet we were never mixed, one never saw the others undress at all . . . and no boy slept in the same room as the girls."[120] Mrs. Milton, born in Lancaster in 1914, said, "There was no fear of sex, m'mother used to frighten us to death. They were very strict upbringings in those days. 'You know what trouble it brings if you go with the fellows.' We wasn't allowed to wash in front of our brothers."[121]

Large families, often with unequal numbers of boys and girls, required creative sleeping arrangements. Mrs. Masterson, born in 1913 in Preston, remembered: "It was hard, because we were a big family and there were only three bedrooms. It meant that all the boys were in one room and I had to sleep with mum and dad and they [brother and his wife] were in the other room. . . . You would get three sleeping at that end of the bed and two or three at the front of the bed. Every space was made available for use. They were really happy times and children were innocent. You would get them in the bed and that, but there was no such thing as sex as you know it today."[122]

Similarly, Mrs. Melling, born in 1917 in Preston, said that as a child she slept in the same room as her father and stepmother:

> I remember quite plainly sleeping on a settee in their bedroom. A high-backed settee, an old-fashioned thing, but it was turned round with the back here and me facing the wall, so I couldn't see nothing else. I was the only girl and they only had two bedrooms besides and there was six and stepmother had a son so there was seven young men. My brothers slept in a double bed. They had the front room, the big bedroom, and there was two double beds in that, and all the brothers would be in that room, all seven of them. How they slept I don't know, possibly three in one. Now the elder brother had the back bedroom and he was the oldest and he got the bedroom, but it was only like a box room.[123]

Informants also remembered efforts to create separate sleeping quarters for their sons and daughters. Mrs. Peterson, born in 1899, said that

120. Mrs. S2B, 22, 49. See also Mrs. M3L, 17; Mrs. S4L, 68.
121. Mrs. M5L, 16.
122. Mrs. M1P, 57.
123. Mrs. M3L, 16.

when her children were small, she had had a boys' bed and a girls' bed. However, when her husband returned from service in World War I, he decided that the family's sleeping arrangements should change: "They had to be in the same room until the war was on, she [youngest daughter] was only born before the war, but when my husband came home from the war he said that we would have to do something different because the eldest girl, she was ten years older than her. He said that he would go in the back room with the boys and the girls had to go in here. So we had to move the beds. It isn't right when they are growing up and they are starting with their periods and all that. But I must say that in them days they didn't think of anything bad."[124] Mr. Best, born in 1897, built a divider in a bedroom to separate his son and daughter.[125] This was both the moral and the respectable thing to do.

REPUTATIONS AND RESPECTABILITY

As we have seen, sexual behavior and reputation, although important for both sexes, particularly defined female respectability. A girl's innocence about sex and avoidance of premarital pregnancy were core elements of that quality. Time-keeping was a conventional way for parents and unmarried girls to protect their reputations.[126] Mrs. Needham, born in 1919, remembered, "They were very suspicious of you when you went out. You had to be in at a certain time, and if you wasn't in at that time, it was God help you."[127] Mrs. Peel, born in 1921, said, "I'll tell you how strict my mother was. My godmother's daughter was 21year old, and I was engaged to be married, so I was 19. And I went to the house to the party, and it was just on nine o-clock, and it was my mother coming to take me home."[128] This means of protecting a girl's reputation continued into the 1950s and '60s. Mrs. Lucas, born in 1943, remembered: "Well, probably many girls acquired a bad reputation which wasn't deserved. They may have had a lot of different boyfriends, maybe were allowed to come in later at night than other girls and word soon got around. Really, I think probably you preserved your reputation by having a steady boyfriend and getting yourself in on time when your parents asked you to come in."[129]

Of course, as this example suggests, it was also important how girls behaved with the boys they met when they were out. Mrs. Emery, born in 1937, who was pregnant when she married, said, "I never went round with

124. Mrs. P1P, 71.
125. Mr. B1B, 111. See also Roberts, *A woman's place,* 15–16.
126. See Roberts, *A woman's place,* 73.
127. Mrs. N3L, 14.
128. Mrs. P6B, 39.
129. Mrs. L3B, 30.

anybody. He [future husband] was the first boy what ever touched me, because I can remember once I went to a dance hall and somebody wanted to take me home. . . . And somebody shouted across, 'Don't bother to take her home, because wherever you take her, you'll not get nowt.'"[130]

To some extent, male respectability was also related to sexual behavior. Mr. Peel, born in 1909, remembered telling his sons, "If you are going to go out with a girl, look after her. Do not mess about with people. . . . Behave yourself."[131] However, male informants recognized the double standard. Mr. Needham, born in 1921, observed, "I think people tended to talk about a woman more than they do a man. . . . Because he was able in many aspects to keep it quiet, whereas a woman can't keep it quiet indefinitely, eventually, when she starts having a baby, the world knows."[132] Mr. Morris, born in 1933, said, "You didn't see many women smoking, yes, they would have been classed as a bad lot. Promiscuous women, they would be classed as not very nice, really, probably as lads you were probably looking for them, but a different point of view, as I say. Yes, everybody wanted to marry a virgin, but they wanted a good time as well."[133]

It is difficult to exaggerate the importance of respectability in early- and mid-twentieth-century working-class neighborhoods. As we have seen, it was the key to the social and mutual aid that was particularly important for women and children, who lived in streets where everyone knew everyone else's business. Along with factors including housekeeping standards and dress, respectability was inextricably linked to sexual demeanor and communication.

TRANSFORMATION OF WORKING-CLASS SEX CULTURE

In the middle of the twentieth century, sex culture in working-class Barrow, Lancaster, and Preston changed. Parents began, unwillingly, to talk about sex with their children, and reticence about sex began to be viewed as a parental shortcoming rather than a virtue. Schools began to offer sex education lessons. Premarital sex became increasingly acceptable, and childbearing outside of marriage gradually lost its stigma. As the bonds between sex and respectability loosened, sex communication lost its power and danger so completely that, as we have seen, several informants expressed disapproval of their mothers' reticence about sexual matters, displaying collective amnesia about the necessity for that reticence.

After about the 1930s, conversations about sex between parents and children began to be recommended by educational and medical authori-

130. Mrs. E2P, 41.
131. Mr. P6B, 21.
132. Mr. N3L, 128.
133. Mr. M12B, 40. See also Mr. F2L, 64; Mr. P5B, 61.

ties. Informants indicated that although working-class parents found this communication difficult, they also felt it was something they should do. Mrs. Barlow, born in 1928, explained her own discomfort about talking with her children about sex: "The older one [her son] was very keen on biology and I think he just picked it up. To be quite honest, I don't know whether his father ever spoke to him about it, I think he must have done at one time. But we are not the sort of people that talk about that sort of thing. You know, I thinking working-class people don't so much, do they, and we are older. The girl I talked to about it, but she never showed a great deal of interest. . . . I think I was probably more explicit than my mother was."[134]

Similarly, Mrs. Lucas, born in 1943, described her mother's embarrassment about this duty:

> I can remember my mother obviously screwing herself up one day to broach this subject of puberty with me, and she had chosen a moment when the house was empty, just the two of us it, and said, "Now, come and sit here a minute, I would like to talk to you," and I can't even remember which facts she told me now, but certainly didn't tell me things I wanted to know. She probably told me about the onset of periods and odd facts about what happens to a woman during pregnancy. What she didn't tell me was how you got pregnant, which was what I really wanted to know. I would probably be about 13 at the time. . . . She was obviously very embarrassed and didn't really want to take it any further.[135]

Other younger informants' accounts document growing parental ease with these conversations. Mrs. Adderley, born in 1932, said, "My mum told me about starting periods and things like this. We just used to sit and talk, with my aunties, about people being pregnant and all this and that happening, it was just . . . they never kept anything from us, really, you know."[136] Mrs. Harrison, born in 1945, at age 14 was advised by her mother to use a tampon if she wanted to swim while she was menstruating.[137]

A few informants remembered parents referring children to books as a way of easing communication about sexual matters—an approach that was still unusual at a time when authors of such publications faced the possibility of obscenity charges. Mrs. Peterson remembered that in the 1930s

> I sent away for a book because I used to read a lot because my mother didn't. There were adverts in about telling your children this that and

134. Mrs. B3B, 58.
135. Mrs. L5B, 20.
136. Mrs. A4L, 30.
137. Mrs. H9P, 22–23. See also Mrs. J1B, 50.

the other. I sent for this book for our Freda and I said to her that when she was quiet on her own in bed she had to read it and it would tell her something and that it would save me telling her. I told her not to let the boys see it and she had to keep it in her own room. Years after when we were talking about something I told one of my husband's sisters that I had sent for this book. One of his sisters said there was no need to send for a book as she would get to know at school. But I didn't want her to know like that. I had to get to know through other people talking and I wanted my family to be a bit different. I sent for this book and when I got talking to her as she got older she said, "Mother I couldn't understand it." I said to her, "Well, you are a dunce! It was plain enough," I didn't like talking to her.[138]

Other informants remembered consulting books on their own. Mrs. Jenkins, born in 1932, said she learned "a little bit from a doctor's book my friend Ginger had, and we sort of secretly looked at this, and she said, 'Oh, look at this!' you know. And there was a little bit and that was all the knowledge I knew."[139]

Of course, books with sexual content could also be a source of embarrassment and shame. Mrs. Hunt, born in 1885 in Barrow, borrowed a library book recommended by another patron:

I got it and when I got it home I was waiting for them coming in for their tea and I sat down and thought I'll have a look at m'book. I just opened it haphazard at a page, and I hid it in the bedding chest. . . . It was thirty years ago. Bob said to me on the Sunday, "I thought you went to the library yesterday, have you not got a book." I said, "No, I didn't get anything that suited me," and I didn't tell him why until the next day. He was going out at dinnertime and I said, "I'll come out with you at dinnertime and change m'book." He said, "I thought you hadn't got one." I said, "Well, I had but it has been hidden in the bedding chest." I'd have been ashamed for anybody to know that I'd had a book like that in the house.[140]

Mrs. Maxwell, born in 1898 in Preston, said her husband never discussed sex. However, "I can find you books and books that he has on sex and I don't think they have ever been opened. In fact, I took a lot out to the dustbin. I don't want the kids to see them." She commented, "It had just been a mania because he wasn't allowed them when he was a child."[141]

138. Mrs. P1P, 43. See also Mr. R3B, 21; Miss C3B, 24. See Porter and Hall, *The facts of life,* 260–63.

139. Mrs. J1B, 74. See also Mrs. B4L, 60; Miss C3B, 24.

140. Mrs. H2B, 28.

141. Mrs. M3P, 13, 53.

While no informants born before 1920 remembered receiving information about sex at school, some informants born in the interwar period remembered having school-based sex education—an approach first undertaken in the study cities by the National Committee for Combating Venereal Diseases.[142] Mr. Christy, born in 1928, provided a very early account of a lesson: "I was in the sixth form when this thing happened, and it was an Army Major, I think he was. He was called in to give the first sex lesson that had ever been given at Preston Grammar School. . . . Well, I presume he was a medical officer. The only thing I can remember was the uproar from his first statement. He started off by saying, 'Sex is a very sticky subject.'"[143]

Girls learned about menstruation at school. Mrs. Burrell, born in 1931, said, "I think it was the PE teacher, Miss Samson, I think she used to talk to us about different things, facts of life. Because you had to tell her if you had your periods and you couldn't have your showers."[144] The oral evidence suggests that some school-based sex education was hampered by the same normative reticence that affected home-based communication about this matter. Mr. Whiteside, born into a Catholic Lancaster family in 1940, remembered:

> We didn't get no sex education as you call it. . . . Well, you just learned yourself, you know, aye. The only reference I seem to recall was—and it was described as sin then—and that was Mother Mary Agatha, the old nun who run the junior school was before I went for my first confession. And she was telling me about sin and that was, that made a lasting impression on me, did that. . . . We had to go—I'll never forget it—we had to go and stand in the corridor and we went in one at a time. And the exact terminology I don't know, but I remember her telling us it was sinful to do this and it was sinful to do that, you know. It was awful, and these are the sins that you will have to confess.[145]

Regardless of its quality, school-based sex education relieved many working-class parents of an uncomfortable responsibility. Mrs. Atkin, born in 1944, remembered, "I could always go home and whatever I'd learned at school I would chat on about it to Mum. But Mum isn't the best of people to talk about [sex]. I think in her own days it was a taboo subject and she finds it very difficult even now. So I think I would just possibly repeat whatever we'd been told and she would okay it."[146] Similarly, Mrs. Harrison, born in 1945, said, "I think the school did it [sex education] via the rabbit. I think it was a rabbit, and my mother tried, but she couldn't express her-

142. See Roberts, *Women and families*, 59–62; Preston MOH Report, 1920, 63.
143. Mr. C8P, 113. Also quoted in Roberts, *Women and families*, 61.
144. Mrs. B2B, 26.
145. Mr. W5L, 52.
146. Mrs. A3L, 44.

self. I can see her now at the old house . . . ironing . . . continually ironing at this cloth and telling me to keep myself nice. . . . I must have been about 11 or 12."[147] Many informants said that although they did not have sex education at school, their own children did. According to Mrs. Peel, born in 1921, "It saves a lot of embarrassment at home."[148]

Informants' accounts illustrate both dramatic change in sexual behavior of adolescents and willingness of those born after about 1930 to talk about these matters; after World War II, sexual knowledge and experimentation before marriage declined as a barrier to respectability. Mrs. Lonsdale, born in 1947, remembered heavy petting that would have been unheard-of for an earlier generation:

> I can remember when I worked at Nelson's, this particular lad, and I fancied him rotten. He was a bit of a Romeo, and he was renowned for—he would kiss a girl and get what he wanted and run away, sort of thing. But he used to . . . fetch me home from Morecambe, but he was one of these lads, as soon as he started kissing you, he was round your neck. And the next day you wouldn't just have one mark, you would have about six all round your neck. And wake up in the morning and, Oh my God, look at my neck! Bloody big polo neck sweater on, you know, and they must have known, you know. Because, say, you went out on a Friday night, every Saturday morning you would get up in this bloody big thing, and keep pulling it up, you know.[149]

Mrs. Jenkins, born in 1932, remembered an intense game of "postman's knock" at her engagement party in the early 1950s: "One of my friends and her future husband were there, all the lads were going mad because [husband] said she had upset all his friends because she had got them turned on and just started screaming. That was it, and they reckoned she was a hot bit of stuff, and then when they started getting passionate, she started screaming and it spoilt the party."

The same informant revealed changes in the way people thought about premarital pregnancy: "Most of the people I knew met their husbands when they were about 15 or 16 and went steady. And it was just a case of you didn't get a bad reputation, it was just how long you could go without having a baby before you were married. And, I mean, I would say fifty percent of people I knew had to get married, including myself, and it was normal. But you didn't get a bad reputation because you only had one boyfriend. . . . Even when I was courting at sixteen, I didn't know much about sex, I didn't know much about babies."[150]

147. Mrs. H9P, 22.
148. Mrs. P6B, 113.
149. Mrs. L3L, 45.
150. Mrs. J1B, 74–75. See also Mrs. B11P, 69.

Mr. Simpkins, born in 1932, commented about his first wife, who was pregnant when they married, "We had been going out I think possibly about six or nine months before intercourse ever occurred. And that was because of the way we felt about each other at the time, you know. It was a natural spontaneous reaction. The chemistry was right."[151] Perhaps most telling, Mr. Ingham, born in 1930, said, "Well, I think I educated my daughter to be honest and to respect other people and also to have some respect for herself. And then to have relationships with a young man, certainly, if she thought that it was a lasting thing, yes, go ahead. It's nature, isn't it, you see."[152] It is worthy of remark that the moral language used about sex by older informants had become scientific language among younger informants: right and wrong became nature and chemistry.

Informants also described change in the ways women who had babies out of wedlock were treated. In response to the question, "How did people round about feel, how did they treat a girl who had become pregnant out of wedlock?" Mr. Priestly, born in Barrow in 1950, said:

> It wasn't as bad as it had been, they were sort of looked down on, not as a sort of loose woman and all the rest of it, I think that had occurred maybe ten years before my time. Like an in-between stage really, nowadays it didn't matter a great deal, even though it's not particularly liked or, you know, still frowned upon, but then it was just starting to become acceptable as something that didn't quite destroy the rest of your life. Lasses were looked down upon, you know, "The silly bugger getting pregnant," even though it wasn't her fault.[153]

Mrs. Britton, born in 1936, commented that nowadays women who have an illegitimate baby "can keep it and bring it up because they get help off the State, which they never got years ago—they usually had to put them out for adoption if their parents wouldn't look after them."[154] Dr. Armstrong, who began his general practice in Lancaster in 1948, remembered that as the stigma of unwed pregnancy declined, more unmarried mothers kept their babies rather than giving them up for adoption.[155]

In addition to these changes, informants revealed alterations in the ways people thought about sex. Increasingly, it was accepted that sex was for pleasure as well as reproduction and that it could be enjoyed by both men and women. Mr. Boyle, born in 1926, said of his mother, "She was brought up a good Roman Catholic, the purpose of marriage was the procreation of children, therefore she would do her bit. But I don't sense there

151. Mr. S7L, 87.
152. Mr. I2L, 38.
153. Mr. P5B, 62.
154. Mrs. B4L, 96.
155. Dr. A5L, 15–16.

was any more to it. There was no human loving side to it."[156] By contrast,
summarizing the changes he observed in his own generation, Mr. Morris,
born in 1933, commented, "I think there has been a big sexual revolution
for women, who were supposed to put up with sex, if you like, but now they
realize that there is as much in it for them as there is for blokes."[157]

FAMILY LIMITATION

In the late nineteenth and early twentieth centuries, working-class families
were large. Nine or ten children were born to 13.5 percent of marriages
celebrated during the 1870s in Britain, while only 12.5 percent of that
decade's marriages produced one or two children. Although this situation
had altered dramatically by the period 1900–9, when only 4 percent of marriages produced nine or ten children and 45 to 50 percent of marriages
produced one or two children, working-class families remained larger than
middle- or upper-class families until after World War I.[158] This study's oral
history evidence reflects this situation. Thirty-three informants born before
1920 came from families with ten children or more; one of these, Mrs.
Dalkey, born in Barrow in 1896, was one of 21 children born to a single
mother.[159] However, only three informants born after 1920 came from families of ten or more children, and none of the interviewees had families of
their own with more than six children.

How can we account for this change? Elizabeth Roberts compares the
fatalism and respect for tradition that resulted in the large family sizes
of the oldest informants with "modern" outlooks and smaller numbers of
children among younger informants, which she argues was motivated by
desire for a better quality of life and concern about the potentially negative
impact of childbearing on the mother's health.[160] Richard Allen Soloway
maintains that "the desire of both men and women to avoid the physical
and financial burdens of too many children coincided with a continually
expanding network of contraceptive information and a rapidly changing social, political, cultural, and religious environment."[161] Diana Gittins
underplays the role of birth control information and technology, writing,
"It seems probable . . . that the decline of family size among the working
class during the first four decades of this century was not so much a result
of increased knowledge and availability of reliable birth control methods,

156. Mr. B9P, 9. See also Roberts, *A woman's place,* 84.
157. Mr. M12B, 42.
158. Soloway, *Birth control,* 8, 13; Seccombe, *Weathering the storm,* 157–58. See Roberts, *A woman's place,* 85, for fertility rates for Barrow and Preston.
159. Mrs. D2B, 1–2.
160. Roberts, *A woman's place,* 92–93.
161. Soloway, *Birth control,* xviii.

but was a response to their changing relations to the socioeconomic system."[162] Wally Seccombe supports this perspective, arguing, "The major impetus, in my view, was the underlying shift in the family economy, inducing a convergence in the reproductive interests of men and women. In the traditional family wage economy, children worked from an early age and their contribution was obvious to parents. . . . The next generation of parents would arrive at the opposite conclusion. When referring to children in economic terms, they treated them as a net cost."[163] The oral evidence suggests that changes in working-class family size had as much to do with shifting expectations and attitudes regarding children as they did with knowledge and use of birth control techniques. Reduced infant mortality and child employment combined with strengthening value for companionate parent-child relationships, lengthening compulsory education, and rising lifestyle and upward mobility aspirations all arguably stimulated working-class desire for smaller families and use of contraception.

Generally speaking, older informants remembered fatalism about family size before World War I. Mr. Townley, born in 1897, whose mother gave birth to 17 babies, 13 of whom survived, said, "Well, they never bothered. They [babies] just came along. People had more then. Next door, they had about six or seven and further up there would be another six or seven. Same as North Road [Preston], they would have so much and then another half a dozen. They were very big families in my younger days."[164] Providing a comparatively late example of traditional attitudes, Mrs. Fleming, born in 1921, said that after her husband returned from service in World War II, "Yes, that's when my trouble started. One [baby] every year, 15 months and 18 months. . . . I don't know as I felt anything, they just arrived. Except the last one, I think, when I thought, 'Crickey! Have I to go through that again?'"[165] This informant had six births and one miscarriage between 1939 and 1952. Mrs. Preston, born in 1907, said her grandmother had had 17 births: "In those days, they had babies as an insurance. They [children] had to keep the old people."[166] Mrs. Shelby, born in 1892, linked large families with religious affiliation: "Mrs. Gardner had twenty-four on West Road. . . . She was Catholic and the nuns were good to her."[167]

Other respondents remembered frequent and numerous births less philosophically, associating them with high infant mortality and maternal health problems. Mrs. Masterson, born in 1913, said: "They had such big

---

162. Diana Gittins, *Fair Sex: Family Size and Structure in Britain, 1900–39* (New York: St. Martin's Press, 1982), 164.

163. Seccombe, *Weathering the storm*, 176–77.

164. Mr. T1P, 42. See also Mr. P6B, 53.

165. Mrs. F1L, 56.

166. Mrs. P2P, 21.

167. Mrs. S1L, 27.

families and the mothers never seemed to get their strength back. Thirteen children was nothing! I had an aunt that had 23 children, but they didn't all live. Sometimes they would lose as many as seven of them. They just couldn't stand the pace. In those days there was no birth control methods. If you were unfortunate enough to be caught, then you were caught! There was no way that you could avoid it, it had to be! Some would probably be caught every nine months."[168] Her metaphor for pregnancy, to be "caught," which was common among informants, reflected both women's sense of powerlessness over this matter and the frequent implication that conception was unwelcome. Mrs. Wilkinson, born in 1881, whose mother had twelve babies, four of whom died, said, "None of them lived to more than three months. . . . They come so quickly, one after the other, they cannot have a lot of stamina."[169] Similarly, Mrs. Mallingham, born in 1896, said her mother would not talk about the many infants she lost: "They died, say three months, five months. She did bring one boy up to eight year old and she did talk of him. I think the idea was they were born too quickly. One every year and I suppose she hadn't the stamina to produce healthy children. She always said that they came too often. She often used to joke and say they didn't know enough in those days."[170] Mrs. Garvey, born in 1888, said that her mother had had sixteen pregnancies: "In those days there was no contraceptives. . . . She used to say that she'd had sixteen good and bad and she brought up eleven—six girls and five boys and they've all done well." This informant frequently repeated that her mother could not cope, was often ill, and required older children to do housework and help with younger children. "She said that she always had one in her arms and one in her basket."[171] Mrs. Hampton, born in 1911, said her father hated children, although there were ten in her family:

> My mother had as good as 15 and I don't know just where they came. There must have been some more between me and the twins because there was 3 years and 8 months between us and that was the longest period she had. She had three lots of twins, only one lot born living. Two were stillborn and she was about six or seven months with the others, she was sat on the window-sill cleaning and the sash-cord broke and the babies were born dead, but whether that was in between my mother never said. . . . I was the seventh and then the twins were eighth and ninth. Then when she come to be having the last one she moved to

168. Mrs. M1P, 47.
169. Mrs. W1L, 7. See also Mrs. D2B, 19; Mrs. M1P, 47.
170. Mrs. M6B, 53.
171. Mrs. G1B, 8. See also Mr. G1P, 76, for an account of Mrs. G1P's mother, who had her last baby at age 40 and was "not fit to have it," paying it no attention and expecting her older daughters to look after it.

Preston and our Alice was born here. She died at 2 years 11 months.[172]

Mrs. Peel, born in 1921, said succinctly, "Well, they had the babies, they didn't know. Let's face it, they didn't know how not to have them. . . . So they just had them."[173]

These accounts suggest that an important reason for frequent repeated pregnancies was ignorance of contraception—an explanation that counters Diana Gittens's contention that certain family limitation methods (e.g., abstinence, *coitus interruptus,* abortion, and condoms) had been known and used for centuries, but working-class motivation to use them changed in the early twentieth century.[174] It is certainly possible that informants' parents knew more about methods of contraception than they told their children but saw little reason to limit family size. It is likely that the association of barrier birth control methods with dirty sex limited respectable people's awareness of and access to these techniques. It is also possible that normative silence about sex, which arguably increased in the late nineteenth and early twentieth centuries, actually decreased collective knowledge of birth control in some communities. Regardless, an important element in many marital relationships that influenced the number of pregnancies was the husband's control over sex and contraception. Mrs. Preston, quoted above, whose grandmother had had 17 babies, said, "My mother had six, but they thought they had to, they were ignorant. The men thought they had to get drunk or they weren't men. It was a general attitude, it was tradition, and people lived that sort of life. Same as today, if you have your hair cut one way, everybody else has the same. It was just the usual thing."[175] While this account indicates some women's complicity in what might be called the custom of large families, Mrs. Winder, born in Lancaster in 1910, suggests a variation on the theme: "They used to have children pretty quick then because there was no birth control. In fact, she [elderly lady who lived next door] used to tell about her husband who was a stonemason and which was often the thing in those days, they went on the booze and she never got pennies for weeks on end. She said that many a night she daren't get into bed with him and sat on the window ledge until he went to sleep. The young ones today say, 'Serve you right, you had a big family,' but they hadn't a clue what went on."[176]

Did couples in this period attempt to limit family size? Some oral history informants suggested that family planning was possible, responsible, and

172. Mrs. H1P, 2.

173. Mrs. P6B, 28.

174. Gittins, *Fair Sex,* 164.

175. Mrs. P2P, 22. This account is also quoted in Roberts, *A woman's place,* 92. See also Mrs. H4P, 31.

176. Mrs. W2L, 14. This account is also quoted in Roberts, *A woman's place,* 96.

within the husband's control. Mrs. Dent, born in 1908, was an only child. She said, "My dad wasn't a lustful man. He could have had more [children] if he wanted."[177] Her comments reflect both the perspective that a married man's frequent demands for sex were irresponsible and the inference that her family's small size was attributable to her father's virtuous self-restraint. Mrs. Smith, born in 1895, whose parents had ten children, indicates both a similar point of view regarding male responsibility for sex and understanding of the consequences of unrestrained lust for the wife, who typically took charge of family finances: "You cannot understand people having so many children when there was so little money to keep them. Yet my father was the easiest going man, he didn't worry whether m'mother could pay her way or not. He was too easy going."[178]

Family size was decreasing in Barrow, Lancaster, and Preston from the beginning of the study period. Annual MOH reports reveal that in 1880, Barrow's birthrate had been 44.1 per 1,000 births; compared to 31.7 in 1900 and 23.7 in 1910. Preston's birthrate declined from 42.35 per 1,000 births in 1878 to 28.67 in 1900 and 23.58 in 1910. Comparable rates are unavailable for Lancaster; however, at 20.63 per 1,000 births in 1910, that city's birthrate was the lowest of the three study cities. The comments of MOsH reveal contradictory perspectives about this issue. For example, in 1882 Barrow's MOH, Dr. John Settle, wrote, "Our continual high birth rate is the principal cause of so many deaths in infants and young children. . . . I have frequently reported to you on the subject of infant mortality, and will simply remark here than an improvement in the social and moral habits of the people would effect more than anything else the preservation of infant life."[179] However, with declining death rates, the same MOH commented in 1884 that the high birthrate "presents most unmistakable evidence not only of natural vigor in our population, but of the sound sanitary conditions affecting our local community."[180] In 1894 Dr. Settle presumed local causes for the drop in Barrow's birthrate to 32.6 per 1,000:

> The fact of our somewhat low birth rate of late years is in a large measure explained by the numbers of unmarried men, and of men married, but having their wives in Scotland, employed at the works of the Naval Construction and Armaments Company. The lowering of our birth rate from this cause we need not lament did it not mean also that a large

177. Mrs. D1P, 31. See also Mrs. H4P (born 1903), whose mother refused to sleep with her father after discovering his infidelity (46).

178. Mrs. S2B, 29. This account is also quoted in Roberts, *A woman's place*, 91. Mr. R3L (born 1890), one of only two children, said his father "didn't want a big family due to economic conditions of the day." He associated larger families with poverty (57).

179. Barrow MOH Report, 1882, 213–15.

180. Barrow MOH Report, 1884, 200.

sum of money was every week sent out of the town, which robs our shopkeepers and business people of a considerable portion of the wages
paid at these works, and which ought to circulate locally.[181]

However, in 1897, when the city's birthrate had dropped to 28.5 per 1,000,
the MOH commented, "There is a steady decline in our birth rate, but this
is not confined to our Borough, but is more or less general throughout the
Kingdom."[182] Similarly, Lancaster's MOH saw the city's decreasing birthrate as part of a national trend, in 1912 linking it to ongoing concerns
about infant mortality: "A declining birth-rate is general, and is to be found
in most highly civilized communities. If a remedy cannot be discovered
more strenuous effects must be made to check the present waste of infant
life."[183]

Preston's birthrate, having been unusually high, began to fall, attracting
notice in 1898 from its MOH, who by 1903 was speculating that birth control was responsible for the continuing decline.[184] Dr. Pilkington believed
that family limitation by either contraception or abortion was both immoral
and contrary to the national interest. In 1903 he attributed the declining
birthrate to "a growing desire in the case of some parents—from economi-
cal or other motives—to keep their families within certain limits. In doing
this they receive instruction from books, pamphlets, and lectures, generally
of American origin, and assistance from unprincipled charlatans, and from
the black sheep that may occasionally be met with in the Medical Profession. But such proceedings, like all violations of Nature's laws, recoil upon
those practicing them, and often result in sickness and disease, sometimes
in death."[185]

Dr. Pilkington believed that "The success—and indeed the safety—of
a nation cannot depend so much upon its wealth as upon the production
of children capable in manhood not only of protecting it at home, but of
upholding its power and dignity in distant lands, so any of which form an
actual part of this mighty Empire."[186] He revealed a eugenicist perspective,
writing in 1909 that "One unsatisfactory feature is that there is reason to
believe this limitation of family does not so much occur amongst the careless, intemperate, and therefore poorest classes, but rather amongst the
thrifty and fairly well to do, the families most likely to produce and rear
a healthy offspring."[187] However, by 1918 he commented that the working
classes had also been corrupted by the selfishness motivating family limita-

181. Barrow MOH Report, 1894, 199.
182. Barrow MOH Report, 1897, 146.
183. Lancaster MOH Report, 1912, 9, 84.
184. Preston MOH Report, 1898, 11–12; Preston MOH Report, 1903, 15.
185. Preston MOH Report, 1903, 15.
186. Preston MOH Report, 1913, 12.
187. Preston MOH Report, 1909, 9; see also Preston MOH Report, 1911, 12.

tion, thus endangering the Empire's labor force. While Pilkington believed birth control to be unpatriotic, he also thought it was immoral and danger-ous to the health of mothers and infants:

> The illegal methods employed to prevent or limit the responsibilities connected with a family of children too often act in the desired direc-tion, but not infrequently if even the main object is not attained they exercise a disastrous effect upon the health of the mother and child exposed to their influence. The honor and nobility connected with motherhood appears to be no longer recognized, home life has lost its charm, and pride in household management is swamped by a feverish desire for liberty, excitement, and an unrestricted round of pleasure. Nor is this condition confined to one class of society, and the luxury formerly supposed to be confined to the wealthy is, under the stimu-lus of shorter hours of labour and vastly increased earnings, gradually invading the homes of the working classes.[188]

As the first line of this quotation suggests, Pilkington was most concerned about abortion, illegal between 1861 and 1967, which was the main form of birth control controlled by women. In contrast to the interwar and post–World War II eras, when abortion was increasingly discussed as a last resort to protect an unmarried pregnant girl from shame, in the years before World War I, abortion tended to be used by married women with large families and small means to space rather than to prevent all births.[189]

Medical Officers of Health believed that women regularly induced abor-tion to limit family size. For example, in 1907 Lancaster's MOH reflected on possible reasons for the large number of premature births in the city: "One is undoubtedly the employment of pregnant women in laborious occupations, but beyond this is the number of cases to which this explana-tion does not apply. After allowing for various forms of disease and mal-formations as a cause of abortion, there are a large number of cases which cannot be explained except on the assumption that they are due to inter-

188. Preston MOH Report, 1918, 11.
189. See, for example, Barbara Brookes, *Abortion in England 1900–1967* (London: Croom Helm, 1988); Seccombe, *Weathering the storm,* 158–59; Ross, *Love and toil,* 104–6. In *A woman's place,* 97–100, Roberts discusses informants' recourse to abortion, indicating that "the evidence about abortion comes entirely from Preston, as the interviews in Barrow and Lancaster did not include questions on it (and perhaps significantly no information was volunteered)" (97). My reading of the evidence is somewhat different owing to my more extensive use of MOH reports and my inclusion in the interviews conducted in the period 1987–89 of questions about family planning and birth control. However, the preponderance of the oral evidence about abortion *is* from Preston, a fact that might be explained by the city's higher poverty rates and larger number of women who worked outside their homes after marriage. However, Preston also had the highest number of Roman Catholics of the study cities and, thus, arguably provided least access to birth control information and materials.

ference with the course of gestation. It is only very occasionally that such interference can be proved, but I am of opinion that it largely exists."[190] Preston's Dr. Pilkington linked abortion with continuing high infant mortality and declining birth rates in 1902, 1911, and 1914.[191]

The likelihood is that many women viewed abortion as, if not entirely respectable, more focused and less immoral than contraceptive methods, which might be regarded as a way to indulge in sexual pleasure without fulfilling the primary purpose of respectable sexual activity—reproduction. Since a "good" woman would not plan to have sex, she could not plan to prevent conception; however, she might use abortion to space her pregnancies. Oral history informants remembered women's attempts to both self-induce abortion and procure abortion services from others.[192] As Barbara Brookes suggests, informants "regulated their fertility in a number of ways primarily oriented round menstruation rather than intercourse. Experience suggested that not every act of intercourse led to pregnancy, whereas late menstruation for a woman whose periods were regular was a sure sign of something amiss. Emmenagogues of many kinds and increasing potency had traditionally been used to ensure regularity, to 'cure' late menstruation and prompt problematic menstruation."[193]

Mrs. Havelock, born in 1903, whose mother had ten births, suffered routine spousal abuse, and died at age 44, remembered buying quinine from the chemist for her mother when she was "worried about her periods."[194] In answer to the question, "I know some people must have planned their families because they would only have one or two?" Mrs. Maxwell, born in 1898, said:

> A lot of people brought on miscarriages. Oh yes, they did! I could tell you all sorts, what they did and what they didn't do!"
>
> *Interviewer:* Did people talk about it amongst themselves?
>
> *Informant:* Women did. I'm not saying about men, because I don't know. I can always remember when I came to have this one after seven years, a neighbor saying, "You should have come to me and I would have shifted it." It was that sort of thing. I said, "Look, I've a long time

190. Lancaster MOH Report, 1907, 49.

191. Preston MOH Report, 1902, 11; Preston MOH Report, 1911, 12; Preston MOH Report, 1914, 12.

192. According to Brookes, *Abortion in England,* "Most women did not equate the restoration of menstruation by means of drugs, douching, or instruments, as a serious offence. Neither did they regard a self-induced abortion, or one achieved with the help of friends, as a violation of the criminal law. The term 'abortion' was usually reserved for a surgical procedure seemingly unrelated, in the words of women themselves, to attempts to 'bring me round,' 'put me on my way' or to 'put me right.' Although the Act of 1861 made all abortion a crime, it was only commercial operators who were popularly judged to be criminal" (8).

193. Brookes, *Abortion in England,* 3.

194. Mrs. H4P, 31, 38.

to live I hope, and I'm not going to ruin my inside." I remember saying that to her. I know she had a terrible time. She is dead now. She must have moved one herself.

    Interviewer: What did they used to do? Have you any idea?

    Informant: Do you know what slippery elm bark is? They pushed that up. I don't know what it did. They pushed needles up. Take washing-soda, quinine, all that sort of thing. But life isn't worth living if you are going to do that sort of thing.

Despite awareness of their danger, however, she said about these practices, "I agree with them planning their families."[195]

Mrs. Dorrington, born in 1905, who had six children, reported trying abortion to limit her family's size: "If you had two or three children in three years, you took all sorts of things they told you to take. . . . We used to take Epsom salts and gin." Mrs. Meadows, born in 1904, added, "There used to be a shop in Moor Lane that did supply bottles of stuff." Reflecting on the unreliability of such means, Mrs. Dorrington said:

No. I tried to stop one or two, I took my salts.

    Interviewer: And it didn't work?

    Informant: No. . . . If you were strong. If you were weak and you hadn't had good food when you were young, and strong inside, it would work. There was one or two other things, hot baths and things like that. But if you were strong it would make no difference. No chance whatever.

    Interviewer: So they just came along.

    Informant: Everybody tried. In our station they tried.

    Interviewer: Did your friends try?

    Informant: Everybody tried.

    Interviewer: But there was no success?

    Informant: No.

    Interviewer: They don't seem to have done as much about preventing it either, do they.

    Informant: There was no prevention, was there. . . . The doctor wouldn't help you. You daren't mention it to the doctor.

    Mrs. Meadows: He would just tell you that that's what married life was all about.[196]

In the eyes of oral history informants, the respectability of abortion depended on the woman's circumstances; a poor mother of many children born close together was thought to have a better excuse for seeking abor-

---

195. Mrs. M3P, 13, 53. See also Mr. W6P, 1; Mrs. P1P, 68; Mr. M10L, 67–68.
196. Mrs. D3P, 30.

tion than a woman with financial resources and few children who repeatedly prevented her pregnancies from going to term. Mrs. Hill, born in
1903, said about her two sisters-in-law:

> I had a sister-in-law, she is dead and gone now. . . . [S]he stopped I don't
> know how many children. She wasn't having any children, but she had
> one son and he's living today. My brother was a policeman, our Joe.
> Now, this is between you and me, I only got to know this after I was
> married myself, they have another girl, Jenny, she is fifty-odd now. My
> brother said to his wife, "If you don't let this baby go through, I'll report
> you to the Chief Constable." So she had Jenny and that was the last one.
> They said she had stopped, they didn't know how many. I had another
> sister-in-law, my eldest brother's wife, she had had eight children, but
> she only kept three.[197]

One reason informants may have indicated disapproval of abortion, been
reticent about it, and talked more often about others' experiences than
their own was awareness both that the procedure was illegal and that it
might damage the health of mother or baby. Women whose attempts to
abort were detected risked prosecution and shame as well as disability and
death. Informants remembered doctors and midwives suspecting attempted
abortion. Mrs. Washburn, born in 1900, recalled an unusually frank conversation with her mother:

> She told me when I got married, "If you are having babies and you don't
> want them, don't take any stuff, because I did." . . . One woman said, "I
> wouldn't keep having them children. You wait and I will get you some
> stuff." So she did. When the doctor came, he said, "Now, what have you
> been taking." She said, "I haven't been taking anything." He said, "I can
> tell, and I think I know who's getting it for you.'" He said, "I'll tell you
> something, this baby will die and so will your next one." And there were
> two boys, Daniel and James, who died in infancy. So she always told us
> not to take any stuff. She had ten altogether and I was the youngest.[198]

Similarly, Mrs. Maxwell said:

> I remember when one of my sisters was born, my mother telling me that
> the doctor came and he was in a temper when he came. He said, "I've
> just been with a woman that has had a child born covered with eczema!
> She tells me she has kissed somebody with eczema, but she hasn't. She
> has been taking some stuff. That's what she has been doing!" I always

197. Mrs. H8P, 36. This account is also quoted in Roberts, A woman's place, 99.
198. Mrs. W4P, 1.

remember my mother telling me this tale. So probably I had a fear of taking anything like that for fear if I didn't move it, what would happen to the child? I might have damaged the baby which would be worse![199]

Neighbors also sometimes reported self-induced abortion to the authorities. Mrs. Hill remembered:

There was one woman and she was a lovely person, she had two sons and a lovely husband, she's dead and buried now. She was old enough to be my mother, were Polly, she served three months' prison sentence. I'll not tell you her name. She had done something to herself to stop a baby and one of her neighbors was watching through the window and reported it. That woman didn't have another day's luck after. Polly nearly died and she was a broken woman after and yet she was a good woman. She said she had her own idea of why she did what she did, but nobody else suffered for it.[200]

Known recourse to abortion could damage reputations in the neighborhood. Mr. Danner, born in 1910, commented, "As a younger man, I have heard scathing comments about miscarriages like, 'I bet she has brought it on herself.' They were very unkind about each other, you know. That could be a killer too, couldn't it?"[201] Also, neighbors could find themselves unwilling participants in legal proceedings. Mr. Grove, born in 1903, said that his mother-in-law had served in a line-up in an abortion investigation:

She was stood at the door waiting for her husband coming home and a car drew up in the street. It was a little back street at the side of the Technical College. They come and asked her if she knew the lady next door but one. She said she didn't as she had only moved there. He said she was just the person that they wanted. He took her in this here house and took her upstairs and she said it was a spare [room], there was nothing in. In the end, an identification took place, and they had about three or four ladies and they walked them round this bed and the lady were laid in bed and she was dying. There were about four doctors there and they asked her to point out which one. She pointed to this lady. This lady said, "Oh no! Don't give me away!" To Ella's mother they said, "Right, you have done what we wanted." She must only have been in her twenties or something like that. So it must have been an ordeal for her, and that was what happened in them days.[202]

Informants remembered people procuring abortions from both ama-

199. Mrs. M3P, 13.
200. Mrs. H8P, 36.
201. Mr. D2P, 29.
202. Mr. G1P, 68.

teurs (unpaid helpers doing the pregnant woman a favor) and experts (paid abortionists). Their accounts indicate that they knew this activity was illegal and felt it was not completely respectable, but sympathized with both the desperate women who sought help and, sometimes, with the people who provided it. Mrs. Drake, born in 1899 in Barrow, said, "Of course, abortions, goodness, it was terrible. Some were paying twenty-five and thirty shillings to get rid of children, but of course we didn't think of anything because we didn't know anything at all. That was terrible and if anybody told the police they were fined heavily, and now they don't think anything of it."[203] Mr. Danner remembered:

> Oh yes, there was a little person had a little shop and their daughter, she was a very good woman, but the rest of the family were mentally backward in some respects, and one of these daughters had two or three of a family, and was having another, and the eldest sister was a churchgoing type of woman. Accordingly, she used to use a hook or something and her sister died. She got six months for it. I have heard people saying that the person went fat and then thin again. The "old mother had been seen again," that sort of thing. . . . But that was a prison case too, and it was really out of the decency of the sister. She wasn't getting money for it. It was because of the plight of this mentally backward man and woman who had married and had a lot of children.[204]

Mrs. Preston said:

> I have had personal experience of people who did abortions. It was common. One particular friend, the sister-in-law that's died, it's her brother's wife had a sister who killed a girl and did time in Strangeways. It was during the last war and she did it out of sympathy. This girl had got in trouble with a sailor and she was from a very upper-class family. She lived on the outskirts of Preston and she was so disgusted and frightened of embarrassing her family and she came to Lily and Lily did the abortion. I don't know what she did, but the girl died. She [Lily] did time in jail but I just forget how many years she did. But it was a very common thing, it was an accepted thing.[205]

Similarly, Mr. Grove recalled: "We did know of a lady that had done an abortion and it was a friend of ours and it were his sister-in-law and she did two years. She was caught and this girl died, somebody had taken her, and she died. She was sent to prison for it. It was a shame because I think these people as went to them, they would plead. They would give you away as easy

---

203. Mrs. D1B, 35.
204. Mr. D2P, 29.
205. Mrs. P2P, 21–22.

as anything. They had done a good turn, hadn't they? I think it was a poor do for them to be let down. I know they were doing wrong."[206]

Informants remembered stereotypical (and demonized) female abortionists. Mrs. Dorrington told of her mother's experience in Wigan with "an abortionist, as I got to know later on. She had a shawl on and she was a dirty old thing."[207] Mrs. Havelock knew of a similar abortionist in Preston: "It was an old woman in Plungington called Mrs. Oldfield, and she was one of them as went from house to house. I think she was a certified midwife, but she would have had a woman helping her. . . . I remember old Mother Oldfield and her funny-shaped black bonnet. She had a shawl round her neck and she was a very ordinary woman. They didn't take it [abortion] as serious as they do now."[208] Dr. Armstrong said of Lancaster in the days before abortion was legal, "There was back-street abortionists, of course. . . . Now well there was a woman in—hopefully it's been knocked down now—in Hood Street in Lancaster who was a well-known back-street abortionist."[209]

Informants also remembered herbalists, druggists, and doctors assisting women with abortions. Mrs. Meadows, born in 1904, said there was a Preston druggist "in Moor Lane that did supply bottles of stuff."[210] Mrs. Fleming, born in 1921 in Lancaster, said, "I mean them days, it would be these back-street abortions. I think really more of that went on Victorian, than when we were younger. . . . We hardly every heard of it, did we? . . . The old herbalist, old MacGregor's . . . they would go there and get pills and what-have-you. They never worked."[211] Mr. Cranston, born in 1884, remembered knowing a Preston general practitioner who was prosecuted and served time for doing abortions.[212]

Before 1967, one of the few justifications for legal abortion was tuberculosis in the mother. Mrs. Jenkins, born in 1932, found herself in the anomalous position of opposing her doctor's advice to terminate her first pregnancy in the 1950s. "Yes, well, because I'd had TB, oh, they nearly took my first baby away because I'd had TB, and I said I didn't want it taken away anyway, but anyway they decided to let me keep it, but they said I'd had it too quickly, I'd had it within one or two years of coming out of sanatorium."[213] However, it was far more common for women to want abortions but to be unable to obtain them legally.

It is noteworthy that older informants had more to say about abortion

206. Mr. G1P, 68.
207. Mrs. D3P, 26.
208. Mrs. H4P, 31. See also Mrs. P1P, 68–69.
209. Dr. A5L, 19.
210. Mrs. D3P, 27.
211. Mrs. F1L, 31.
212. Mr. C1P, 75.
213. Mrs. J1B, 10. See also Mrs. T3B, 3.

than younger informants, despite (or perhaps because of) rising official concern about this issue during the interwar period.[214] However, evidence from a few informants born after 1930 indicates that traditional practices continued. Mr. Monkham, born in Lancaster in 1948, said that women tried to self-abort: "Hot mustard baths was common, gin or drink was thought to be a common one. There was a lot of talk . . . about knitting needles." He also remembered "some sort of gossip about a girl that lived on Cedar Road when I was a child, who was commonly thought to have visited an illegal abortionist. It was quite the gossip for a long long time, and I remember the speculation if the police or the doctor found out."[215] Mr. Simkins, born in 1932 in Lancaster, remembered knowing a divorced woman who became pregnant and had an abortion in Preston; after returning home, she hemorrhaged and was taken to the Lancaster Royal Infirmary for transfusions.[216] These informants indicated that women sought abortions for reasons similar to those in earlier periods. Mr. Simpkins recalled his sister becoming very depressed when she became pregnant. He believed that an abortion would have spared her a life of mental illness and institutionalization.[217] Mr. Monkham said of abortion attempts: "I think the biggest factor of all was financial, most of them were working-class women, very often with large families anyway, and the addition of another mouth and the burden on the finances was very often a great fear. . . . The common thing was, 'I don't know how I'm going to manage with this one, I don't know how we are going to keep another mouth.'"[218]

Abortion was legalized at the end of the study period, in 1967. Only one informant discussed personal experience of legal abortion. Shortly after her divorce, Mrs. Howard, who already had three children, became pregnant with her lover's child. Her account reveals traditional preoccupation with respectability, the medicalization of abortion and huge power of general practitioners and consultants, and ongoing support from informal female health authorities:

> Well, my doctor was great. He was a family doctor that knew all about you because he had been my doctor for so long. . . . And of course he knew how you had got on, he knew that your husband had left you. He knew that I had got this other guy living with me. And he thought

214. See, for example, Brookes, *Abortion in England;* Jones, *Health and society in twentieth-century Britain,* 67; James Thomas and A. Susan Williams, "Women and abortion in 1930s Britain: A survey and its data," *Social History of Medicine* 11, no. 2 (1998): 283–309. Mrs. H5L (born 1931) was the only respondent to talk about having had an early legal abortion in 1971 (111). Mr. P5B (born 1950) said he "never heard of any abortions or anything like that. . . . I might be wrong because obviously if they got an abortion they wouldn't advertise it, particularly then" (62).
215. Mr. M10L, 67.
216. Mr. S7L, 84–85.
217. Mr. S7L, 81–83.
218. Mr. M10L, 68.

that mentally I could have that [pregnancy] terminated, as far as he was concerned, the kids had to adjust to a new fellow so they wouldn't take too kindly. What would I say to them, I wouldn't be able to hold my head up to the neighbors, all these things went towards being traumatic enough for him to give permission to have it terminated. So he just had to get another doctor to okay it and then the two doctors sign it and then it's okay. But I went to see one of—this is one of the most terrible things I have ever had to do—is going to see this other fellow at the Infirmary. . . . And he made me feel as though I was a loose woman. He threw all sorts of questions at me, I was in tears and he said, "And, okay, if we get rid of this," he said, "If we have this terminated, how do I know that you are not going to be in next year for the same thing?" Well, I was absolutely flabbergasted, because I was not like that, I hated being classed as that kind of person. I was so upset I nearly threw myself under a bus when I came out, you know, I was that upset. I cried all the way home on the bus. And I know I sat next to a lady who used to be a nurse there . . . and she saw me crying and she came and sat next to me . . . and we had a right good talk about him, and she said, "Take no notice of that Mr. T—, he will do the same to everybody, he just has got to be so sure that you really want to get rid of it, to have this terminated, you see."

Mrs. Howard went on to have the abortion. "And at that time I was glad I was having it done. But I think anybody who had had a pregnancy terminated always looks back and thinks, 'Would that have been a boy or would that have been the girl I always wanted?' And every year think, 'How old would it have been now?' you know."[219]

Although few informants had personal experience with abortion, many, regardless of family size, discussed both the trend toward smaller families and their parents' or their own desires and decisions concerning this matter. Some who had had many children wished it had been possible to control numbers. Mrs. Peterson, born in 1899, said she was afraid of abortion: "I would never, although I could have done with less children, done a thing like that. I am not religious, but I should have thought that God would have paid me back, he would either do something to me or the baby. If I had had a baby that had anything wrong with it through that, I would never have lived. You might as well be poor as see your child a cripple or something like that." However, when during their delivery she found out she was having twins when she already had two young children at home, she remembered:

219. Mrs. H5L, 113–15. See also Mrs. T2L, 86. She talked to her GP about having an abortion when her last pregnancy was confirmed in 1971. However, since she was already 16 weeks pregnant, he advised against termination.

I couldn't think of anything to say because I had two at home. Our George was three and our Freda was six and them two. And no extra money. Every baby you had, there was no extra money and I had that on my mind. . . . After that it was four years before I had Margaret and I went to the Infirmary again. It was a young doctor, and he said, "I can't fathom this." They sent me for an x-ray as they thought it was twins again. There must have been tears in my eyes because I was thinking about keeping them. . . . I loved children, but it was the thought of keeping them. You want them to be as nice as others as well as feeding them. He [doctor] said, "It's no good crying now, it's too late!" I felt like saying that it wasn't the woman's fault all the time. You are married and you have got to abide by these things, you know. He [husband] once said that if anybody had seen this squad in here, they would think that we had a wonderful time, but they don't know what I have gone through to try to avoid it, you know. But we never would take anything in them days. God had sent them and they had to be there.[220]

Mrs. Peterson gave birth to six children, although two did not survive. Her account indicates resignation regarding family size, unwillingness to try abortion to end unwanted pregnancies, her husband's control over their sex life, and lack of support (or sympathy) from a young male doctor who apparently viewed her fertility as irresponsible.

By contrast, Mrs. Black, born in 1916, whose paternal grandmother had had 17 children while her parents had had two, explained successful family planning in terms of marital communication and cooperation, saying, "She [mother] was just quite satisfied with me and my brother. . . . They were people that thought things out first. They wouldn't go rash bang into anything. Even when they were going on holiday. It would be, 'Should we go here? Or what do you think?' They would sort it out between themselves."[221] Mr. Glover, born in 1913, was one of three children. He commented: "During my parents' time the large Victorian family had gone by that time. My maternal and paternal grandfathers, they both had somewhere in the region of nine or ten children, but my parents had only three and that was about normal at that time, although there were a lot of people with more children. But that was normal at that time because you were coming on to the First World War then."[222] Asked when people started limiting family size, Mrs. Masterson, born in 1913, responded: "I reckon it was round about 1929. They would start with five or four children and if they had six that was excessive. They gradually began to realize that there was nothing for them. Then all this social reform came in and started with this

220. Mrs. P1P, 12. See also Mr. M10L, 30.
221. Mrs. B2P, 29.
222. Mr. G3P, 1.

family allowance, that was the beginning. Then there was the doctor and all this. It helped them to realize that there was nothing in having these big families. When these methods came out they found they could do something about it."[223] This account illustrates Mrs. Masterson's association of the expanding welfare state and working-class dependence on professional medicine with changing perception of both ideal family size and potential control of conception.

Informants suggested a number of reasons for limiting family size. Supporting Dr. Pilkington's pre–World War I speculation about selfishness and pleasure-seeking, Mr. Ford, born in 1906, said that people limited family size in the 1930s because "things were becoming so much fun, so much pleasure around, after the time we had been through, that they were more interested in what they could get out of life than starting families. And they had seen so much with big families that I don't think anyone would attempt it. We had learnt sense and we had better education than our father and mothers had."[224] Many couples practiced birth control for economic reasons. Mrs. Harrison, born in 1945, said she had a brother ten years older than herself. "My mother lost a child before I was born, two years before me I think, a premature child. But I think there was family talk that my dad had insisted on not having a big family because he couldn't survive business-wise. He was building up from nothing I suppose." Her father had a market garden.[225] Mrs. Adderly, born in 1932, began her family in the 1950s. She said, "I didn't want too many, I didn't want a right big family, but I wanted more than one. . . . Well, it's just keeping them decent, you know. I mean, you like to think they are getting what they want, what they need and keep them nice and everything. Whereas, when you have a big family, it is hard, isn't it?"[226] Similarly, Mr. Boswell, born in 1920, said he wanted no more than three children: "Well, it was hard work and not only that, you can't really cater for more than three." Mrs. Boswell added, "You can cope with them, can't you, give them a decent start in life?"[227]

By the post–World War II years, it is clear both that large families were associated with poverty and that smaller families were considered more respectable than bigger ones. Mrs. Boyle, whose five children were born during the 1950s and 1960s, remembered of her Preston neighborhood:

They were all working-class people, they had all worked in the factory. They worked on the railway or cotton mills, you know, all like that. And they were all big families, you know. All family. There weren't many in them streets that didn't have families, were there.

223. Mrs. M1P, 47.
224. Mr. F1P, 69. See also Mrs. P2P, 22.
225. Mrs. H9P, 2.
226. Mrs. A4L, 43.
227. Mr. B4B, 10, 55.

Mr. Boyle: But they still had one street that were more upper class than the next street.

Mrs. Boyle: Harrison Street were like that, weren't it?

Mr. Boyle: They classed themselves better.

Mrs. Boyle: Because, like, some of them had bathrooms, you know, which were great then. Because there weren't many, because I mean, like, we hadn't. . . . We used to have to go to Saul Street baths, local baths, you know, for ours. But they used to look down on. . . . There were some that only had one or two children, you know, in other streets. They could, of course, afford better things for themselves and for their kids, you know.[228]

Associated with this shift was a change in norms about appropriate family size. Mrs. Wheaton, born in 1933, recalled: "I said I wanted three, three lads actually . . . when I was in my teens, but I think perhaps if we'd had two lads, I would've gone on and had three, whatever it was, but we got a boy and a girl and that was it . . . never felt like a proper family . . . with Derek, but as soon as I got Janet, suddenly we felt like a family . . . just felt complete, yes, so I had no ambitions to have any more after that."[229] It is also apparent that changes in marital relationships and male attitudes regarding women's obligation to bear children may have influenced family size. Mr. Ingham, born in 1930, said his ex-wife did not want more than one child. "I think it's all right if I was saying, 'I want a baby, I want another son.' But really I wouldn't demand it of a woman, you know. Some people did, I suppose, but I don't think I would. No, it's too big a thing to take off a woman, five years, six years. Or even more, isn't it, having a baby?"[230]

The oral evidence reveals that some couples were more successful than others at planning family size. In addition to the occasional desire for many children or traditional fatalism about conception and family size, as we have seen, barriers to family limitation included ignorance of birth control techniques. For example, Mrs. Becker, who had had a very bad first birth, described the way her family grew: "Well, I was seven years before I had another, you see. Then I sort of wanted one, you know, she was at school, and we got another daughter, like, and then it was only three years after when we had another and then I went another seven and a half years, and then this one came along, so my husband said, really, you've been tied all your life, all your married life, with babies, he said. Instead of us having them all . . . but we were so ignorant, we were, really."[231] This account suggests a successful attempt to space pregnancies, but inability to prevent them confidently. Some informants indicated distaste for contraception,

228. Mrs. B11P, 49.
229. Mrs. W5B, 22.
230. Mr. I2L, 53.
231. Mrs. B1P, 44.

associating birth control (particularly barrier methods) with sexual vice. Mrs. Dent, born in 1908, had a friend who was a hospital Sister. This friend told Mrs. Dent about prostitutes who were "fumigated" for venereal diseases and treated for botched abortions. Then the sister described a diaphragm: "She told me what you could buy in the chemist shop, they were like a woman's womb, made of rubber, and they put that in, and that man just believes . . . and then they take it out and wash it. She said, 'How dirty can they get?'" Asked, "And you had never heard of that before?" Mrs. Dent responded, "Never in my life. I was 49 when I got to know that."[232]

In addition to lack of knowledge or inclination regarding birth control methods, religious beliefs and clerical influence continued to influence family planning and the use of contraception. Mrs. Peterson commented:

I've said many a time that I would get locked up if the priest heard me. I said that there was many a woman in her grave today through having a big family and didn't want to. The priest used to come round and they used to be terrified of the priest and they used to make such a fuss of them, treated them like God. I never did that, I never made a fuss of them. . . . Why should a young fellow old enough to be his grandmother nearly, come and tell you what you should and what you shouldn't do in your married life? They have never been married and they don't know what it is like.[233]

Mr. Thomas, born in 1903, commented, "The people at that time were so religious conscious that the church had a lot to do with what they were doing. If the church said it was wrong, it was wrong. Even if it was right, it was wrong. There was a certain amount of fear. . . . I don't think the church is in favor of family planning now."[234] According to Mrs. Musgrove, born in 1886 in Barrow, religion also influenced information and services provided by doctors:

I worked voluntary for a couple of years at a clinic that was held on Barrow Island. The mothers used to come and see the nurse and the doctor and I was asked to help. I charted the babies' weights, nurse weighed the baby, and I saw a great deal there that would have made me a suffragette if I hadn't felt like it. One mother came, and I said to someone what a poor bedraggled person she was and they said, "Yes, that's her twentieth child and she's going to have another." She died, of course. I saw the husband pushing a pram and you never saw such a miserable, wretched shrimp of a creature. That was her twentieth child she brought, no wonder she looked miserable. They wanted the doc-

232. Mrs. D1P, 54.
233. Mrs. P1P, 88.
234. Mr. T2P, 43. See also Mr. S4P, 28.

tor to teach family planning and she refused. It was her principle, she was an RC and wouldn't teach family planning. Of course, the Roman Church doesn't approve, not now, and of course then it was absolutely tabooed.[235]

Several other older informants mentioned that they were unable to get birth control information or help from physicians.[236] However, increasingly doctors led the way in helping working-class women to limit family size. Mrs. Fleming, who had a miscarriage in the early 1950s after having had six births quite close together, was advised by her doctor to be surgically sterilized: "Well they (doctors) said it more than me really. I mean, if I had have gone on, I might have had sixteen or seventeen."[237] Dr. Armstrong said of his Lancaster practice, "We were quite interested in contraception from an early stage, much before, you know, any of the clinics were established. We are talking, I mean, about fitting diaphragms and that and general advice, a long time before the pill, or it was a long time before communities pushed so much." He said during his career he gave birth control advice

> to my people without any hesitation whatsoever. I was a bit reluctant if you are talking about girls under sixteen. . . . What I used to do was, I used to say, "Well, have you discussed it with your mother?" And if they said, "No," I said, "Will you discuss it with your mother, and or your father?" And if they said, "Well, no, I don't want to do it." And then you just had to ask them what were the chances were of getting an unwanted pregnancy, and if you thought there were chances of them getting an unwanted pregnancy, you just went out and gave them advice. We never questioned religion.[238]

Before 1950, the main ways informants prevented conception were abstinence and *coitus interruptus*—techniques that were also usual in other parts of the country, arguably because they were controlled by men, did not involve artificial and embarrassing barrier methods, and were private and comparatively respectable.[239] Simon Szreter observes "the importance of 'a culture of abstinence' in providing the principal means for birth control in British society throughout the period in which fertility fell."[240] Although few oral history informants explicitly discussed using either abstinence or withdrawal to space pregnancies, they implied use of these methods or

235. Mrs. M3B, 13.
236. See, for example, Mrs. D3P, 30.
237. Mrs. F1L, 110. See also Mrs. T2L, 86; Mrs. J1B, 12.
238. Dr. A5L, 14–15.
239. In "'She was quite satisfied with the arrangements I made,'" Kate Fisher argues that scholars have underestimated male influence over family planning, but she stresses the importance of that influence.
240. Szreter, *Fertility, Class, and Gender*, 420.

used metaphors to describe them. As we have seen above, even among older interviewees, a "good" or "responsible" husband was one who limited his sexual demands, thus also reducing both the number of his wife's pregnancies and the number of children they produced.[241] Sometimes couples stopped having sex for health reasons. Mrs. Hopkins, born in 1903, had a bad time with her first delivery, and her doctor advised her not to have more children.[242] Mrs. Maxwell, born in 1898, remembered her husband being ill in the 1930s: "After he was ill, the doctor at the time said that we would have to have separate beds because my husband wasn't well for a long time after. . . . We had no sex for awhile until he got better."[243] Mrs. Washburn, born in 1900, said she only had one child because "I didn't feel strong enough to have any more." She felt contraception "is up to your husband" and used a metaphor for *coitus interruptus:* "Don't forget, always get off the bus at South Shore, don't go all the way to Blackpool. That was how they kept their family down. It was just that the men had to be careful."[244] Mrs. Maxwell, born in 1898, recommended abstinence to prevent pregnancy: "I can remember my eldest daughter and her friend coming to ask me how to manage not having any more children. . . . It was really Lily that said it, Margaret's friend. Mind you, she had no mother and she lived with an auntie who had never been married. She said that she didn't want another one [baby]. I said, 'Well, you'll have to behave yourselves then.' What could I tell them? I didn't know anything."[245]

In the mid-twentieth century, contraception became both increasingly respectable and medicalized, although older interviewees still found it difficult to talk about this subject. Working-class people began to use barrier methods. The oldest informant to report using a condom for birth control in marriage was Mr. Danner, born in 1910, who was untypical in many respects, not least in his tendency to base family decisions on research and reading. When he and his bride arrived for their honeymoon in Blackpool in the 1930s,

> I realized now we were married that I would have to do something about birth control, so I went along to Boots the chemist. I was surprised how busy these shops were. I stood outside for ages waiting while a male assistant was free. Then I dashed in and asked for my requirements. I was answered, I thought, in a very cultured, "We don't sell them." I dashed out of the shop with my face red. I had another long

241. See, for example, Mrs. D1P, 31; Mrs. S2B, 29.

242. Mrs. H8P, 36. See also Mrs. H2P, 20; Mrs. L3B, 26.

243. Mrs. M3P, 12.

244. Mrs. W4P, 19. The bus metaphor was common among informants. See also, for example, Mr. W6P (born 1887), 19; Mrs. H5L (born 1931), 112. It is worthy of remark that Mrs. W4P said she disapproved of the Pill because it encourages "badness." However, she may have confused the birth control pill with abortifacients, because she also commented, "I never took any pills, but I never had any more babies" (12).

245. Mrs. M3P, 53.

wait outside another chemist's. This time I wrote my requirements on a piece of paper. The male assistant laughed and asked me what size I required. I was stunned and muttered, "Average." He was joking and put me at ease: "They sold thousands."[246]

Mr. Danner's experience was not unusual at a time when condoms and diaphragms were associated with deviant sex and sold in brown paper packages, by mail order, under the counter in chemist and barber shops, or in "rubber shops" specializing in sex-related goods.[247] However, particularly after World War II, younger informants reported having prevented pregnancy by means increasingly supplied by official health care providers, including the cap (diaphragm), sheath (condom), coil (intrauterine device [IUD]), Pill, and surgical sterilization and vasectomy.[248] It is possible that the dominant male experience of military service in World War II, when men were routinely issued condoms, helped to spread their use among the civilian population.[249] Alternatively, it is also arguable that the shift from moral to scientific conceptualization of sex, observed above, changed the cultural context of contraception and removed barriers to both communication about and use of birth control methods, while the related growing cultural authority of physicians increased their influence among working-class patients. Thus, for example, Mrs. Gerard, born in 1958, said that with her mother's knowledge her doctor put her on birth control pills as a teenager to control her periods, and that her husband had a vasectomy once they felt their family was complete (with three children). She also reported that her mother, who had had five children in the 1950s and '60s, had controlled her family size with "Durex" (condoms)—information an older woman would be unlikely to have known about her own mother.[250]

Rising use of barrier and surgical birth control technologies arguably accompanied a shift in normative responsibility for contraception from men to women. Mrs. Jenkins, born in 1932, described having had three babies in quick succession, despite her recent recovery from tuberculosis:

> We didn't do anything, no, my husband wouldn't do anything and he said it was up to me, and I used to go to the doctor and, I don't know, things were very sort of . . .
> *Interviewer:* You didn't talk about it a lot, did you?
> *Informant:* No, no, and you were very embarrassed with the doctor, and my husband never used anything, he didn't like, he said, but

246. Mr. D2P, 50. Also quoted in Roberts, *A woman's place*, 97.
247. See Leathard, *The fight for family planning*, 5, 23, for brief discussion of "rubber shops."
248. Roberts, *Women and families*, 76–81. See, for example, Mrs. H5L, 113; Mrs. L3L, 54.
249. See, for example, Mr. M10L, 30.
250. Mrs. G5P, 48–49.

he said it was up to me not to have any, so he'd, I mean you've got to have your husband's permission when you're sterilized and immediately jumped at it. . . . I'm always glad I did because those three children all went on to university, so I mean if we'd had a big family we couldn't have done that, it was a struggle as it was.[251]

Medically managed birth control did not always prevent conception. Mrs. Turnbull, born in 1932, became pregnant with her fourth child in 1971 after having been advised by her doctor to "take a break" from the birth control pill and have an IUD inserted.[252] Regardless, the oral evidence indicates that after World War II, women became dependent on professional medicine for birth control advice and materials.

Despite concern about sustained high infant mortality rates, study city Medical Officers of Health did not mention birth control as a way of improving either maternal health or the prospects for infant survival and vitality before the interwar period. Indeed, Barrow was apparently the first of the three study cities, beginning in 1938, to officially offer family planning services, while, as we have seen, there was a voluntary birth control clinic in that city before World War I.[253] While Lancaster's MOH recognized as early as 1907 the likelihood that abortion accounted for the large number of premature births, nowhere in that city's available annual reports are birth control services mentioned. Preston's public health officials were hostile or neutral to birth control until the 1960s, although the Family Planning Association began offering services there in 1950. In 1966 the city's MOH recognized the changing attitudes toward contraception: "The altered outlook in birth control and family planning has enabled the Council to give active support to the local Family Planning Association to an extent that would not have been dreamt of some years ago and there is building up a close liaison with the health visitors which is resulting in the facilities of the Association being utilized by a wider section of the population."[254] This evidence suggests that working-class people received very little professional medical help with limiting family size until after World War II, when birth control became increasingly respectable. Indeed, it is possible that consumer demand drove provision of professional birth control services in Barrow, Lancaster, and Preston and that the development of medical dominance over access to contraception was a by-product rather than a cause of this process.

251. Mrs. J1B, 11.
252. Mrs. T2L, 57. See also Mrs. Y2P, 7.
253. Barrow MOH Report, 1938, 18; Mrs. M3B, 13.
254. Preston MOH Report, 1966, 5.

CONCLUSIONS

How can we account for the changes in working-class attitudes regarding family limitation? Decline of child employment coupled with lengthy compulsory education changed the role of children in working-class families from contributor to consumer. This, along with decreasing infant mortality and increasing working-class prosperity, helped to stimulate successful family limitation which, in turn, required and rendered respectable knowledge and utilization of birth control methods.[255] As contraception became both respectable and almost universally used, abortion lost its tenuous claim to respectability in working-class neighborhoods and was increasingly associated with back-street, furtive, dirty old women. Only the transfer of legal abortion into the hands of physicians after 1967 rescued the procedure's cultural status as an acceptable way of limiting family size.

Similarly, wider social and economic changes influenced working-class attitudes and communication regarding sex. The smaller working-class families of the interwar and post–World War II periods, living in vastly improved houses with bathrooms, had less reason to worry about incest stimulated by overcrowding and, thus, reduced the need to keep information about bodies and sex from children. In those smaller families, there was an increase and alteration in parent-child communication about sexual and other matters, which was fostered by external influences including the theories of Freud and Spock. In addition to these authoritative theories, as I have argued elsewhere, working-class families developed increasing dependence on professional experts to manage health, illness, and childbearing.[256] As informants' references to consultation of "doctor's books" for information about sex suggests, sex and reproduction were also being medicalized—removed from the sphere of lay knowledge and control.[257]

In addition, younger informants' experience of sex education suggests that sex was joining subjects that were respectable enough to be discussed at school. One can speculate that inclusion in the curriculum both demystified and "scientized" a topic that may have been more interesting when it was secret. It is also possible that this process moved at least some aspects of sexuality (e.g., menstruation) out of the powerful realm of the social and moral into the same rational, safe, useful, and rather dull sphere as nutrition and dental hygiene. The same process consigned some traditional ideas, such as the prohibition of hair-washing during menstruation, to the disreputable realm of old wives' tales.

What about the importance of respectability? I do not mean to suggest

255. See Seccombe, *Weathering the storm*, 157–58, 177; Leathard, *The fight for family planning*; Soloway, *Birth control*.

256. Beier, "'I used to take her to the doctor's and get the *proper* thing,'" 221–41; Beier, "Expertise and control," 404–9.

257. See, for example, Mrs. A3L, 44. See also Oakley, *The captured womb*.

that working-class individuals and families stopped caring about their reputations or that sexual behavior ceased to affect those reputations. However, as working-class dependence on mutual aid declined as a result of increasing prosperity and expansion of the formal social safety net, the importance of respectability within the small world of the neighborhood arguably also declined. Furthermore, the components of working-class respectability changed. Instead of the intense focus on sexual demeanor within an enclosed social world, other elements, including educational attainment, occupation, and income became factors in individual and family reputations.

Chapter Six

❧

"With having my mother, I didn't need any advice off anybody else"

Bearing and Caring for Children

INTRODUCTION

Of all health-related processes, childbearing and infant care have historically been the most strongly associated with and controlled by women.
While in Britain male practitioners began taking an interest in midwifery
in the seventeenth century, working-class women continued to depend
mainly on neighborhood-based social childbirth until the mid-twentieth
century.[1] Traditionally attended by their female relatives, friends, and
informally trained midwives, they called in a doctor only for emergencies.
Only the very poor gave birth in charitable lying-in hospitals or workhouse
infirmaries, institutions that also sometimes offered training to medical
students and midwives.[2] While professional outpatient maternity services
were offered and welcomed in some cities, in general working-class women
avoided institutional care, preferring to give birth at home when possible,
assisted by neighborhood midwives.[3] This tradition both projected and pro-

---

1. See, for example, Adrian Wilson, *The making of man-midwifery: Childbirth in England,
1660–1770* (Cambridge, MA: Harvard University Press, 1995); Lucinda McCray Beier, *Sufferers
and healers: The experience of illness in seventeenth-century England* (London and New York:
Routledge and Kegan Paul, 1987), 15–19, 186–87, 233–35; Lucinda McCray Beier, "Expertise
and control: Childbearing in three twentieth-century working-class Lancashire communities,"
Bulletin of the History of Medicine 78:2 (2004): 379–409.

2. Brian Abel-Smith, *The hospitals 1800–1948: A study in social administration in England and
Wales* (Cambridge, MA: Harvard University Press, 1964), 14, 23.

3. See, for example, Lara Marks, "Mothers, babies and hospitals: 'The London' and the
provision of maternity care in East London, 1870–1939," in Valerie Fildes, Lara Marks, and
Hilary Marland, eds., *Women and children first: International maternal and infant welfare 1870–1945*

tected family respectability, building participants' reputations for appropriate behavior and limiting outside intervention in private matters.

Similarly, child care was considered the natural and primary responsibility of all women, but was especially central to the identities of working-class mothers who, unlike their middle- and upper-class counterparts, did the work themselves without relying on servants. Knowledge of child development and management passed between generations and among neighbors. As we have seen, mothers routinely dealt independently with serious childhood ailments; it was rare for children outside of major cities to be treated in a hospital for any but notifiable contagious diseases before the interwar period.[4] Babies were born—and frequently died—at home, often without professional medical attention or ascription of blame to caregivers. However, it was continued high infant mortality, in contrast to declining overall mortality rates, that attracted official attention toward the end of the nineteenth century, stimulating the infant welfare movement that shifted expertise and authority from mothers to health care professionals and the transition of birth and the care of sick children from home to hospital.[5] In Barrow, Lancaster, and Preston, as elsewhere in Britain, childbearing women made the transition from mothers to patients, their pregnancies increasingly monitored, their deliveries orchestrated and managed through mounting levels of intervention and technology.[6] Children, no longer the sole charges of their parents (who, in any case, tended to be viewed as inadequate guides and caregivers), became the responsibility and, to some extent, the property of the state, which empowered experts

(London and New York: Routledge, 1992), 48–73.

4. Some cities also had hospitals providing care for chronically ill and crippled children, although these were unusual and admission to them was a distinctly minority experience. See, for example, Bruce Lindsay, "'Pariahs or partners': Welcome and unwelcome visitors in a British children's hospital, 1900–1950," unpublished paper on the Jenny Lind Hospital, Norwich, presented at the American Association of the History of Medicine's annual meeting in Halifax, Nova Scotia, May 2006; Andrea Tanner, "Come all, cure few: The diseases of the in-patients at Great Ormond Street Hospital, 1852–1900," unpublished paper delivered at the Social Science History Association Conference, November 2005, Portland, Oregon.

5. See, for example, Deborah Dwork, *War is good for babies and other young children: A history of the infant and child welfare movement in England 1898–1918* (London and New York: Tavistock Publications, 1987); Richard Allen Soloway, *Birth control and the population question in England, 1877–1930* (Chapel Hill and London: University of North Carolina Press, 1982); Wally Seccombe, *Weathering the storm: Working-class families from the Industrial Revolution to the fertility decline* (London and New York: Verso, 1993); Porter, *Health, civilization and the state,* chapters 8 and 10.

6. See, for example, Ann Oakley, *The captured womb: A history of the medical care of pregnant women* (Oxford: Basil Blackwell, 1984); Edward Shorter, *A history of women's bodies* (Harmondsworth: Penguin, 1984); Judith Walzer Leavitt, *Brought to bed: Child-bearing in America, 1750–1950* (New York and Oxford: Oxford University Press, 1986); Jan Williams, "The controlling power of childbirth in Britain," in *Midwives, society and childbirth: Debates and controversies in the modern period,* Hilary Marland and Anne Marie Rafferty, eds. (London and New York: Routledge, 1997), 232–47.

such as doctors, health visitors, and teachers to direct and support their development.[7]

While it is indisputable that infant and maternal mortality rates dropped as the medicalization of pregnancy, birth, and child care gathered steam, it may be incorrect to presume a cause-effect relationship between these developments.[8] The same factors that extended expectation of life at birth from 46 for men and 49 for women in 1901 to 68 for men and 74 for women in 1961—factors that included improved wages, diet, housing, and sanitation, as well as medical prevention and intervention—also arguably reduced infant and maternal mortality.[9] Furthermore, focusing on whether or not medicalization "worked" begs the questions of why and how it developed and ignores its social and cultural impacts.

Feminist scholars have interpreted the medicalization of pregnancy and birth in gendered terms, as the hijacking of midwifery by medical men from laywomen.[10] While there is no denying that the theft occurred, this new orthodoxy obscures both female collusion in the process and its class dimensions and implications. Middle-class mothers and female health care providers, governmental officials, and members of advocacy groups embraced the medicalization of childbearing and infant welfare, and became its agents.[11] They shared the social status of physicians and were early and enthusiastic converts to professional health culture, which reinforced their sense of propriety and authority over ways to bear and care for children.

The medicalization of child development was rooted in the turn-of-the-century panic about national fitness and competitiveness and rising enthusiasm for efficiency. Regardless of orientation, whether eugenicist or Fabian, imperialist or socialist, conservative or liberal, there existed both broad consensus that children would benefit from greater medical supervision and care and an increasing tendency to identify as medical prob-

7. See, for example, Roger Cooter, ed., *In the name of the child: Health and welfare, 1880–1940* (London and New York: Routledge, 1992); Bernard Harris, *The health of the schoolchild: A history of the school medical service in England and Wales* (Buckingham and Philadelphia: Open University Press, 1995).

8. This relationship is presumed in recent works including Lara Marks, *Model mothers: Jewish mothers and maternity provision in East London, 1870–1939* (Oxford: Clarendon Press, 1994), 9.

9. Helen Jones, *Health and society in twentieth-century Britain* (New York: Longman, 1994), 196; Roy Porter, *The greatest benefit to mankind* (London and New York: W. W. Norton, 1997), 691–93.

10. See, for example, Oakley, *Captured womb;* Leavitt, *Brought to bed;* Jean Donnison, *Midwives and medical men: A history of inter-professional rivalries and women's rights* (New York: Schocken, 1977); Doreen Evenden, *The midwives of seventeenth-century London* (Cambridge: Cambridge University Press, 2000).

11. See, for example, Jane Lewis, *The politics of motherhood: Child and maternal welfare in England, 1900–1930* (London: Croom Helm, 1980); Judy Giles, *Women, identity, and private life in Britain, 1900–1950* (New York: St. Martin's Press, 1995).

lems conditions that might previously have been considered hereditary or environmental.[12] Since middle-class mothers were already routinely seeking doctors' attention for their children, this shift had comparatively little impact on them but instead validated their behavior.

By contrast, medicalization of childbearing and child care was, to a large degree, imposed on a working-class population that maintained lay management of these matters well into the twentieth century. Inevitably, this process had the greatest impact on women as bearers of babies, traditional family health authorities, and (along with children) those who inhabited the very bottom of the food chain in a male-dominated and class-stratified society. As we have seen, public health policymakers and local health authorities held working-class mothers and informal female health authorities responsible for infant and maternal morbidity and mortality. Those agents tended to advocate adoption of healthy habits and medical treatment as solutions to the problems they observed—rather than other possible, but more costly and politically charged alternatives including reduction of poverty, family size, and labor exploitation.[13]

The history of childbirth in the twentieth century is often told as the history of maternity care—midwifery, obstetrics, and clinic and hospital provision. The history of infant welfare tends to focus on the activities of interest groups, policy development, and institutional implementation. Following the work of Jane Lewis, this chapter takes an alternative approach, observing through the contrasting voices of public health professionals and working-class women and men the processes by which pregnancy, birth, and childcare were medicalized, regulated, and institutionalized in Lancaster, Barrow, and Preston. It also considers the relationship between those processes and the norms governing working-class respectability, which was intimately intertwined with sex, pregnancy, birth, and childrearing.

INFANT MORTALITY AND PUBLIC HEALTH SERVICES IN BARROW, LANCASTER, AND PRESTON

Before World War I, it was not uncommon for babies to die within their first year of life, and for mothers to die during or following childbirth. Such deaths were particularly frequent in working-class communities, where they both stimulated and measured the effectiveness of public health services.[14]

12. Dwork, *War is good for babies*, 3–21.

13. See, for example, Lewis, *Politics of motherhood*, 27; Dwork, *War is good for babies*, 19.

14. See, for example, R. I. Woods, P. A. Watterson, and J. H. Woodward, "The causes of rapid infant mortality decline in England and Wales, 1861–1921," Part 1, *Population Studies* 42:3 (1988): 343–66, and Part 2, *Population Studies* 43: 1 (1989): 113–32; Carol Dyhouse, "Working-class mothers and infant mortality in England, 1895–1914," *Journal of Social History* 12:2 (1978):

Infant mortality attracted a host of explanations. Preston's Dr. Pilkington blamed female employment, early marriage, failure to breastfeed, unsanitary preparation of feeding bottles, infants sharing parents' beds, female drunkenness, consultation of local female health authorities, and the small profit arising from insurance.[15] While the language was modified and greater awareness voiced about the challenges facing working-class mothers, the general tenor of these comments is echoed in public health reports throughout the study period. In 1969 Preston's MOH wrote:

> There would seem to be too ready an acceptance that babies are expected to die. There still remains, to a slight extent, the echo from the past when a mother was asked how many children she had, the reply would be, "ten, and I buried four." Insufficient public concern is manifested at this loss of infant life. It is clear that babies' lives can be saved if parents, or those responsible for the care of young babies, recognized the early signs of disease and took their children promptly to their doctors, or asked their doctors to visit early. It is sad to see children lose their lives because a doctor has not been called in time, or in some cases, not called at all.[16]

By contrast, working-class mothers themselves blamed their own ill-health, overwork, and lack of support, as well as diseases that could be neither prevented nor cured.[17] Maternal mortality attracted increased attention during the interwar period, when rates rose, contrasting with declining infant deaths.[18]

Approaches to the problem of infant mortality were linked to philosophical and political orientations. Eugenicists took the Malthusian ("better dead") line that survival of the weak or degenerate undermined the health of the population as a whole; thus, provision of infant welfare services was counterproductive.[19] This perspective was undermined by the shocking mortality of World War I and a growing consensus on the left and right that civilized nations attended to the health and welfare of their children. The contrasting imperialist pronatalist view advocated public support of a large healthy working-class population to enhance British strength and

---

248–67.

15. See, for example, Preston MOH Reports for 1896 (10), 1898 (7), 1899 (14), 1900 (13), 1902 (10–12), 1906 (8–9), 1911 (10–11). See also, for example, Dyhouse, "Working-class mothers," 251–44; Lewis, *Politics of motherhood*, 61.

16. Preston MOH Report, 1969, 4.

17. See, for example, The Women's Co-operative Guild, *Maternity: Letters from working-women* (New York and London: Garland Publishing, 1980. Reprint of the 1915 ed. published by G. Bell); Margery Spring Rice, *Working-class wives: Their health and conditions*, 2nd ed. (London: Virago, 1981). See also Mrs. B1P, 49.

18. Lewis, *Politics of motherhood*, 117–19.

19. Lewis, *Politics of motherhood*, 29–30; Dwork, *War is good for babies*, 3–21.

success in the competition with rising powers such as Germany, the United States, and Japan.[20] Medical Officers of Health for Barrow, Lancaster, and Preston tended toward the latter perspective, advocating the infant welfare services that attracted increasing public support and broadened their own responsibilities and resources, particularly after World War I.

Infant mortality rates in the study cities justified MOH concern about the issue. In 1896 Dr. Pilkington wrote, "During the past ten years the infantile mortality (as estimated by the number of deaths under the age of twelve months to each thousand births), has been for the whole of England and Wales 142, for the large towns 169, and for Preston, always remarkable for its high infantile death rate, not less than 232."[21] In 1910 rates for Barrow (124), Lancaster (137), and Preston (158) remained high compared to that for England and Wales (102). Medical Officers of Health saw working-class infant mortality as an unnecessary waste that could be remedied by maternal education and expert intervention. Working-class people, however, viewed infant death as inevitable, though unfortunate, and rarely held mothers responsible.[22]

More than MOH statistics and commentary, the oral history evidence documents the cultural context and emotional toll of infant mortality. Many older informants said that one or more of their siblings had died as infants or young children. Mrs. Oxley, born in 1902 in Preston commented:

> Well, I had four brothers and four sisters, of course, only six of us lived to be brought up. . . . Well, Olive, they said she was a lovely baby, she was nine months old, the undertaker said it was shame to put her in her coffin, she died of convulsions. They used to have convulsions then. Then another baby, Alice, I think she was only a month old and Mother had us all down with whooping cough and the doctor said, "Be careful of that baby, it doesn't catch it," but it did and it choked with whooping cough. She was only about a month old. Of course, then there was no such thing as an injection for a baby if they got whooping cough or measles. You were just meant to keep them warm and such-like. There was no real thing that they could do.[23]

Like this informant, many blamed such deaths on illnesses that could later

20. Anna Davin, "Imperialism and motherhood," *History Workshop* 5 (1978): 9–65; Harris, *The health of the schoolchild*, 7–8.

21. Preston MOH Report, 1896, 9.

22. This fatalism was sometimes supported by family doctors. For example, Mrs. Crest (Mrs. C3P) (born in Preston in 1897) gave birth to only one child, who died at birth. She said, "I asked the doctor, 'Why did my baby die when I wanted it so much?' He said, 'You never know. You could have many more because physically there's nothing wrong with you.' Poor child, but I was rightly constituted, so he said. But it never came my way again" (12).

23. Mrs. O1P, 3. See also, for example, Mr. B1B, 15; Mrs. C2L, 16; Mrs. H8P, 1, 10; Mr. L1L, 1; Mrs. M3L, 14; Mrs. M3P, 4; Mrs. S5P, 21.

have been prevented or cured—although they did not necessarily favor medical intervention. For example, Mr. Glover, born in Preston in 1913, said his mother thought vaccination caused the death of his older brother at 12 months, and Mr. Ackerman, born in 1904 in Barrow, attributed the death of an infant sibling to medicine prescribed for his mother when she was breastfeeding.[24] As we have seen, some interviewees thought babies died if mothers had too many pregnancies too close together. And several informants agreed with the social investigator B. Seebohm Rountree: "Lots of babies died because of the poor homes."[25]

Ellen Ross describes the attachment of poor London mothers to their newborns in the years between 1870 and 1918 as "tentative," saying these babies "were not officially viewed as persons and were not always loved as children."[26] This observation was also true of some working-class mothers in Barrow, Lancaster, and Preston before World War I.[27] In families with many children and few resources, there might even be relief when an infant did not survive, as well as minimal effort to support the live birth of a baby that appeared "not right." For example, Mr. Peel, born in Barrow in 1909, said it was common to lose newborns: "Oh, a lot of people did, a lot of people. But they just never brought them [the babies] to, did they, they just left them. If it wasn't right, they just left them, they didn't smack its bum or anything like that. . . . Like they used to say in the old days, 'Put it at the bottom of the bed.' And that was it, it was finished, it wasn't right."[28] However, it is also clear that, despite poverty and the fragility of new life, many parents mourned the loss of an infant. Mr. Townley, born in 1897, whose mother gave birth to 17 babies, 13 of whom survived, said, "She was always upset. She had cried many a time. To think she had gone through all that, nine months. She never liked losing any."[29]

The oral evidence reveals that children knew far more about infant death than they knew about sex, pregnancy, or birth. Several informants remembered small bodies being prepared for burial. Mrs. Havelock, born in Preston in 1903, said stillborn babies "were put in a box and put under the bed until this man came and took them somewhere. . . . I think the child's birth had to be registered, but after a couple of days somebody would call and take the box away. There was a rumor at the time that they were buried in paupers' graves."[30] Mrs. Addison, born in 1892 in Barrow,

24. Mr. G3P. 1; Mr. A2B, 14.

25. See, for example, Dwork, *War is good for babies*, 14–15; Mrs. R1B, 19. See also, for example, Mr. F3B, 12; Dr. K1P, 6; Mr. L1L, 1.

26. Ellen Ross, *Love and toil: Motherhood in outcast London, 1870–1918* (New York and Oxford: Oxford University Press, 1993), 184.

27. Elizabeth Roberts, *A woman's place: An oral history of working-class women 1890–1940* (Oxford and New York: Basil Blackwell, 1985), 165.

28. Mr. P6B, 27–28. See also Mr. T2P, 37.

29. Mr. T1P, 42. See also Mrs. G1B, 19.

30. Mrs. H4P, 30.

recalled as a twelve-year-old being asked by her mother to stay home from school and deliver a stillborn infant to the gravedigger for interment in the "public grave." Rather than reacting with horror, this informant expressed both pride in being given an adult responsibility and confidence about accomplishing it.[31]

Nonetheless, respectable families felt shame about consignment of infants to paupers' graves. Mr. Danner, born in 1910 in Preston, remembered his "brother who had died at birth and had been buried in a pauper's grave. My mother had told me this. She was bitter about it. In her time, a child that had not been baptised was not even buried in consecrated ground."[32] To prevent this possibility, families sometimes requested emergency baptism of an infant thought to be in danger of death.[33] In addition, most parents purchased burial insurance for their children to cover the cost of a respectable funeral and interment. Mr. Carson, born in 1902 in Lancaster, said he and his siblings "were insured at birth for death. There were a lot of epidemics, things that you don't hear about now. I had the lot—scarlet fever, measles, ringworm and whooping cough."[34] Mrs. Masterson, born in 1913 in Preston, said her mother bought burial insurance for children "as soon as we were born. I still pay mine and I'm 66. As soon as you were born you were put in the Shelley Insurance and you paid a penny each week and I still pay that penny. I only get £12 when I die. . . . That was the thing, in those days they didn't depend on charity like them today."[35] This effort, expense, and the dismal reality that required it renders particularly callous Dr. Pilkington's 1896 comment that "Amongst other causes [for infant mortality] must be mentioned that of Insurance, by which the death of a child brings a monetary gain to the parents."[36]

PREGNANCY AND ANTENATAL CARE

To combat, first, high infant mortality rates and, after 1920, high maternal mortality rates, public health agencies advocated notification of births, home visits by health visitors, antenatal care, provision of child health clinic services, employment of licensed midwives or physicians for deliveries, and, ultimately, hospital birth—measures emphasizing the importance of professional advice and institutional care.[37] Their targets were the unhygienic

31. Mrs. A3B, 3. This event is quoted at length in Roberts, *A woman's place*, 21.
32. Mr. D2P, 53.
33. See, for example, Mrs. M3P, 4.
34. Mr. C1L, 10. See also, for example, Mrs. A1P, 38; Mr. B7P, 40; Miss C2L, 16; Mrs. C5P, 37; Mrs. C7L, 51; Mrs. D1B, 11.
35. Mrs. M1P, 50.
36. Preston MOH Report, 1896, 10. See also Lewis, *Politics of motherhood*, 77.
37. See Lewis, *What price community medicine*, for an overview of public health provision in

conditions surrounding working-class birth and infant care and the ignorance and negligence of traditional "handywoman" midwives and working-class mothers. Their message was clear: if working-class mothers could
only be persuaded to emulate middle-class mothers, their babies would
not die.

Increasingly, professional supervision was thought necessary during
pregnancy as well as after delivery.[38] Each of the study communities opened
publicly supported antenatal clinics after World War I. Pressure for public health authorities to provide, and pregnant women to use, antenatal
services was linked to development of biomedical laboratory and diagnostic techniques. It is noteworthy that accurate laboratory diagnosis of
pregnancy became available only in the 1920s. Routine testing of urine
for the albumin that, with other symptoms, indicated possible toxemia of
pregnancy, began during the same decade.[39] Public health professionals
expected antenatal care to detect obstetrical abnormalities, enable referral
of at-risk mothers to doctors or hospitals, and reduce the number of premature babies born. Clinic attendance, interviews with uniformed health
care providers, examination, and diagnostic testing paved the way to the
medicalization of pregnancy and birth for both caregivers and what could
now be described as patients (e.g., pregnant women).

Preston's Health Authority opened its first antenatal clinic in 1919. By
the early 1930s, the city's clinics were routinely seeing between 346 and
482 new patients each year—less than one-third of expectant mothers.[40]
The clinics offered pregnancy tests and checked blood pressure, weight,
urine, and presentation of the fetus. The MOH commented in 1934, "Most
women appreciate the value of regular supervision, and seriously regard
the advice given. Our difficulty is to reach the diffident, the unintelligent,
the careless and the overburdened." The main abnormality detected at
the antenatal clinics in that year was tooth decay (109). Other problems
included transverse presentation (98), albuminuria (44), anemia (34),
varicose veins (33), constipation (18), contracted pelvis (16), breech presentations (16), heart disease (13), and high blood pressure (6).[41] Official

---

the period. Ann Oakley (*The captured womb*) remains the authority on antenatal care. Irvine
Loudon's research on infant and maternal mortality assesses factors contributing to incidence,
including socioeconomic conditions and quality of assistance at deliveries. See, for example,
"On maternal and infant mortality 1900–1960," *Social History of Medicine* 4:1 (1991): 29–74. The
term "antenatal" is used throughout this chapter because it appears both in official sources and
in oral history accounts, rather than the term "prenatal," which is more familiar to American
readers.

38. See, for example, Barrow MOH Report, 1913, 282; Lancaster MOH Report, 1913, 88.

39. Oakley, *Captured womb*, 17, 277–79.

40. Preston MOH Report, 1933, 93. Beginning in the 1930s, Preston's expectant mothers
also attended antenatal clinics at Preston Royal Infirmary and Sharoe Green Hospital. Oral
history accounts indicate that women increasingly received regular antenatal care from their
GPs as well.

41. Preston MOH Report, 1934, 98. It is noteworthy that these free clinics detected a range

provision of antenatal care changed with the introduction of the National Health Service in 1948. After this time, women received care at no charge from their general practitioners. In addition, with growing numbers of consultant obstetricians, after the mid-1950s pregnant women were increasingly seen by specialists as part of routine antenatal care.[42]

Few informants born before 1920 said that either their mothers or they themselves (or their wives) had had professional antenatal care.[43] The traditional pattern was for a woman to plan for her confinement by "booking" the midwife. The mother remained firmly in charge of the process. According to Mr. Priestly, born in 1909, "They used to do the time [i.e., experience their pregnancy] and then, when everything was right and they had an idea of how long, they would go and book the midwife. And then the midwife when the time was coming would come round on a bicycle . . . and do what she had to do, you see. Examine them and say, oh well, when you're ready, give me a call."[44] A few interviewees remembered receiving traditional advice about caring for themselves in pregnancy to ensure an easier delivery. Mrs. Sykes, born in 1927, was advised by her aunt to drink raspberry leaf tea: "Your inside will be like jelly and you will have no trouble."[45] Mrs. Wallington, born in 1923, remembered, "My mum told me to take liquid paraffin and I took liquid paraffin every day, twice a day. And of course when the baby was born I didn't . . . have any pains or anything."[46] Only informants who were ill during their pregnancies sought medical help.[47]

Part of the challenge in persuading women to use formal antenatal services was traditional working-class modesty and shame regarding pregnancy because of its association with sexual activity. Respectable pregnancy was a very private matter, discussed only with close relatives and friends and concealed from children, acquaintances, and strangers. Mrs. Carter, born in 1919, spoke for many. She had no regular antenatal care, although she was examined twice in nine months. "I never went out when I were pregnant, not till it was over with. I used to feel ashamed, because I knew they would think what I'd been doing and I used to think it was terrible."[48]

---

of health problems widely present in the working-class female population of the time and offered pregnant working-class women health screening that their nonpregnant contemporaries often could not afford before the introduction of the National Health Service. See Margery Spring Rice, *Working-class wives,* 2nd ed. (London: Virago, 1981), for information about working-class women's health collected by a survey begun in 1933.

42. Preston's consultative antenatal clinic opened in April 1954.

43. According to Lewis, *Politics of motherhood,* 155, little antenatal care was being given outside of London before the 1930s.

44. Mr. P6B, 51. See also Mrs. D3P, 29.

45. Mrs. S3B, 75.

46. Mrs. W4L, 38.

47. For example, Mrs. S1L, born in 1898, had her first baby in 1929. She said, "I was very ill and Dr. Kay was coming sixpence a week. He sent a bill for one pound one" (28).

48. Mrs. C5P, 30. See also Mrs. M6P, 31; Mrs. P2P, 23.

Preston's public health authorities ran into this problem in 1931, when they opened a new neighborhood antenatal clinic: "Working-class mothers will not attend an antenatal center near their own homes owing, in the earlier months, to a desire to keep the knowledge of their pregnancies a secret from their neighbors. A considerable proportion have objected to attending a clinic where schoolchildren are also present. Those mothers who were told that Cuttle Street was their center simply did not attend at all."[49] Pregnancy was also concealed from other children in the family. Mrs. Dorrington, born in 1905, remembered, "In those days, there was no maternity clothes, you just had a big piece of tape with a safety-pin here when you were expanding, and my brother said, 'You want to get yourself a new skirt, Mum. You figure's gone terrible.' He didn't know there was a baby on the way. He was 19 nearly. . . . She just cried with shame."[50]

Despite normative concealment of pregnancy, for working-class mothers in the late nineteenth and early twentieth centuries this condition was both "normal," in the sense that it was expected, appropriate, and common for married women, and "special," in that it was attended by risks not encountered by people who were not pregnant. Although pregnancy was not considered an illness, expectant mothers perceived dangers including overwork, special vulnerability to injury, and having babies too close together.[51] However, birth and the lying-in period were considered a much more perilous time, when the life and future health of the mother hung in the balance. Thus, traditional working-class management of childbearing focused on confinement rather than pregnancy.

Many informants reported that their mothers did not have professional antenatal care, but that they or their wives had received regular attention during pregnancy from a doctor, midwife, clinic, or hospital.[52] The experience of Mrs. Jenkins, born in 1932, was typical of the younger age group: "You came and spent nearly the whole day at Risedale Maternity Home Hospital, and when I say the whole day, you were there from about 9 in the morning, I think everybody got the same appointment, from about 9 in the morning 'til say about dinner-time or 2 o'clock sometimes, and they did check everything, blood, blood pressure, weight, if there was any problems at all . . . they immediately took you into the Annexe [inpatient facility]."[53] Informants whose children were born after about 1955 remembered attending childbirth preparation classes provided through the National Health Service.[54]

49. Preston MOH Report, 1931, 85.

50. Mrs. D3P, 31.

51. See, for example, Mrs. H7P, 4; Mrs. P1P, 93.

52. See, for example, Mr. R3B, 57; Mrs. H6L, 43; Mrs. L3L, 52; Mrs. W6L, 82; Mrs. C8P, 151; Mrs. G5P, 44; Mrs. K2P, 106; Mrs. R1P, 65.

53. Mrs. J1B, 12. See also Mrs. M1P, 50.

54. See, for example, Mrs. P5B, 40; Mrs. C7L, 34; Mrs. C8P, 151; Mrs. J1B, 12; Mrs. T2L, 54;

Formal antenatal care led to increased medical management of and intervention in deliveries. For example, Mrs. Lewthwaite, born in 1920, was hospitalized for 14 weeks before the birth of her only child. "It was high blood pressure I was troubled with, and I went in at the Whitsuntide, which was the end of May. . . . And he was born on the last day of August, and then I had to do a fortnight after that, so it was the 14th of September when I came out." An obstetrician, nurse, and "lady doctor" were present for the birth, during which Mrs. Lewthwaite was given both "gas and air" and a general anesthetic. "I was very small . . . and that was the trouble. So, of course, afterwards I had clips in, I was torn slightly, and I had clips in for awhile."[55]

HOME CONFINEMENT

Before 1920, almost all Barrow, Lancaster, and Preston births took place at home. The birth environment, people present, and management of delivery were controlled by the mother, her female relatives, an informal neighborhood health expert (who sometimes served as a monthly nurse), and tradition. The majority of working-class babies were delivered by informally qualified midwives (called "handywomen" by MOsH). All but the poorest mothers stayed in bed for two weeks after delivery; female relatives and neighbors assumed their housework and child care responsibilities.[56] Indeed, in the oral evidence childbirth was among the most commonly mentioned times when working-class families called upon their mutual aid networks. Mr. Clarke, born in Barrow in 1900, remembered, "When my mother had all her [four] babies at home, the neighbors helped and you didn't have to pay anybody. . . . Everybody helped, they came in and did your washing and looked after the rest of your children."[57] Mrs. Washburn, born in 1899 in Preston, whose mother had nine births, explained, "The neighbors did a lot for each other because there was no district nurse. There was no National Health and so the doctors were very rarely called upon because they made charges. Often people would come and borrow things for a birth."[58]

Appropriate care in the lying-in period was considered crucial by both informal and professional attendants, although it became less common

Mrs. H3P, 43.

55. Mrs. L3B, 24.

56. See, for example, Roberts, *A woman's place*, and *Women and families*; Giles, *Women, identity, and private life in Britain*; Beier, "Expertise and control."

57. Mr. C1B, 25.

58. Mrs. W1P, 11. See also Mrs. B11P (born 1936) who compared a long, lonely stay in hospital with her first birth to neighborhood management of her subsequent four confinements (47).

after World War II for women to be confined to bed, fed a special diet, or told to wear a belly binder. The consensus was that rising too soon after delivery was terribly risky. Mrs. Drake, born in Barrow in 1899, remembered that midwives made mothers stay in bed for at least ten days: "They wouldn't let you get up because they said that your bones, the backbone where the child is, they have to knit together."[59] Mrs. Martin, born in 1914, remembered that she was "in [hospital for] a fortnight for Geoffrey, during which you never put your feet to the floor for ten days, and the old wives' saying was that if you put your feet to the floor you drop down dead."[60] Mrs. Critchley, born in 1926 in Lancaster, said of her mother's confinements, "They used to keep them in bed a long time as well and they used to bind them up, you know, afterwards, very tight to get the stomach flat."[61] Mrs. Fleming, born in 1921, stayed in bed for ten days after each of her six home deliveries. Her mother would not let her eat anything for three days after a birth because "you couldn't stand a substantial meal."[62]

The lying-in period was protected by memories about new mothers who had violated the warning to stay in bed. Mrs. Melling, born in 1917, said she lost her mother for this reason:

> I remember this very plainly, and Mother was in bed, and he [Father] was downstairs and she needed him, she needed to get out of bed and we'd no bathroom, and she called him, "John, John," I can hear her now. He was busy and he got a bit irritable when he was busy and he shouted, "All right, I'll come." She'd had the baby then. It was three weeks old when she died. But she had to stay in bed, so she shouted for him and it seems to me she needed to get out of bed, or she would have marked the bed. She gets out of bed and pulls the jerry from under the bed, and she was in a long white nightdress. . . . She pulls the jerry out to use it and as she comes to sit on it, it cracks, and I can hear this distinctly in my mind, this jerry cracking. I heard her say, "Oh, John," and he hadn't come up, and I [age 4] scrambled out of that cot and went to her and the last words my mother said in this world, she looked at me and said, "Oh Peggy," and then when m'dad had got upstairs, she'd gone. She had a white leg and with getting out of bed it killed her. That is how she died.[63]

59. Mrs. D1B, 19. See also Mrs. B1P, 46.
60. Mrs. M11B, 7.
61. Mrs. C7L, 57.
62. Mrs. F1L, 85.
63. Mrs. M3L, 33. The online *OED* defines "white leg" as "Swelling of a limb; *esp.* (for fully *phlegmasia alba, phlegmasia dolens*) phlegmasia alba dolens. . . . Phlegmasia is a rare but potentially limb-threatening vascular emergency caused by thrombosis of the deep and superficial veins of the leg." Several informants mentioned this complication of childbirth. See, for example, Mrs. H2L, 4–5; Mrs. H5L, 55.

Because of this danger, help from relatives, neighbors, and monthly nurses—unqualified women who were paid for their services, was necessary and arguably gave working-class mothers respite from otherwise unremitting toil, as well as cementing mutual aid relationships. The lying-in period also provided training for young daughters who normatively took on a larger than usual share of the housework and child care at this time.

Most older oral history informants' mothers were attended by unqualified midwives. Mrs. Addison, born in Barrow in 1892, whose mother had nine births, remembered "an ordinary woman with a white apron on. They didn't call them nurses, you called them 'missus.'"[64] Mr. Thomas, born in 1903 in Preston, whose mother had had seven births, remembered, "Midwives are people that are special . . . always scrubbed clean. They were always heavy-looking women, never slim . . . and they always had a white apron on."[65] Mrs. Hampton's mother's six babies were delivered by "Mrs. Dixon . . . Number 4 Rawlinson Street [Barrow], and if there was anybody in an interesting condition in the street she was always the woman to go and deliver." She was not qualified, "only that she'd had ten of her own."[66] Mrs. Parke, born in Lancaster in 1898, said, "The doctor would come if he was called, but midwives used to like to deliver on their own if they could. They weren't specialized people, only women that had a bent that way."[67] Informants understood the difference between formally and informally trained birth attendants. Mrs. Garvey, born in 1888, was delivered by a midwife who "wasn't fully qualified. . . . The doctors told her what to do and what not to do, but she couldn't read a thermometer, but she brought babies into the world. There are hundreds of women in Barrow who've had to go under the gynecologist through her."[68] Similarly, Mrs. Dorrington, born in 1905, commented, "You didn't go in [to hospital] then, there were midwives all over the place. Some were midwives and some were old butchers. . . . I had Nurse Green, she was qualified, some kind of qualification."[69]

The 1902 Midwives Act required local authorities annually to register midwives in their districts. Untrained ("bona-fide") midwives who had been practicing for at least one year previous to 1902 could be registered after the Medical Officer of Health's approval of their applications; only those new midwives who had certificates from either the Central Midwives Board in London or a recognized training institution could be added to the register after that date. Henceforth, local health authorities were responsible for inspecting midwives and reporting those found to have been negligent or to have caused harm. In 1905 Preston's MOH reported 53 midwives

64. Mrs. A3B, 4.
65. Mr. T2P, 37.
66. Mrs. H3B, 60.
67. Mrs. P1L, 77.
68. Mrs. G1B, 13. See also Mrs. D3P, 28; Mr. T3P, 45.
69. Mrs. D3P, 28. See also Mrs. H3L, 62; Mr. K1L, 33.

on the register, 5 with certificates from recognized institutions: "All [53 of] these [midwives] have attended before me at the Health Office and have produced for inspection their Registers, Case Books, instruments, and other necessary appliances. Such an inspection, however, admits of preparation, and in future I propose to carry it out more in the line of a surprise visit. These midwives vary very much in character, experience, and education; some being absolutely illiterate, whilst other perhaps with less actual experience, have had more education, and some scientific training."[70] Barrow's MOH wrote in 1910, "A better administration in midwifery means the clearing out of the Sariah [sic] Gamp midwife—less meddlesome midwifery and cleaner domestic habits and sanitation all round. The old midwife is dying out gradually."[71]

Despite the medical officers' disdain, unqualified midwives continued to practice, and until the 1930s many working-class women kept consulting them instead of doctors or the rising number of trained midwives.[72] Cost was undoubtedly a factor in this decision. Mr. Grove, born in 1903 in Preston, remembered the doctor charging four guineas for a home delivery. Mrs. Grove wept over the bill when it arrived on Christmas Eve.[73] Mrs. Harte, born in Lancaster in 1889, whose mother had eleven births, said, "Martha used to come, the midwife. . . . She wasn't certified or anything, but she was one of the good old midwives and it was only a few shillings for a confinement. I've heard m'mother say that she used to give her sixpence a week until she got it paid off."[74] Mr. Madison, born in 1910, also remembered this midwife:

> Children weren't born in hospital same as today in maternity wards. They were all at home. Martha Blezzard was the midwife. Martha Blezzard brought most of my generation into the world in that district in Lancaster. She was a very nice person and worked day and night.
>
> *Interviewer:* Was it usual to have the doctor, or was he only called in an emergency?
>
> *Informant:* Emergencies. Martha used to deal with the lot. Then the neighbors used to be around getting hot water. Martha used to get them organized. People used to come, "So-and-so is having a baby and

---

70. Preston MOH Report, 1905, 33. For an account of the process of registering and examining midwives in another northern English community, see Joan Mottram, "State control in local context: Public health and midwife regulation in Manchester, 1900–1914," in *Midwives, society and childbirth: Debates and controversies in the modern period,* Hilary Marland and Anne Marie Rafferty, eds. (London and New York: Routledge, 1997), 134–52.

71. Barrow MOH Report, 1910, 250.

72. This was also true elsewhere in Britain. See, for example, Marks, *Model mothers,* 98; Robert Dingwall, Anne Marie Rafferty, Charles Webster, eds., *A Social History of Nursing* (London: Routledge, 1988), 145–47.

73. Mr. G1P, 67. See also Mrs. N1L, 2; Mrs. W2L, 14; Mrs. W1P, 7; Miss T4P, 39.

74. Mrs. H2L, 39.

Martha's gone in. Martha, can we do anything to help?" "Yes, make sure there is plenty of hot water." The neighbors used to stop with you until the baby was born with Martha. Then they used to be running in with gruel for the mother. Washing a few dirty nappies or any bedding. The doctor was only brought in as a last resort. Again, the expense of bringing the doctor in and that was avoided if possible, so you were very careful with the birth and everything.[75]

This account suggests that avoiding the doctor's bill was an important reason for working-class loyalty to bona-fide midwives.

Another possible factor in working-class women's decision to continue consulting unqualified midwives, according to Elizabeth Roberts, was that such midwives "were generally thought to be friendlier, and less 'starchy'; and they were certainly less likely to tell the woman what to do, being more likely to cooperate both with her and her female relatives. It is an example of working-class women rejecting the invasion of their homes and lives by the professional."[76] Medical Officers of Health were aware of this attitude. Dr. Pilkington commented in 1918: "It might be expected that the work will gradually pass into the hands of the fully trained midwife, but there still remains an astonishing predilection for the members of the old school, many of whom possess only the merest rudiments of general education. This due to their 'motherly' character and to the fact that they are bound by long acquaintance, and in some cases by relationship, with the members of their clientele."[77]

With the advent of National Health Insurance in 1911, insured women and wives of insured workers obtained coverage for the services of qualified midwives. In some families, this served as an incentive to employ them. According to Mr. Grove, born in 1903, "Previous to 1911, the midwife was anybody that could do it. Some charged 5s. or something like that. Then it come 1911 and there was a grant of 30s. for every child that were born. Then they compelled them to have a registered nurse. Now, her fee was 30s., so the patient was not better off. But you got better treatment because you had a fully trained nurse instead of an amateur."[78] Nonetheless, many families in the study communities continued to use unqualified "handywomen." Nationwide, in 1920, 80 percent of practicing midwives were trained, while the figures for Lancaster and Preston were 46 percent and 47 percent, respectively.[79] In that year, one Lancaster handywoman delivered 137 (14 percent) of the 963 babies born in the community; there were

75. Mr. M1L, 81.
76. Roberts, *A woman's place*, 107.
77. Preston MOH Report, 1918, 12.
78. Mr. G1P, 7. See also Jones, *Health and society in twentieth-century Britain*, 27.
79. Lewis, *Politics of motherhood*, 128; Lancaster MOH Report, 1920, 27–28; Preston MOH Report, 1920, 73. The figure for Barrow is not provided in the MOH report for 1920.

then 15 midwives on the register.[80] Regardless of growing legal pressure, unqualified midwives practiced until the 1936 Midwives Act put them out of business. Lancaster's MOH reported in 1926: "Our enquiries show that a number of women were attended during confinement by handywomen who are debarred by the Act of 1926 from attending 'except under the direction and personal supervision' of a doctor. Unless they can satisfy the Court that such 'attention was given in a case of sudden or urgent necessity they shall be liable on summary conviction to a fine not exceeding ten pounds.'"[81]

The 1936 Midwives Act required that all practicing midwives be formally qualified. By 1937, 24 months of training was needed for certification. At the same time, municipal domiciliary midwifery services, run by local health authorities, were established. This employment was attractive to midwives because it provided compensation and equipment and a regulated time commitment.[82] By the end of World War II, most midwives in study communities were employed either by hospitals or as municipal midwives; establishment of the National Health Service eliminated fees. Few midwives continued in private practice, and those who remained on the register handled declining numbers of births. For example, in Barrow in 1951, municipal midwives attended 444 births (98 percent of domiciliary cases); private midwives managed 9 cases. Of the five private midwives on the register, only three delivered babies in that year.[83] Midwifery was standardized, medicalized, and increasingly institutionalized; midwives had made the transition from traditional community-based participants in a normal event to agents of official state-sponsored medicine managing a pathological process.[84]

It is clear that despite the repeated experience of infant death, many early-twentieth-century working-class women were happy with and loyal to traditional neighborhood midwives. Their perspectives on home confinements were more mixed. Many working-class homes provided inadequate facilities for confinement. Mr. Burrell, born in 1897, remembered: "In a very small house . . . they only had two bedrooms and if they had what they called a bigger family house, it would have two bedrooms and a box room making three bedrooms. Now, you see, the baby was born in the house, there was no electric light, there was only a little gas light and in some

---

80. Lancaster MOH Report, 1920, 28.
81. Lancaster MOH Report, 1926, 42.
82. Preston MOH Report, 1937, 106.
83. Barrow MOH Report, 1951, 12. See also Preston MOH Report, 1947, 47; Preston MOH Report, 1948, 40.
84. See Williams, "The controlling power of childbirth in Britain," 232–47, for a useful discussion of trained midwives' participation in the power structure of official institutionalized medicine.

cases not even gas in the house."[85] A home birth could require a major upheaval in household arrangements. Mr. Thomas, born in 1903, said of his mother's last confinement in 1915, "The bed came downstairs, the front room had to be fitted up and everything else."[86] Home confinements also required imaginative improvisation in cases when the birth did not go as expected. In 1932, Mrs. Turnbull's widowed 22-year-old mother gave birth in her own mother's front room: "But like I said, my mother didn't know she was having twins until we were born. . . . No, didn't know. Got the shock of her life, my granny: I couldn't tell you what she said. No, shock of her life, you know, being left with two of us, just little things. They couldn't put real clothes on us, so they had to wrap us up in olive oil and cotton wool, they put us in a jug, you know, to keep us warm at the fireside."[87]

In complicated cases, midwives would send for a doctor. Mrs. Musgrove's mother had ten babies, five of whom survived. She said, "When I was being born it was very difficult in 1886 and the midwife sent my father looking for a doctor and he found one. He had a look at mother and he sent for another doctor and then he sent him for another one. . . . When they were all there, they turned to my father and said, should they save the child or the mother. . . . My father naturally said that he'd have his wife."[88] Mrs. Anston, born in 1900 in Preston, had very difficult pregnancies and births:

> It was terrible, I dreaded it. The last one I had, the doctor said I must go to hospital and they wanted to terminate it. I said no, and he was stillborn, a lovely boy. It hadn't to be, but I was sorry for my husband because he would have liked a boy, after three girls.
>
> *Interviewer:* And they didn't tell you why they thought he would be stillborn?
>
> *Informant:* Yes. They couldn't separate the cord, it was round his neck.
>
> *Interviewer:* And what happened to the other one that you lost?
>
> *Informant:* That came before time. It was after my first one and it came before time. I had an awful time. They didn't know what to do in those days.
>
> *Interviewer:* And that would be at home, was it?
>
> *Informant:* Yes.
>
> *Interviewer:* Did you have a doctor and a midwife or just the midwife?
>
> *Informant:* I had to have the doctor every time, but I had a midwife and I always had a woman to stay for about a month to do the work, till I got on my feet again.

85. Mr. B1B, 24.
86. Mr. T2P, 37.
87. Mrs. T2L, 27.
88. Mrs. M3B, 3.

Mrs. Anston said about her contemporaries, "A lot didn't have the doctor, did they? I was obliged to because things weren't straightforward."[89] There is some evidence that even when problems arose, women sometimes resisted calling the doctor, not only to save money, but because they thought they should be able to do without medical help. Mrs. Hill, born in 1903, remembered that her midwife "wanted to send for the doctor earlier but I said I would manage. She said that I wouldn't. In the end, I was living with Father then, she went downstairs and told Father he was going to lose both of us if I didn't let them send for the doctor. Father said, 'You send for the doctor, never mind her!' Afterwards she asked me why I had held out on her. I told her that none of my sisters had needed a doctor, but she said that was nothing to do with me."[90]

Oral evidence indicates that calling in a general practitioner for normal home deliveries became more usual as time went on, as did people's awareness of regulations regarding management of birth. Mrs. Chase, born in 1887 in Barrow, compared her own experience to her mother's: "When I had our babies I had a midwife and a doctor. I'd suppose the neighbors would come and do what they could but she'd [mother] always had to have a nurse or midwife. They didn't have doctors and there was no maternity homes, nothing like that, just home and stayed in bed for ten days. Oh, you'd to have a nurse, neighbors weren't allowed to do. They'd come in and cook for you, make a meal or anything like that, but they wouldn't be allowed to undertake the medical part."[91] This is not to say that general practitioners were necessarily better equipped than experienced midwives to handle complications. Dr. Kuppersmith, who did a lot of home deliveries in his Preston practice that began in 1920, said: "I remember when I came to Preston and I was only newly qualified, the midwife sent for me and this was an emergency. Very often the midwife used to act on her own, but would send for the doctor if she was stuck. Well, this was a breach. I had never had any experience of a breach, so I went home and got my textbook in front of me and I made a perfect delivery."[92] Furthermore, calling the doctor did not guarantee a good result. Mrs. Lincoln, born in 1900, said:

> Well, to me, I think they interfere with nature too much but still, it's a good thing. If I had been going there [clinic], they would have known about my first child, he was fast, you see, and I had a bad time. They didn't take you to the hospital in them days. I had to have two doctors with my first. The doctors came and they said they couldn't do anything but they would come back in two hours and they said so which life it

89. Mrs. A2P, 19–20.
90. Mrs. H8P, 27.
91. Mrs. C2B, 13.
92. Dr. K1P, 2. See also Mrs. L1P, 8–9, 39.

took, it would have to be done. . . . Anyhow, we both survived. They hurt his head, but anyway he is here today.[93]

There was a marked difference among the three study communities in the extent to which doctors delivered babies. In Preston, midwives delivered the majority of infants, whether at home or in hospital, throughout the study period. In Barrow after World War II, midwives attended most deliveries, although a growing proportion of home births were also "booked" with GPs. In Lancaster, doctors managed 45 percent of total births in 1916—a proportion that declined to 25 percent in 1938, the last year for which figures are available. During the same period, the proportion of babies delivered by trained midwives in that city rose from 42 percent to 72 percent. Although GPs' midwifery training improved during the study period, and their role in antenatal care was institutionalized after the establishment of the National Health Service, the proliferation of obstetricians, hospital employment of trained midwives, and increased hospitalization of birth pushed GPs out of the delivery room after World War II.[94]

Before hospital facilities were available and used, because of a lack of appropriate facilities in their own dwellings some women gave birth at relatives' homes. Mrs. Becker, born in 1900, remembered her sister-in-law, Lily, delivering at her stepmother's house in Preston in 1919: "I walked home with her [Lily's] friend part way to where this friend lived and she said, 'How was your Lily?' And I said, I didn't see her at dinnertime, she was in the toilet all the time; my mother had made her go and sit in there because she was in pain, you see, and she was in labor. My mother was very hard, my stepmother, she had had 13, my stepmother, made her stay in there while we had had our dinner and got back to work."[95] Mrs. Fleming, born in 1921, remembered her sister-in-law giving birth at her family's home when she herself was pregnant with her first child: "She made a right performance, she literally walked a hole in the floor. . . . God! And she was down on her hands and knees and this that and the other, and I was having one as well. I thought, 'My God! Have I got to go through this?' And of course, nothing like it, was it. . . . I don't know why she was there. Anyway, perhaps she had come to have the baby the night before, you did, didn't you? And she literally walked a hole through the kitchen floor. And down on her knees and screaming."[96] This account suggests the inconvenience of some home deliveries, the potential impact of one woman's birth experience on other women, and the implication that there were respectable and disreputable ways to give birth.

Of course, as we have seen, women also had bad deliveries in their own

93. Mrs. M1P, 8–9.
94. See, for example, Lewis, *The politics of motherhood*, 140–41, 146–47.
95. Mrs. B1P, 45.
96. Mrs. F1L, 58

homes. Mr. Emery, born in 1895, said that his wife was delivered at home by a doctor and an unqualified midwife. "We were downstairs and I had this here wireless [radio] going and I could hear screaming upstairs and I put this wireless on as loud as I could so as her [wife's younger] sister couldn't hear it. . . . It was on a Sunday night was that. I always remember going upstairs after and the bed was here and when I looked at the wall there was blood all over it. I had to get it all decorated again."[97] Furthermore, many informants remembered as children being sent out of the house and waiting outdoors or at a neighbor's house while their mother gave birth.

Despite inconvenience, throughout the study period many informants chose to give birth at home. Mr. Norton, born 1931, said his wife had the option to have her four babies in hospital, but decided to have them at home, explaining:

> I don't know, possibly the freedom of access for visitors and that sort of thing. She felt more comfortable, I think, I don't think any of our generation, I think even now, don't enjoy hospitals. Because, I think, of the regimentation and . . . restriction and that sort of thing. I suppose it's part of our inbuilt way of life, that we don't like regimentation, we just don't like it. And the children have been born at home, well since dot, so why on earth change it? Thank goodness, we were very lucky, there were no complications. We were advised before the birth that there were no complications. She did visit the doctor. She did have visits from the midwife prior to the birth and we were told that everything was going to be natural, sort of thing. As indeed it was.[98]

Mrs. Kennedy, born in 1936, had both home and hospital deliveries for her six children. She commented:

> Well, I had three of them at home, so like I just got into my own routine, you know. But the midwives would come and then . . . the district nurse would come just for a couple of days, you know. . . . I used to like being at home. I enjoyed it in hospital, but I don't know, I think it brought us closer together somehow, you know, altogether. . . . Well, I had my first one, which is natural enough, in hospital, but when it came to Martin and Clifford I had reached, I had turned thirty. And I think when you have turned thirty you are getting on in they like to keep an eye on you, you know. And I had Martin in Sharoe Green and I enjoyed it and I had Clifford in the old PRI [Preston Royal Infirmary].[99]

97. Mr. E1P, 42.
98. Mr. N2L, 60. See also Mrs. T2L, 55; Mrs. B11P, 47; Mrs. C8P, 150.
99. Mrs. K2P, 105.

Dr. Kuppersmith observed, "Quite a lot of people would prefer to have their babies born at home," even though he found private dwellings ill-equipped for birth. "We had to improvise quite a lot. For instance, some of the houses didn't have running hot water. . . . We had to improvise, the boiler was boiled up a lot."[100]

HOSPITAL BIRTH

With declining infant mortality rates, in the years immediately following World War I, public attention shifted to maternal mortality, which actually rose in the 1920s and early '30s.[101] According to Jane Lewis, "Research into the clinical causes of maternal deaths led to a call for the medicalization of childbirth. Obstetricians and departmental committees advocated, first, techniques for the management of labor developed for use in hospitals rather than in the home . . . and, second, for more scientific care by better trained doctors, midwives and medical officers working in local authority clinics."[102] Led by national trends, study city MOsH argued local need for maternity hospital accommodation in terms of medical and social factors; after 1929, they took responsibility for administering and reporting on municipal hospitals.[103] In 1919, Preston's MOH wrote: "There is a great need in Preston of a Maternity Hospital, especially for abnormal cases of confinement, as in many instances life could be saved if any operation necessary could be performed under the aseptic conditions prevailing in Hospital and with the skilled assistance available there. Maternity Homes and Hospitals are recommended by the Ministry of Health in the Act of 1918 and it would be well to consider the advisability of establishing such an institution in the near future in Preston."[104] In 1921 the Preston Royal Infirmary opened a maternity ward, and by 1928 many mothers were also delivered at Sharoe Green Hospital (the former Poor Law institution).[105] In Barrow, where Risedale Maternity Home opened its doors in 1922, the MOH indicated "the need of some place where cases of confinement could be attended to with, at least, ordinary decency. . . . Owing to the congestion in the town, these cases could not be adequately dealt with in the homes of the people."[106] In Lancaster, the earliest institutional accommodation was

100. Dr. K1P, 2.
101. See, for example, Enid Fox, "Powers of life and death: Aspects of maternal welfare in England and Wales between the wars," *Medical History* 35 (1991): 328–52.
102. Lewis, *The politics of motherhood,* 117, 119.
103. Lewis, *What price community medicine,* 1.
104. Preston MOH Report, 1919, 43.
105. Preston MOH Report, 1928, 107–8. Babies had been delivered at Sharoe Green Hospital since 1926, although the number of deliveries was not reported before 1928.
106. Barrow MOH Report, 1922, 346.

at the Poor Law Hospital; need for additional beds was justified in terms of circumstances "where danger to the mother or child is anticipated" (1925) and reports from health visitors that "Many women are confined in overcrowded and often insanitary dwellings" (1928).[107] In 1932 the Royal Lancaster Infirmary expanded to accommodate 18 maternity beds.[108]

With increasing resources and facilities devoted to institutional childbirth, use of hospitals for antenatal inpatient care and delivery began to rise. In 1938, of 868 Barrow births, 281 (32 percent) occurred in institutions; by 1947, 54 percent of Barrow births were in Risedale.[109] In Lancaster, of 731 births in 1943, 301 (41 percent) were in institutions.[110] In Preston, of 1,711 births in 1940, 790 (46 percent) occurred at Preston Royal Infirmary; by 1957 only 19 percent of Preston babies were born at home.[111]

Many working-class parents welcomed the opportunity for hospital confinement. For some, a home delivery would have been inappropriate or inconvenient. Mrs. Burrell, born in 1931, who was living with her mother in a two-bedroom house during her first pregnancy, was told by her mother, "You can't have the baby here." Her three children were born in North Lonsdale Nursing Home.[112] Mr. Boswell, born in 1920, said: "The first instance, when Robert was born, we lived in rented rooms, and the war was still on of course, and we lived in a place over town and it wasn't convivial to have it at the home, you know. And it was better off to go to the hospital, so we did do. When Christine was born, we did have our house . . . but again she [wife] decided she would go to hospital to have it, you know. If she had been at Wigan, where she hails from, near her own mother, I should imagine she would have had it at home."[113]

Rising awareness of biomedical arguments and pressure from physicians, health visitors, and trained midwives affected some people's decisions about where to give birth. Mrs. Howard, born in 1931, said, "I think they realized, the health service, that everything was there if there were complications. And I think you were quite happy to go and be there where if anything did go wrong you were in safe hands. I know I wanted to go in hospital. . . . There was no way I wanted to stay at home."[114] Mrs. Barlow, born in 1928, also had her three children in hospital. "It never occurred to me to have them at home." She went on to explain, "My doctor, when I came to have my children . . . definitely pushed me towards hospital to

---

107. Lancaster MOH Report, 1925, 24; Lancaster MOH Report, 1928, 37.
108. Lancaster MOH Report, 1931, 10–11.
109. Barrow MOH Report, 1938, 4, 17; Barrow MOH Report, 1947, 8, 10.
110. Lancaster MOH Report, 1943, 10.
111. Preston MOH Report, 1940, 38–39; Preston MOH Report, 1957, 33.
112. Mrs. B2B, 49. See also Mrs. R3B, 55; Mrs. G1B, 13.
113. Mr. B4B, 54.
114. Mrs. H5L, 65. See also Mrs. B4L, 66.

have it. . . . They had all the antenatal care laid on at hospital."[115] Dr. Armstrong, a Lancaster general practitioner who dealt with many maternity cases beginning in 1948, remembered:

Yes, well, first of all facilities became more available, it isn't terribly long since we had a maternity hospital here, and for awhile we hadn't very much in the way of beds available to us as general practitioners. But then of course, you see, the advice of the consultant obstetricians was, all right, then, don't have a first birth at home, once you get to four, come and tell us. So deal with basically your second and third children if there is no hint of trouble. . . . And I had no objections to that at all, I mean, I was no obstetrician. I didn't deal with anything abnormal, just into hospital and of course we are not very far away from the hospital here, it worked very well. So I was quite happy when the general advice came to put your midwifery people into hospital and let them get on with it.[116]

Some mothers viewed a hospital or nursing home delivery as being something of a luxury. Mrs. Owen, born in 1916, who felt she "couldn't" deliver her only child at home, said, "I could have gone into Risedale Maternity Hospital, but you had to pay then, it went on your husband's wages. And it wasn't much difference me going up there than in the nursing home, so we decided to go in the nursing home. . . . You paid five pounds extra, I think, to have your own doctor in the nursing home."[117] Mrs. Becker, born in 1900, had her fourth baby in a hospital: "That was private. . . . [I thought] I'm going to spoil myself a bit."[118]

Other informants remembered the change in expectations accompanying the transition from home to hospital birth. Mrs. Calvert, born in 1919 in Preston, who had her first baby in 1940, when asked, "Did most people go to the hospital then, or did they have them [babies] at home?" responded:

I don't know. I always thought I would never go away. My sister-in-law, she went away. I think then, you were only supposed to go for your first baby and after that you were supposed to stop at home if you had somebody to look to you. I sat at home with our Ann. I think you had to pay £4 at the Infirmary or Sharoe Green then, and at home it was only 30 shillings.
Interviewer: That was for the doctor and the midwife, was it?
Informant: Oh no, you didn't have a doctor. There again, I had to

115. Mrs. B3B, 63.
116. Dr. A5L, 13.
117. Mrs. O1B, 24–25.
118. Mrs. B1P, 25.

have a doctor with my first one to be stitched, but my insurance paid
for that. I had three good confinements, so it didn't bother me that
way.[119]

With hospital confinement, it was not only the place but the personnel, management, and control over birth environment and processes that
changed. Mr. Danner, born in 1910, recalled the hospital birth of his first
child:

> My wife had gone to her mother's as usual on a Monday, which was about
> one and a quarter miles of a walk. She took her washing, as this was
> done with her mother, a joint effort. Grandmother and my wife walked
> to the Infirmary when they felt sure deliverance was due. I learned of
> this on my way home from work. . . . I phoned the hospital, but nothing
> was then doing, so I went to Grandmother's. My word, she was in a state,
> she had aches and pains, she was "feeling for her daughter." I was called
> a great clown, it was all my fault. If men had to have babies, no family
> would be greater than three, one from the man, two from the woman.
> I'm not sure it was all my fault, as it takes two to make a bargain. Visiting
> time was 7 p.m., husbands only. This annoyed my mother-in-law, she felt
> equally as important as a husband. However, she would come along with
> me and wait outside. But I could not see my wife as she was up in the
> labour ward, and I reported to my mother-in-law immediately. As soon
> as I mentioned labour ward, she developed a pain (this I believe to be
> genuine) and a groan, and had to sit on the boundary wall. Again I was
> wished for a turn of baby-having, and in turn I wished I'd left the old
> woman at home. David was born about 10 p.m., and I was told I could
> see my wife for a few minutes with my son. I was shown the latter first,
> what a creased-up business new babies are. I was most concerned. The
> nurse said he was lovely. I said, "Looks like he's got a bad heart to me.
> He's blue and how little he is." I was comforted by being taken to see
> other babies for comparison. Good old nurse, I was comforted. I think
> the most wonderful sight to a man is to see his wife just after childbirth,
> they are then at their bonniest. They are elated and relieved, they are
> thankful, they want to share. It really is ours. I of course was able to
> say that I had seen our son, and that he was a beauty. Up to then Mum
> herself had not seen him. He was brought in shortly afterwards and for
> a few minutes we three were together. Oh, happy day![120]

This account illustrates a traditional relationship between a young pregnant
woman and her mother; that mother's exclusion from the hospital birth

119. Mrs. C5P, 36.
120. Mr. D2P, 59.

process (a situation where previously she would have been a dominant participant); the authority of the trained nurse; the new hospital-imposed separation of newborns from parents; and the accommodation of new parents to an alien institutional environment.

In the 1940s and '50s, particularly after establishment of the National Health Service eliminated both charges for hospital delivery and the traditional stigma of delivery in the workhouse, demand for hospital beds outstripped supply.[121] In 1946 Preston's MOH reported:

> One of the features of the year has been the increase in the number of births in the Borough, which reached the highest total since 1923. This post-war increase was not unexpected, and it did prove a strain on the resources of the town to deal with the problem. The modern expectant mother, quite rightly, expects a higher standard in the surroundings for her confinement, and owing to the unsatisfactory housing conditions and other factors, which has led to an increased demand for confinements in hospital. This, in turn, has led to a very great strain on the maternity accommodation in the local hospitals, which has been increased by shortage of staff. There is no quick and easy solution to the problem.[122]

Similar conditions existed in Barrow and Lancaster in the postwar period.[123]

Preston's MOH reports show a commitment to home delivery that was supported by assiduous efforts to recruit domiciliary midwives in the 1950s. In 1936 the MOH wrote: "The financial and practical advantages to be gained by entering a maternity home for confinement and the enthusiasm and loyalty engendered in supporters of these institutions should not blind us to the fact that, for the majority of women, home is the natural place for normal childbirth and that our efforts should be directed towards securing for these women all the facilities in the way of medical and nursing help that are required in their particular case."[124] In 1960 the MOH celebrated the fact that 29.27 percent of births in that year had taken place at home—up from 19.24 percent.[125] 1963's report described the situation that had

121. Mrs. N3L had her first child out of wedlock in the Lancaster Workhouse. When, after marriage, she chose to have her second baby in the same facility, her husband was furious, feeling she had shamed him. Mrs. N3L, 65; Mr. N3L, 136–37.

122. Preston MOH Report, 1946, 3.

123. See, for example, Barrow MOH Reports for 1938, 1944, 1946, and 1947. Hospital deliveries rose from 279 in 1938 to 822 in 1947. See also Lancaster MOH Reports for 1940 and 1942. In 1940, 184 births occurred in the Royal Lancaster Infirmary; 254 births occurred there in 1942—an increase which "led to a greatly increased strain on the accommodation available" (6).

124. Preston MOH Report, 1936, 6.

125. Preston MOH Report, 1960, 35.

stabilized by the end of the study period (1970):

> This service is organized on the basis of a highly efficient antenatal service with selection of cases for hospital confinement in the hands of the consultants who not only work in the hospitals, but also carry out regular weekly consultative sessions on behalf of the local health authority. Mothers having their first babies and those who already have had four pregnancies are encouraged and persuaded to accept hospital delivery whilst the remainder are carefully reviewed to determine whether, in the light of the clinical conditions, the past history and the social conditions home or hospital delivery is indicated.

In that year, 30 percent of deliveries took place at home.[126] Not until the 1970s would Preston follow the nation in hospitalizing virtually all births.[127] Nonetheless, it is fair to observe that home births had also become medicalized by the post–World War II era; officially trained and licensed midwives took birth technologies and drugs to parents' homes and either called physicians or transported mothers to hospital according to conservative risk protocols.

As we have seen, the oral history evidence does not romanticize home birth. However, it does reveal both some negative aspects of institutional delivery and a growing awareness of the implications of whatever choice was made. Some women who had had a bad birth experience at home chose hospitalization on later occasions.[128] Others found that hospital birth experiences varied. Mrs. Marley, born in 1914, chose to have her son in Ulverston Cottage Hospital, for which she and her husband paid £20—a fortune at a time when her husband's weekly wage was £3. She remembered having considerable control over this birth: "We got to the hospital and the nurse said, 'Oh well, you've been a straightforward case, so Dr. Smith might say Matron can attend to you.' And I can remember saying he better hadn't, he's been paid for this child, he had better come. Anyway, he came."[129] By contrast, Mr. Kennedy, born in 1930, said that his first four children were born at home and his last two in hospital:

> You get different hospitals. I mean to say, one of my lads was born in Preston Infirmary, and they was very very strict. I was told off for picking

126. Preston MOH Report, 1963, 24.

127. In *The politics of motherhood,* Jane Lewis provides an excellent discussion of mid-twentieth-century trends in official thinking about the desirability of hospital versus home birth (119–41). Enid Fox argues that the medicalization and institutionalization of midwifery changed midwives' professional identity and relationships with both patients and physicians ("Powers of life and death: Aspects of maternal welfare in England and Wales between the wars," *Medical History* 35 [1991]: 328–52).

128. See, for example, Mrs. P1P, 18; Mrs. Y2P, 7; Mrs. B11P, 39.

129. Mrs. M11B, 7.

the baby up when I went to see the missus, you know. I told the nurse, you know, there's no way I'm putting him down, he's my baby. And she said, you are not allowed to touch him, you'll have brought germs in. I said, well all the others that were born at home, I said, they've survived and there was no bother. People came in to see them and they brought germs in. Now, the other hospital where I think it was the fifth one was born, they were fantastic, you know. You could get hold of the baby and nurse him. You could feed him, actually, if he were on the bottle.[130]

Mrs. Hocking, born in 1933, had her first child in hospital and the last two at home, "Because I thought it was more personal." She also said that her husband was present for the home deliveries, but not for the hospital birth, "Because it wasn't done in those days." Informants who delivered in hospital experienced more medical intervention, including anesthetics, instrument deliveries, and surgery.[131] After World War II, hospital delivery became the norm among working-class residents of Barrow, Lancaster, and Preston, joining routine consultation of general practitioners and use of public health clinics.

INFANT AND CHILD CARE

The same public concern about infant mortality that favored medicalization of pregnancy and birth stimulated early-twentieth-century infant and child welfare initiatives including health visiting, clinics, and school medical services. As we have seen, each of the study cities appointed health visitors and opened infant welfare clinics before World War I. In response to the establishment of the School Medical Service in 1907, each also initiated school-based health services that by the interwar period included medical inspection, "treatment for minor ailments, dental defects and defective vision," and physical training, while Barrow and Preston established open-air schools for frail children.[132] During World War II, each city

130. Mr. K2P, 13.

131. Mrs. M11B, 6; Mrs. O1B, 25; Mrs. W5B, 22; Mrs. W6B, 80; Mrs. H5L, 65–66; Mrs. L3L, 52. Barrow's Medical Officer of Health noted dramatic increases in "surgical work" performed in the late 1940s. At Risedale Maternity Hospital in 1947, there were 467 normal deliveries, 91 caesarean sections, 51 inductions, 45 forceps deliveries, 5 sterilizations following delivery, and 4 hysterectomies (Barrow MOH Report, 1947, 12–13).

132. Bernard Harris, *The health of the schoolchild: A history of the school medical service in England and Wales* (Buckingham and Philadelphia: Open University Press, 1995); Charles Webster, "The health of the school child during the Depression," in *The fitness of the nation: Physical and health education in the nineteenth and twentieth centuries*, Nicholas Parry and David McNair, eds. (Leicester: History of Education Society of Great Britain, 1982), 70–99. See also John Welshman, *Municipal medicine: Public health in twentieth-century Britain* (Oxford: Peter Lang, 2000); David Parker, "'A convenient dispensary': Elementary education and the influence of the school medical service 1907–39," *History of Education* 27:1 (1998): 59–83, which provide studies of school medical

opened free nursery schools. All of these amenities were established with altruistic intentions. However, as in the related case of contagious disease control, they combined free or low-cost advice and care with surveillance and enforcement, extending what Jacques Donzelot called "the policing of families" and what Judy Giles observed as the proliferating intervention of officials and experts in working-class domestic life.[133] Because infant and child welfare programs viewed working-class mothering as the primary cause of child health problems, they sought either to change working-class mothers or to replace them as decision makers and caregivers. In response, working-class women either resisted advice and services, thus confirming experts' negative opinions of them, or, by deferring to the authority of professional public health and medicine, lost confidence and agency regarding the responsibility that was most central to their identities and roles—child care.

In the late nineteenth and early twentieth centuries, study city MOsH considered approaches to preventing infant illness and death including crèches for the infants of working mothers, milk depots (resources for low-cost, safe milk), schools for mothers, domestic science classes for schoolgirls, and appointment of health visitors.[134] As we have seen, health visiting led local infant welfare efforts, followed closely by establishment of clinics. In 1913 Lancaster's MOH described the first of these facilities in his city:

> A "School for Mothers," or Infant Consultation Centre, a name which more accurately expresses its nature, was inaugurated about the middle of the year. Mothers of infants are invited to bring their babies to this center, which is held in the Parade Room at the town Hall every Tuesday afternoon. The babies are stripped and weighed and the mothers are given charts showing the progress made from week to week. The center is in charge of the Medical Officer and the Health Visitors, who give advice as to the feeding, clothing and general management of the infant. No attempt is made at treatment. Where the services of a medical man are required, the mother is advised to consult her own doctor. In addition to the baby, the mother often brings her children who are under school age, and advantage is taken of their presence to inquire into their state of health. Many remediable conditions are discovered as a result of such enquiries, and examination of these older infants, and

---

services in Leicester and Hertfordshire, respectively.

133. Jacques Donzelot, *The policing of families* (New York: Pantheon Books, 1979); Judy Giles, *Women, identity and private life in Britain, 1900–50* (New York: St. Martin's Press, 1995), 101. See also George K Behlmer, *Friends of the family: The English home and its guardians, 1850–1940* (Stanford, CA: Stanford University Press, 1998).

134. See, for example, Barrow MOH Report, 1885, 201; Barrow MOH Report, 1913, 282; Lancaster MOH Report, 1907, 22; Preston MOH Report, 1901, 17; Preston MOH Report, 1915, 22.

the mothers are exhorted to have these attended to without delay. The only difficulty we have experienced in connection with this branch of the work of preventing infant mortality has been to get the initial visit paid. It is very encouraging to note the increasing interest which the mothers take in the health of their children afterwards.[135]

Preston's MOH, Dr. Pilkington, placed such activities in a broader context, writing in 1915, "The State is keeping a watchful eye upon all children from—and even before—the time of their birth until after the completion of school life, and much is being done to safeguard their health, and ensure their growing up to strong and vigorous adolescence."[136]

The oral history evidence indicates that while the oldest informants had no experience of health visitors or clinics, people born after the turn of the twentieth century were aware of these services and remembered hostility to them, either due to their association with the hated Poor Law, or because health visitors were seen as either intrusive or useless.[137] Mr. Boyle, born in 1927, said his mother would not have attended a child health clinic, because "It was all linked somehow with welfare. It wasn't quite the same thing as the workhouse but the same sort of tradition of public help for individuals, it used to be avoided if you tended to keep your self respect and all the rest of it. . . . She would rather have been seen dead, I think."[138] Mrs. Lincoln, born in 1900, said she went to a clinic once, "but I didn't like it. I don't know why. I have never been used to anything like that, and getting something given me, I would rather be the other side. It doesn't do to be too independent. They were very nice, but with having my mother I really didn't go. There were ten of us." She disapproved of others going to clinics to "get something for nothing"—behavior she regarded as not quite respectable—and reiterated, "With having my mother, I didn't need any advice off anybody else."[139] Similarly, Mrs. Maxwell, born in Preston in 1898, said:

> I always remember the Health Visitor when she came because I never had a Health Visitor with the first one. She came when the second boy was born and when she saw Margaret she asked how I had managed to bring her up without going to the clinic. She said, "What have you done?" I said, "I breastfed her!" I breastfed the second one with abscesses all round my eyes. I asked the doctor if I should take him off the breast. He said, "No. Get the food down yourself and it won't do him any harm!" I fed him until he was nine months old. Now they are

135. Lancaster MOH Report, 1913, 85–86.
136. Preston MOH Report, 1915, 14.
137. See, for example, Mr. G1P, 60; Mrs. H4P, 16; Mrs. M1P, 50; Mrs. A3B, 51; Mrs. B5P, 48.
138. Mr. B9P, 10.
139. Mr. L1P, 9, 38.

feeding them on solids at two and three weeks.

Interviewer: Who did you turn to for advice about the children if you ever wanted any?

Informant: My mother.

Interviewer: How far away did she live?

Informant: Only down the road off Water Lane.[140]

Regardless of such resistance, the oral evidence documents gradual working-class acceptance of clinics and health visitors. Many informants remember obtaining free or cheap food and supplies from clinics—despite the opinions quoted above, a much more popular service than the advice that was also offered.[141] Some also regarded clinic attendance as "a social afternoon out."[142] Mrs. Hill, born in 1903, remembered:

When she was born the Health lady came and she told me that if I took her to the clinic I would get my food fresher and cheaper. St. Savior's Room at Manchester Road, that's where they had the baby clinic. It was nothing to do with the hospital or the doctor and they would weigh your baby and they had a nurse that would have a look at it and see if anything was wrong. You had a card with how much she weighed and how much food you got. That clinic was a good thing because there was Mrs. Rainford and she was a JP of our town and she was a lovely person and they had a long chain of butcher shops and I loved that woman and I wasn't the only one. . . . She could play the piano, she could lead games, she could sing, she could teach you things and she had the patience of Job. It was lovely to go because when you had your baby attended to, you went out of the small weighing room into the large room and they gave you a cup of tea, the ladies of the town, and they didn't charge you anything. We would all be sitting round with our little babies discussing all different sorts of things. Mrs. Rainford would come and she would say, "Now, ladies, let's have a sing-song." She would play the piano and the people that could sing, if they could sing above these babies that were nattering. . . . Then when it came holiday time she would make a little fancy cake and sandwiches. I thought it was really lovely. . . . There was among the ladies, second-hand clothes when their babies had grown out of them, they would wash them and bring them here. There was many a lot helped that way. I was lucky enough as I could knit and I could sew, so I didn't need to do that, but many a lot that were poorly was helped in that respect.

Interviewer: Did most of your friends go when they had babies?

140. Mrs. M3P, 14. See also Mrs. B5P, whose husband "didn't believe in vaccination, he didn't believe in clinics or undressing. . . . He wouldn't let me take them to the clinic" (21).

141. See, for example, Mrs. M1P, 50; Mrs. W4P, 20; Mrs. M11B, 8–9.

142. See, for example, Mrs. S3B, 75; Mrs. C8L, 17.

> *Informant:* Of course, nearly all of that neighborhood went. Some
> people were that way, they didn't want to know about anything, but they
> were in the minority. They would give one another hints about their
> babies and you got a lot of help at that place.[143]

This account shows the early association between clinics and private philan-
thropy, as well as social class aspects of the services clinics provided. It also
suggests strengthening links between clinic attendance and respectability,
as opposed to a neighborhood minority who "didn't want to know about
anything" and clung to increasingly disreputable traditional ways.

Mrs. Jenkins, born in 1932 in Barrow, recognized the generational shift
in acceptance of official health advice that was occurring in the mid-twentieth century. She took advice from health visitors herself, but reported
that her mother-in-law, who was also raising a baby at the time, "wouldn't
allow her [the health visitor] in the house. Said she was an interfering busybody or similar. But young people . . . I mean, I went regular to the clinic,
my mother-in-law didn't, so you know."[144] Mrs. Jenkins' comments illustrate both a traditional working-class method of resisting official authority—denying access to the home—and the post–World War II transition to
acceptance of both biomedical information about disease prevention and
intervention of experts in family management.

It is clear that younger informants' reliance on advice from health visitors and clinic personnel reduced their dependence on informal health
authorities. Mrs. Jenkins said: "Yes, I started off by asking, well originally
there was just my mother-in-law, but she had very old-fashioned ideas, but
I took them at first, but I did a lot of reading in the clinic and I gradually
got more confidence, but for instance we had cinder tea when my first
baby, I mean, we were living with them and she was little and she got, she
kept crying, and so we gave her a cinder tea."[145] Infant feeding was a major
battleground. Public health authorities advocated breastfeeding, keeping
babies on a schedule, avoiding bottle-feeding and pacifiers ("dummies"),
consulting doctors, and ignoring the advice of female relatives and friends.
For instance, in 1926 Lancaster's MOH reported:

> The proportion of breast-fed babies in the town is very small. One
> reason for this is that the baby is fed irregularly and, as a consequence,

143. Mrs. H8P, 51.

144. Mrs. J1B, 64. See also Mrs. B2B, 51; Mrs. L3L, 53; Mrs. W4L, 40; Mrs. Y1L, 52; Mrs. G5P,
45.

145. Mrs. J1B, 14. Dr. Armstrong, who began general practice in Lancaster in 1848,
remembered, "There was all sorts of weird and wonderful things with the influence of granny
when I came here, if the infant had colic and was windy and you couldn't get it up by smacking
its bottom, You used to feed it with the ashes from the fire. Now this seems ridiculous, but it
was activated charcoal they were actually feeding it, wasn't it. You see, it was good for the child"
(18).

suffers and cries, whereupon the mother, acting on the advice of a neighbor, immediately alters the method of feeding. Another reason is the facility with which a bottle-feed is prepared from dried milk. It is hoped, however, that by prompt home-visiting or securing the attendance of mothers at the Welfare Centre, and impressing on them the necessity of seeking medical advice before changing the child's food, it may be possible to arrest the decay of breast-feeding.[146]

Short-circuiting traditional role modeling and intergenerational advice was, however, a stubborn challenge. Mrs. Masterson, born in 1913, said she asked her mother for advice about infant feeding: "They were older and they knew what to do. I did it with my daughter with these pobs [bread and milk artificial feeding]. You see, it passed from one generation to another. . . . She didn't believe in this 2-hourly feed and 4-hourly feed. She said to feed them when they cried and were hungry. That was one thing she didn't believe in. Now, I didn't keep to those rules, I fed them when they were hungry. They slept, you see, and they came on."[147] Similarly, Mrs. Marley, born in Barrow in 1914, said:

> I didn't normally go to clinics, I don't think you did in those days, you know. . . . We had a nurse came round. She used to come round every month, didn't she, and just ask a few questions and look at her, you know, because I know came in one day about 2 o'clock in the afternoon and she said when was she fed, and I said 9 o'clock this morning, and she said, "Ooh, you shouldn't . . . leave her so long," and I said, "Look, the last one I had cried every half hour after he'd have been fed," I said, "I'm not waking this one up while she's asleep," I said, "If she's hungry she'll waken."[148]

As this account indicates, mothers, battered by contradictory advice, made feeding decisions based on their particular circumstances. For example, Mrs. Burton, born in 1898, said her mother-in-law had recommended that she bottle-feed her baby: "Well, I nearly starved the kid to death with a bottle so I thought, Oh, here comes. So I breastfed them both. . . . I put him back on the breast and he were poorly and the doctor come and I put him back and I breastfed them both."[149] By contrast, Mrs. Becker, born in 1900, remembered:

> I fed the first one about 4 months. The second one I tried for 6 months but my eldest one was in bed with rheumatic fever and the doctor gave

146. Lancaster MOH Report, 1926, 37
147. Mrs. M1P, 50.
148. Mrs. M11B, 9.
149. Mrs. B5P, 21.

me . . . baby was crying one day and when he came to the other one, he said, "What are you feeding on?" and I said, "Me," and he looked at me and gave me such a thump in my back and he said, "Oh, for God's sake, get a bottle," and so I said, "Well, I did want to try."

Interviewer: Why did he think she ought to have a bottle?

Informant: Well, he knew she wasn't getting enough. I was worried about the other one in bed, you know. She was in bed seven months, and I was worried to death, so she [baby] went on a bottle. . . . And then so my husband said, that's the end, when I came to be having another, he said, "You're not feeding, that's the end." . . . Then the next one, I fed her just while I was in hospital and about a fortnight after, I came home and I thought, oh, it's going to be a battle, because I could see I couldn't satisfy her, and it was wartime. We weren't really getting much.[150]

Mrs. Mallingham, born in 1892 in Barrow, said her sister, who had her first baby in 1909, could not breastfeed. "The first bottles were rounded like that, and they had a screw top and a tube. They weren't hygienic, you know. Then these boat shaped bottles came and a teat on one end and a little cap on the other. They were the bottles that m'sister used. . . . You mixed the baby food and made it into a liquid and put it in. She lost her third baby, and when her fourth one was born in 1915 and he was brought up on National milk. Dr. Weir used to play pop with her—'He'll have this, and he'll have that,' but he thrived on it so she kept him on it."[151] Along similar lines, Mrs. Nance, born in Lancaster in 1899, said: "Doctors advised you then to feed your baby if you could. They were cleaner and smelt sweeter. You could nearly tell a bottle-fed baby. They seemed to have a sour smell. There was long narrow tubes and mothers had a habit of standing the bottle in the pram and the long tube to the baby and they could leave them feeding. That was why a lot had tummy ache, wind and that. They'd be sucking away at that when the bottle was empty."[152] Informants were aware that the tube-style bottles were notoriously unhygienic—a matter often highlighted by MOsH.[153]

While older informants tended to depend on their mothers and other informal authorities for advice on childrearing, they also had more confidence about their child care methods and less guilt about their babies' progress or problems than their younger counterparts who depended more on professional advice. Mrs. Grove, who bottle-fed her babies during the 1920s and '30s, said: "It was terrible how they taught us in those days, cow's

150. Mrs. B1P, 48.
151. Mrs. M6B, 73.
152. Mrs. N1L, 53.
153. See, for example, Mrs. N1L, 54; Mrs. W1B, 51. See also, for example, Barrow MOH Report, 1895, 191; Lancaster MOH Report, 1919, 18; Preston MOH Report, 1916, 8.

milk and so much water. They [babies] did cry a lot because they weren't having enough. We had these books that they gave us at the Infirmary and I went to the clinic and they had the same books. . . . I just felt frightened as it was my first baby. I hadn't had that responsibility because we went to work at 12. So really, I was a bit frightened and I went every week. I hadn't had any experience of young children."[154] Mrs. Hunter, a generation younger, recalled taking her baby to the clinic: "It used to upset me because he never seemed to be gaining as much as they said he ought to be gaining. I fed him myself and of course breastfed babies don't gain like the bottle ones, and it was just across the road really, and I used to get quite upset. . . . They tried to persuade me to put him on a bottle, which I don't think they would do now, would they?"[155] Conversely, Mrs. Brayshaw, born in 1947, said her mother "breast fed me until I was seven weeks old—she only told me this when I had my children—and I didn't gain an ounce in seven weeks. And she said I just looked like a skinned rabbit and everybody else had plump babies, and she had this horrible skinned rabbit. And so she took me to the clinic, I think, for the fourth time, and they said, 'Oh, leave it another week.' And she thought, that's the end. And walked up Fishergate Hill to the chemist and bought some bottles and some Ostermilk, or was it National Dried."[156] This account documents increasing utilization of clinics and acceptance of professional advice while also validating superior maternal knowledge and lingering strength of mother-daughter interdependence.

The oral evidence shows that information from medical authorities was sometimes inconsistent, further undermining the confidence of parents who were trying to make the best possible "modern" decisions about feeding their babies. Mr. Danner, born in 1910, said that while his mother had not attended clinics, he and his wife took their first child, David, to both the neighborhood clinic and a general practitioner:

> I had seen so much and read so much. The rich people took their children and had them vetted with doctors, so I had the idea that if we went to the doctor every week, this could be a marvelous thing. So we went to Dr. Howarth and it cost three shillings a time and he had got a baby the same age as ours, he was a young man. We would go along, and my wife couldn't feed the baby as the milk went away from her, so he told her to use Ostermilk as his child was doing well on that. Every week we went and David never gained at all and after a long while he gained an ounce. We were terribly worried and other people would call him a poor little fellow. They would have a big baby against our little one. So

154. Mrs. G1P, 60.
155. Mrs. H3P, 43. See also Mrs. B2B, 50.
156. Mrs. B10P, 68.

she [wife] went to the clinic and the clinic wouldn't interfere because she was going to the doctor. So I went down to see him and said, "Look, my child has only gained an ounce. Is Ostermilk right?" He said it was doing well for his. . . . He asked me why I was worrying, as it [the baby] hadn't lost weight. I told him that according to the books I had read, it wasn't doing what it should be doing. From this, I said, that I wouldn't come any more. I went home and I told my wife to do what they told her at the clinic. The clinic said that now we weren't under the doctor we had to use tuberculin-tested milk, pasteurized milk sort of thing. They told us to give it to him neat. By the time he had got to a certain age, he had doubled his weight and he was a fine youngster. So the doctor had been proved wrong and my wife had more commonsense than he had and had brought this about. She tried to keep to regular feeding and regular habits and that sort of thing. My mother had been in gentleman's service and she knew there were nicer things in life than slums and that sort of thing and so the whole aim was to give them the opportunity.[157]

In this account, self-consciously modern, upwardly mobile young parents sought information from books, doctor, and clinic. The physician's advice was based not on his scientific training but on his personal experience—the same type of evidence that stimulated the parents' worry about their child appearing to be a "poor little fellow." Nonetheless, the clinic would not provide its alternative feeding recommendation until the father had officially terminated his family's relationship with the doctor—a situation related to tension between general practitioners and public health officials regarding relationships with patients. Ultimately, the informant credits his wife's common sense for the child's improvement, although her choice was of two high-status authorities (the clinic's and mother-in-law's experience of "gentleman's service") as opposed to a third (the general practitioner's)—all of which were presumed to be superior to traditional management of babies in the "slums."

Compulsory education had enormous influence on working-class health culture. Classroom norms for personal hygiene; physical examinations by teachers, nurses, and medical officers; referrals for treatment; physical training; and formal health education provided generations of students with officially endorsed alternatives to informal health traditions.[158] As David Parker argues, "School medical officers accumulated power and came to wield increasing and often decisive influence over a remarkably wide range of educational development."[159] However, like public health

157. Mr. D2P, 20.

158. See, for example, J. S. Hurt, *Elementary schooling and the working classes 1860–1918* (London: Routledge and Kegan Paul, 1979), 101–52.

159. Parker, "'A convenient dispensary,'" 60.

services generally, school medical inspections and their links to contagious disease notification and isolation were initially associated with enforced school attendance and related working-class resistance. For many families, school was an unwelcome alternative to youth employment, and educational authorities contested parents' control of children.[160] For example, Mr. Tasker, born in Preston in 1886, recalled the school inspector coming to his home if he had not been in school that day: "Fathers have been prosecuted many a time for not sending their children to school." Having occasioned this embarrassing confrontation with authority, truants would "get a hiding" [beating] from both teachers and parents.[161] As indicated in chapter 4, teachers were required to report suspected cases of contagious disease, which stimulated a home visit from a health visitor and possible medical consultation, home quarantine, or hospital isolation. In addition, as Bernard Harris observes, the school medical service represented a further invasion into family life.[162]

Medical inspections were resisted and feared because of the negative light they could shed on family hygiene and child care practices. Early-twentieth-century medical officers reported difficulties in convincing parents to support school medical examinations. For example, in 1912 Lancaster's new MOH, also the School Medical Officer, wrote that when inspections were first initiated, he thought it desirable to invite parents to examinations to dispel worries about the process. However, with inspection "no longer a novelty," other challenges had arisen. Either parents sent children to school on inspection day scrubbed and dressed up, thus masking health problems, or the frailest and poorest pupils were kept at home on the date of the inspection.[163] In 1913 the same MOH highlighted the increasing role of teachers in directing and enforcing physical and moral hygiene: "The subject of personal hygiene receives universal attention, and practice is encouraged by daily inspection, at more than half the schools, of the condition of the children as to cleanliness. Regular visits are made to the Public Baths in the case of a number of the schools—as a rule outside school hours. A charge of a penny per head is made. Lessons are given on temperance in all the upper departments, and instruction in baby-care to the senior girls."[164]

Informants remembered shame regarding personal hygiene in relationships with teachers, who were generally perceived as being of superior

---

160. See, for example, Wally Seccombe, *Weathering the storm: Working-class families from the Industrial Revolution to the fertility decline* (London and New York: Verso, 1993), 177; Hurt, *Elementary schooling*, 155–213.

161. Mr. T3P, 55. This same pattern occurred when children got into trouble with the police.

162. Harris, *The health of the schoolchild*, 2.

163. Lancaster MOH Report, 1912, 106.

164. Lancaster MOH Report, 1913, 145.

social status. Mrs. Nance, born in 1899 in Lancaster, said teachers were particularly strict about "going clean. They used to show you up if you were poor. My mother once waited a week for a teacher to give her [the teacher] a good hiding. We'd to wear all my mother's clothes, and this teacher had pulled my sister and swung her round with her hair. My mother went, but she never got hold of her [the teacher] because the schoolmaster knew and when my mother waited at one end he let her [the teacher] out at the other."[165] This shame, closely related to the struggle for respectability, translated to both unremitting efforts to keep children clean and well-dressed, thereby representing and maintaining family reputations, and to invidious comparisons between one's own clean family and those other dirty children who threatened to contaminate the clean. Thus, Mr. Maines, born in 1897 in Barrow, associated lack of personal hygiene with Jewish boys attending his school: "They didn't sit the better class boys and the better dressed boys and girls together, they mixed you up, you sat next to the dirtiest in the class. They smelt, some of them."[166] In this case, hygiene standards inculcated at school supported both anti-Semitism and antagonism between the rough and the respectable.

Similarly, certain children's ailments besmirched family reputations. Mr. Boyle, born into a rough Preston family in 1937, recalled an experience that occurred during World War II:

> Now on Harrison Hill they classed theirselves as different families than what we were. We were scum to them. I'll give you an instance, me, my brothers and sisters all got what they called at the time, impetigo, which is scabies. So you had to go to this place which is called Atkinson Street. . . . And you went there and there were big tin baths and you got in them baths of hot water, and this bloke used to scrub these scabs . . . scrub you until he made them bleed. Then you got out of the bath and . . . they used to cover you from head to toe in this yellow ointment. And then you could put your clothes back on, which you had a woollen vest and one thing and another, and then my mam would walk us back down this street, an then you would see on the other side where these kids were at it, "Don't go up near [Boyles], they've all got scabies, keep away from them, they've impetigo."[167]

Because of the threat of such social sanctions, the effort to keep children looking clean and healthy was an investment in the family's reputation. Mrs. Burton, born in Preston in 1898, remembered a neighbor's struggle to maintain standards: "The woman lower down than me, she used to get

165. Mrs. N1L, 66. See also Mr. H3L, 134; Mr. M1L, 77; Mrs. M1P, 24.
166. Mr. M7B, 27.
167. Mrs. B11P, 17.

the dolly tub [used for laundry] and put her children in to bath them."
Mr. Burton added, "She had a lot of children, didn't she? My mother said
she used to put them in clean clothes every morning and they were in
those clothes till the following morning. They slept in them and the next
morning she put them clean ones on for twenty-four hours. But she had
about 13 children, and I suppose it was the only way she could cope."[168]
This example illustrates both one mother's attempts to keep her children
looking respectable and the power of neighborhood gossip to undermine
reputations.

Concern about children's personal hygiene centered, in the oral evidence, on head lice. Mothers fought endlessly against these nuisances,
which were associated with dirty families and disease and, like bugs in
houses, were unwillingly shared. Schoolchildren found to be infested were
sent home with instructions for cleansing; those who remained persistently
lousy could be excluded from school.[169] Mrs. Addison, born in Barrow in
1892, remembered, "Our mother always tied our hair back or plaited it
because she used to say that if they were hanging on your shoulder, you
might get something off the other little girls next to you, so we always
had plaits."[170] Boys were told not to wear another child's cap.[171] Virtually
all informants remembered mothers or grannies going through their hair
with a fine-toothed comb and using various soaps and solutions to kill
or prevent lice. Because school nurses and health visitors (often collectively personified as "Nitty Nora") regularly searched children's heads for
signs of head lice, the verdict was a public announcement of cleanliness
or shame. For example, Mrs. Havelock, born in Preston in 1903, remembered, "It was very common. The nurse used to come round and if you had
that sassafras [a commonly used remedy for head lice], that told a story.
Naturally, as a child, you dreaded it because it spoke for itself. Oh yes, they
just didn't sit next to you. The thing happened, even to clean folk."[172] Mr.
Madison, born in 1910 in Lancaster, described social class associations with
children's hygiene:

> The middle class and the high class didn't want to know us. . . . There
> was a sort of shying away from you. Keeping a fair distance between you.
> Let's face it, same as working-class today, everybody wasn't as clean as
> one another. You might have had poor clothes on, but you were clean.
> On the other hand you'd get the others that weren't even clean, head
> sores and lice, vermin marks, sores on their face, dirty finger nails.

168. Mrs. B5P, 9.
169. See, for example, Lancaster MOH Report, 1912, 125.
170. Mrs. A3B, 26. It is noteworthy that in his 1913 report, Lancaster's MOH advocated the
"hygienic practice of plaiting the hair" (127).
171. Mr. B1B, 71–72; Mrs. W1B, 11.
172. Mrs. H4P, 41.

These people used to shy away so them that kept themselves reasonably clean had to suffer along with the rest.[173]

Because of the close links between children's appearance and cleanliness, mothers' competence, and family reputations, the school-based inspection of children's heads represented more than public health authorities' efforts to limit the potential for lice-borne infection.

In addition to inspections, as indicated in chapter 4, oral history informants attending primary school after 1920 remembered being given milk and "emulsion" (cod-liver oil and malt) to prevent illness (particularly tuberculosis) and improve dental health. Mr. Norton, born in 1931 in Lancaster, remembered, "We were given emulsion at school and we were given cod-liver-oil capsules at school, but again, this was during the war where again vitamins were in short supply anyway. And we didn't decide to have these things, it was decided for us."[174] Mr. Monkham, born in 1948 in Lancaster, said that this practice continued after World War II:

And I well remember we started off very orderly and very nice, particularly the boys, the girls weren't too bad, but particularly the boys. And we were all told we had got to bring our own spoon to school of course, and in order to identify a particular spoon it was suggested that we wrap a piece of colored wool round it or raffia, so that you knew whose spoon was whose. But of course inevitably we found that seventeen of us were using the same spoon. And it was wiped clean on the jersey and it was passed, you know, behind to the next guy. And we survived, I don't remember an epidemic going through the school, but I probably exaggerated when I said seventeen of us, it was probably only about twelve.[175]

Like head inspections, classroom administration of emulsion was a step toward replacing mothers' traditional responsibility for preventive health care. In addition, it sent health-related messages to schoolchildren that were reinforced by the school's authority.

Schools also delivered information about health through domestic science and hygiene education—a strategy intended to mould the behavior of future mothers. As Elizabeth Roberts points out, the 1876 Education Code required girls to be taught domestic economy, which by the early twentieth century included sewing, cookery, and laundry work.[176] From the late nineteenth century, teacher training included instruction on healthful design, construction, and maintenance of school facilities as well as atten-

173. Mr. M1L, 77.
174. Mr. N2L, 52. See also Mrs. B4L, 63; Mrs. C8P, 89; Mr. M14B, 40–41.
175. Mr. M10L, 53.
176. Roberts, A woman's place, 30–31.

tion to students' health and personal hygiene, although this emphasized the teacher's knowledge rather than instruction to be given students about these matters. For example, *Health in Schools and Workshop* (1888) offered teachers guidelines ranging from appropriate sites, drainage, and ventilation of schools to physical and emotional developmental issues affecting students' health and ability to learn.[177]

The Physical Deterioration Report published in 1904 recognized the opportunity for schools to add health information to domestic science lessons, proposing that schoolgirls be given "social education" comprising "methods of infant care and management, cookery, hygiene and domestic economy."[178] Medical Officers of Health championed this approach. In 1910 Lancaster's MOH advocated establishment of a program

> in which the elder girls in the public elementary schools could be taught the management of infants and how best to bring them up. . . . The amount of ignorance as to the proper management (feeding, clothing, and surroundings) of little children in the families of the poor is absolutely astounding. This is far more marked in the towns than in the country, for in the country mothers still try to teach their daughters something of domestic duties, and when those girls are of a suitable age they go out to domestic situations, and learn in most cases much more. In the towns, however, girls seek employment in many other ways (mills, shops, clerks, etc.) and this effectually puts a stop to all further instruction in domestic matters, for when they reach home in the evening they naturally seek some recreation, or are too tired to take any interest in either recreation or the affairs of the family.[179]

This comment exemplifies Roberts's observation of official belief that there was no meaningful training in housewifery and hygiene taking place in working-class homes.[180] Yet, the oral evidence strongly indicates that most girls and young women both learned and exercised a full range of domestic skills at home. Thus, an alternative interpretation of health authorities'

177. *Health in schools and workshops* (London: Ward, Lock, & Co., 1888). Along similar lines was Arthur Newsholme's *School hygiene: The laws of health in relation to school life* (Boston: D. C. Heath and Co., 1904). By the interwar period, school hygiene and health education had become established parts of teacher training. See, for example, M. B. Davis, *Hygiene and health education for colleges of education,* published by Longmans, which appeared in 11 editions between 1932 and 1967. Its last edition still contained a chapter on eugenics (343–63).

178. Harris, *The health of the schoolchild,* 23.

179. Lancaster MOH Report, 1910, 24.

180. Roberts, *A woman's place,* 33. Some scholars have taken these observations at face value. See, for example, Margaret Hewitt, *Wives and mothers in Victorian industry* (London: Rockliff, 1958); Peter Stearns, "Working-class women in Britain, 1890–1914," in Marsha Vicinus, ed., *Suffer and be still: Women in the Victorian age* (Bloomington and London: Indiana University Press, 1972), 100–120.

observations suggests their desire to replace traditional "old wives'" lore with professionally endorsed knowledge and practices.

Older informants remembered school lessons that mainly dealt with housekeeping skills. Mrs. Peterson, born in 1899, said: "I can remember when we went to school we used to have housewifery classes. This cookery business they said we would have to plan for ourselves. Me and this other girl had to plan what we wanted and she didn't know what to have, but I wanted liver and bacon. We had to go to a big butcher's shop and we had to get 2 ounces of liver and somewhere else for an onion. We cooked them and we were allowed to have it when we had cooked it. Same with buns, we would have those when we had cooked them."[181] However, younger informants remembered instruction in both traditional housekeeping skills and health issues. Mrs. Jenkins, born in 1932, recalled a full domestic science curriculum involving cooking, washing, shopping, and even measuring for floor coverings. However, she also said: "I think we did hygiene at school and I used to follow it faithfully. I think I told you, the first thing I can remember as soon as I started to read was "Don't be afraid of soap and water," and I think the soap was chasing you, you know, and I thought why be afraid of soap and water. That was when I was only about five or six. It was when I first started reading and it was on the wall, a little poster. This is at St. George's, I remember it as if it was yesterday, isn't it funny? I could tell you everything about that classroom as if it was yesterday."[182] Apparently referring to a public health poster, this account shows that school-based health education and propaganda had their intended influence—at least on this informant. In addition to general hygiene, schools helped to disseminate information about contagious diseases. For example, in 1907 Lancaster's MOH reported:

> The Director of Education and I at our meeting agreed that it was advisable that a copy of Vacher's Diagram of Infectious Diseases should be placed in each school, and I think that this is being carried out. Also that a copy of that section of the Public Health Act, 1875, relating to the exposure of cases of Infectious Disease and the penalties incurred by disobedience should be exhibited in a prominent place in each school in order to impress the information upon the minds of the children. I think this would do much to teach the parents of the future that these infectious diseases, although at times simple and mild in character, should be carefully isolated and attended to.[183]

Validating lessons on hygiene and, as time went on, sex, were science classes.

181. Mrs. P1P, 3.
182. Mrs. J1B, 68.
183. Lancaster MOH Report, 1907, 12.

Mr. King, born in 1907 in Lancaster, said, "I liked physiology—lessons on the human body and anything appertaining. I was always interested in that. How many bones is in your body, and blood. That was one lesson I was really interested in."[184] This evidence also supports the argument that the health messages delivered at school were authoritative and remembered.

In addition to medical inspection and health education, during World War I study-city school medical services began to offer treatment—a step that was controversial because of its perceived threat to general practice but believed necessary because of parents' reluctance or inability to follow health authorities' advice to consult a doctor or dentist.[185] Ironically, because of the large numbers of children involved, treatment arguably increased working-class familiarity with professional medicine and aided the transition from informal to professional management of health problems. For example, in 1916 Preston's School Medical Officer supervised 40 schools with an average attendance of 17,620. As a result of "defects" found during medical inspections, the School Medical Service paid Preston Royal Infirmary 300 to treat 462 cases of defective vision, 234 children with enlarged tonsils and adenoids (231 had surgery), 25 diseases of the nose, 86 of the eye, and 44 of the ears.[186] The city also offered a free dental clinic, although the MOH repeatedly complained that parents resisted having children treated or waited too long to save decayed teeth.[187]

Of the treatment provided, oral history informants most frequently remembered attention from school dentists, which was universally feared and disliked. However, they also recalled traditional reactive approaches to private dental care, which involved no attention to teeth until they ached and no treatment but extraction, often performed by the neighborhood chemist. Mr. Ford, born in Preston in 1906, described a common experience: "It was horrifying to go to the dentist in our day. They just pulled them out. They used to say, 'Just pull my coat if I'm hurting you!' You were too petrified with fear to do anything. You just opened your mouth and he yanked it out! And you weren't taught to clean your teeth like they do today. I don't remember toothpaste, anyway. I remember trying to clean them with salt and water, but most people had a mouth full of rotten teeth and I suffered the agonies of hell with pyorrhea until I was eighteen or so."[188] It was common for people to have all of their teeth pulled very young. Mr. Barrington, born in Preston in 1927, recalled, "My mother said

184. Mr. K1L, 35.
185. See, for example, Welshman, *Municipal medicine,* 175. See also, for example, Lancaster MOH Reports for 1912 (141) and 1913 (120).
186. Preston School Medical Report, 1916, 3–4.
187. Preston School Medical Reports for 1917 (6) and 1918 (5). This problem was not unusual. See John Welshman, "Dental health as a neglected issue in medical history: The school dental service in England and Wales, 1900–40," *Medical History* 42 (1998): 310.
188. Mr. F1P, 6. See also, for example, Mrs. A3B, 40; Mr. C1P, 76–77.

she went one day to the dentist to have one tooth out and on the spur of the moment said to the dentist, 'You may as well take them all out!' And he did. I suppose she was just that sort of tidy person, one out all out!" When asked, "How old would she be then?" he responded, "I would think in her twenties, possibly. Like cutting her long hair, quite suddenly it went one day."[189]

The schools played a significant role in educating children about dental hygiene and treatment. Mr. Grove, born in 1903, said that when he was in school:

> I think school dentists were only just coming up in their time. This Dr. Brown said to me, "Do you clean your teeth?" Well, I didn't. There was nobody had toothbrushes or owt. I said, "Yes." He said, "Well, how often?" I just said, "Once a day." He said, "How often do you wash your face?" I said, "About three times a day." He said, "Your teeth are more important than your face." He was a proper old-fashioned doctor.
>
> *Mrs. Grove:* It was through the schools that we got brushes and Gibb's toothpaste. They gave them to us.
>
> *Mr. Grove:* I didn't get that. I only once remember we had a toothbrush in the house and I think everybody had a do with it.
>
> *Mrs. Grove:* I must have went to a better school than you.
>
> *Interviewer:* Did your children have toothbrushes, though?
>
> *Mr. Grove:* Yes. Our children had theirs, but we hadn't. To tell the truth, we were dirty in our way.[190]

Informants remembered school dentists being less concerned about individual children than private dentists. Mrs. Burrell, born in Barrow in 1931, said:

> Oh, when I think back when I used to go to the school clinic, I used to be terrified. They used to nearly pull me in. . . . Well, they weren't very nice, and one was a lady as well, and they weren't very nice at all to children, just like a conveyor belt, going in and out all the time. . . . I think the school dentists, they just used to pull teeth out, although I had quite a few teeth filled. I used to hate fillings because it hurt, I mean, they didn't do injections or anything then. But I think dentists now do tend to try and save the teeth more than they did when I was young.[191]

Informants also remembered school dentists being selective about the children offered treatment—a policy John Welshman explains by the decision,

---

189. Mr. B9P, 10. See also Mrs. H4L, 23.
190. Mr. G1P, 90.
191. Mrs. B2B, 54. See also Mr. R3B, 61, for an account of the same school dentist.

based on resource limitations, to offer dental treatment only to children whose parents had accepted it in the past.[192] Mr. Thomas, born in 1903 in Preston, had an alternative interpretation: "This was where the school people came in. Just about that time the dentist used to come to school, I think it was question of who was recommended, who they were, what contacts the parents had with the teacher or the headmaster. We had two divisions in our school, one with clogs and one with shoes. This made all the difference in the world to selection in our school. . . . I'm not saying for a minute that the upper classes were generally a little bit better than what the rest of them was. . . . But it was question of they got the dentist."[193]

Although access to school dentists improved over time, people did not necessarily take advantage of their services. For example, Mr. Fleming, born in 1917 in Lancaster, said: "Once I went to the dentist to Mr. Smith, the school dentist. He gave me two pennies for not crying. And then after that I never went again until I was seventeen, I think I was. And then I went to a chap that's a friend of the family's. I went to his house one Sunday morning and [he] took the bottom set out. And then the following week, a fortnight after, he took the others out. . . . I was fed up with them, I was getting toothache."[194] Nonetheless, a likely effect of school-related dental education, examination, and treatment was that almost all oral history informants said their children had regular preventive and therapeutic dental care.

CONCLUSIONS

As we have seen, maternal, infant, and child welfare was embraced by local as well as national leaders, appealing to the left, right, and center of the political spectrum. Less controversial than prevention of contagious diseases, initiatives associated with this goal endured throughout the period under consideration, altering with changes in demography, science, technology, and political environment, but continuing into the post–World War II era when the target shifted from working-class people generally to "problem families" and children with special needs.[195] Regardless of techniques used, the objectives of improving the health and moral status of working-class people remained and implied reducing the authority and agency of working-class mothers and their informal advisors.

Statistics validated the success of early-twentieth-century efforts. After World War II, infant and maternal mortality ceased to be major problems in Barrow, Lancaster, and Preston. Given public credit for these and other improvements in health and longevity, formal health authorities completed

192. Welshman, "Dental health," 319–20.
193. Mr. T2P, 76.
194. Mr. F1L, 31.
195. See, for example, Welshman, *Municipal medicine*, 241–47.

the process of medicalizing pregnancy, birth, and child care. Women of all social classes were encouraged to mistrust their knowledge of their own bodies and those of their children and, instead, to "call the doctor" for interpretation of all physical and mental sensations and advice regarding all health-related decisions. This change rang the death knell for lay female management of childbearing and child care. It occurred generationally, with older women resisting the services of qualified midwives, health visitors, and physicians, while younger women learned officially sanctioned health information and behavior, then rejected as "old-fashioned" the advice of their mothers and neighborhood health authorities. As the "modern" generation, born after 1920, came of age, that advice was increasingly regarded as quaint and backward—associated with gendered ignorance and superstition encapsulated in "old wives' tales," and displayed in a variety of unhealthy behaviors. Dependence on the scientific health advice and care delivered by licensed educational, medical, and public health experts became a characteristic of the responsible and respectable parent; none of the informants contributing to this study who reached adulthood after World War II questioned the authority of these professionals—although some members of this group occasionally displayed passive resistance by failing to follow advice.

Chapter Seven

≈

"By gum, we did enjoy it"

Popular Media and the Construction
of Modern Health Culture

INTRODUCTION

The core question of this book is why and how traditional working-class Lancashire health culture was transformed in the mid-twentieth century. Previous chapters have documented the shift of working-class experience from home-based management of health and illness, predominantly controlled by laywomen, to professional management of these matters, increasingly in institutional settings. We have observed what might be called enforcement emanating from professional medicine and public health—factors ranging from the increasing gate-keeping functions of physicians to the surveillance, notification, and isolation required by local health authorities—as well as the attraction of proliferating publicly sponsored services, such as low-cost or free supplies and advice provided by neighborhood clinics. However, we have also considered the sturdy survival into the interwar period of traditional ways of preventing illness and dealing with health events, as well as continuing working-class selectivity about which professional advice and services to accept. It is, therefore, striking that after World War II these traditions became "old-fashioned," and that working-class people belatedly experienced conversion to what Paul Starr identified as the cultural authority of physicians, and what might more broadly be conceptualized as the cultural authority of professional medicine.[1]

Starr explains this conversion, which he dates from the Progressive Era in the United States, by a new popular consensus that specialized scientific training beyond the generalized knowledge of the layman was required to

---

1. Paul Starr, *The social transformation of American medicine* (New York: Basic Books, 1982).

deal with illness, injury, childbearing, and other health challenges.[2] While
this consensus also developed in middle-class Victorian Britain, it evolved
later among people further down the social ladder.[3] As chapter 3 argues,
working-class men and women did not share the social comfort of middle-class patients with physicians and other formally qualified health care
workers. Neither did science and technology always appear as unalloyed
benefits to people who were arguably likely to associate these entities, not
with opportunities or solutions to problems, but with unwelcome changes
in the workplace (e.g., new machines and processes), justification for mandated medical coercion (e.g., vaccination, admission to isolation hospitals
or TB sanatoria), or challenges from teachers and schoolchildren to parental authority. Furthermore, in Starr's narrative, doctors' cultural authority
was imposed from the top down by an active, successful, occupational group
upon a passive, faceless, and undifferentiated public, which automatically
accepted and internalized it.[4] By contrast, the oral history and public health
evidence counter this supply-side, "Field of Dreams" account, revealing a
good deal of working-class resistance to medical authority, as well as considerable diversity in acceptance of official health care advice and attention.
Therefore, it seems clear that, in addition to pressure from professional
medicine and public policy, other factors influenced the transformation of
working-class health culture. Exclusive dependence on the oral and public
health evidence may blinker understanding of the broad cultural environment within which this transformation occurred. This chapter considers
messages regarding "modern medicine" purveyed in the mass media, arguing that these messages stimulated changes in working-class perception of
health care personnel, institutions, and interventions.

The chapter uses evidence drawn from popular magazines, radio programs, and films—media outlets arguably new to working-class consumers
in the early twentieth century that increasingly featured medical themes.
Michael Shortland writes of the cinema:

> After a period during the 1920s during which two or three films were
> released each year on medical themes, there occurred a steady but
> remarkable rise in output during the thirties, compared to the overall
> film output during the period. In the ten years from 1930 to 1939,
> over 100 medical films have been recorded, which signals a remarkable

2. Starr, *Social transformation*, 140–42.

3. M. Jeanne Peterson, *The medical profession in mid-Victorian London* (Berkeley: University
of California Press, 1978); Bernice A. Pescosolido and Jack K. Martin, "Cultural authority and
the sovereignty of American medicine: The role of networks, class and community," *Journal of
Health Politics, Policy and Law* 29 (2004): 4–5, 735–56.

4. John Harley Warner points out the absence of nonphysicians from Starr's social history,
citing, in particular, a review by Susan Reverby that critiqued Starr's silence about patients (769).
Warner, "Grand narrative and its discontents: Medical history and the social transformation of
American medicine," *Journal of Health Politics, Policy and Law* 29 (2004): 4–5, 757–80.

degree of interest on the part of film-makers and audiences alike. The
war years witnessed a steep decline again . . . after which output was relatively steady at four or five films per year during the fifties and sixties.[5]

The same escalating attention to biomedicine appeared in magazine features and radio programs. Coinciding with increasing governmental investment in clinical medicine and public health services, stories with medical
plots and positive characterizations of doctors, nurses, hospitals, patients,
and medical interventions proliferated and arguably helped to construct
new working-class perspectives about these matters. At the same time, in
vehicles ranging from magazine drug advertisements to radio lectures,
media messages projected the authority of science and modern medicine.
While these developments were not initiated by the British medical profession or its powerful social-class, political, and industrial allies, they were
influenced by and benefited formally trained and qualified health care
workers and institutions. They also served an educational function among
working-class people, most of whose personal experience of professional
medicine did not reflect the white-garbed saviors and gleaming chromed
environments of its media representations.

During the interwar years, there was widening awareness of the power
of the mass media to shape public opinion through the employment of
advertising and propaganda methods.[6] Physicians both used and censored
media products to influence the representation and reputation of their
profession.[7] In addition, messages intended to convince or sell, including
public health posters and advertisements for patent remedies, borrowed
from and enhanced the growing authority of biomedicine by using authoritative heroic images of doctors, nurses, and scientists, on the one hand,
and receptive compliant images of newly stereotyped "patients" and their
caregivers, on the other.

Since working-class health care decision-making was highly gendered,
it is particularly important to consider the impact of these messages on
women. Both the volume and range of popular media products and working-class women's access to them increased substantially after World War
I. Furthermore, many media products specifically targeted working-class
women, while others appealed to women because of factors including cost,
the environment in which they were consumed, and the developing reputations of those products and their consumption. The fact that magazine
reading and radio listening, for example, were typically done at home, and

5. Michael Shortland, *Medicine and film: A checklist, survey and research resource* (Oxford:
Wellcome Unit for the History of Medicine, 1989), 10.

6. See, for example, Mariel Grant, *Propaganda and the role of the state in inter-war Britain*
(Oxford: Clarendon Press, 1994), particularly chapter 5, "Health Publicity 1919–1939," 123–93.

7. Ann Karpf, *Doctoring the media: The reporting of health and medicine* (London: Routledge,
1988), 32–33, 42, 44, 110–32; Shortland, *Medicine and film*, 8.

film attendance was both inexpensive and respectable, made such activities particularly attractive to women. In turn, inundation with positive media messages about modern professional medicine and normatively passive and deferent patient behavior supported changes in working-class women's health care choices—including decline of reliance on traditional preventives, therapies, and care providers.

I hypothesize that the information and images delivered by magazines, radio programs, and movies helped support a hegemonic process whereby working-class people adopted professional medicine's valuation of itself and accepted its authority at the same time as they also relinquished traditional lay female authority regarding health matters. Furthermore, an important reason for the comparative success of this process was that, unlike the sometimes painful interference with working-class bodies and daily lives by physicians, nurses, and public health workers, consuming mass media products was pleasurable, embodying the adage that a spoonful of sugar helps the medicine go down.

This chapter focuses on three forms of mass media that were especially popular among working-class women: weekly magazines, radio programs, and feature films. While other media products, such as newspapers, documentary movies, and television shows, had medical content and were produced and widely available during the period under consideration, they are not emphasized here for reasons including overwhelming range and volume of material (newspapers), limited distribution and popularity (documentary films), and comparatively late release (television "doctor" shows). Popular magazines, radio programs, and films projected different, although complementary, perspectives on health, medicine, treatments, doctors, nurses, and hospitals. The health content of women's magazines was diverse, addressing a wide range of goals (e.g., sales, advice, entertainment) and audiences (e.g., young employed women, mothers, wives, older women). Magazines adopted a familiar, cozy tone, more often implying acceptance of readers' customary ways of doing things than overtly challenging those practices. By contrast, radio programs on health issues tended to be didactic and motivational, or, if fictional, reflected middle-class norms. Providing a third alternative, feature films created imaginary worlds with time frames, cultures, and events far different from the day-to-day realities of their audiences. Along with vicarious experience and emotion, the "pictures" delivered medical images with huge authority and power—images that inevitably colored the ways working-class people viewed illness, treatments, nurses, doctors, and hospitals. The common denominator of these diverse media representations was the presumption that modern professional medicine was better than any alternative and offered an altruistic, scientific, safe, and incontestably correct approach to health challenges. That presumption was highly gendered, represented by predominantly male physicians supported by female nurses and doctors'

wives. It also emphasized both the chasm and the partnership between medical professionals and laypeople, demonstrating the almost invariable success of medical management coupled with patient compliance.

This chapter uses oral history and other evidence to support the contention that working-class people regularly read cheap periodicals, listened to the radio, and went to the cinema. It explores the medical content of mass media products, including sampled issues of *Woman's Weekly,* a magazine published beginning in 1911 for a largely lower middle- and working-class readership; feature films with medical themes; and radio programs. Finally, it observes in the annual reports of the Medical Officers of Health increasing official utilization of techniques borrowed from the mass media to transmit health messages.

WORKING-CLASS LEISURE, GENDER, AND POPULAR MEDIA

Working-class men and women engaged in different types of leisure activities.[8] As Claire Langhamer points out, "A conceptualization of leisure as fundamentally distinct from work is unhelpful to the study of women's experiences. In essence, 'leisure' as constructed by many historians is a gendered concept: understandings of the category assume the male wage-earning experience to be normative."[9] According to Andrew Davies, "Drinking, gambling and sport, three of the cornerstones of 'traditional' working-class culture, were all heavily male-dominated, and men were identified by their hobbies or by the pubs where they drank as 'regulars,' as well as by their occupations and political or religious allegiances."[10] In their time off work, Barrow, Lancaster, and Preston men also went fishing, kept garden allotments, and raced whippets. For the most part, women did not participate in these activities; for example, women, who were welcome with their husbands in the saloon bar on a Saturday evening, risked their reputations if they entered pubs alone or with women friends at other times. Working-class leisure activities were customarily sex-segregated.

In addition to gender, participation in leisure activities was affected by age and life stage. In the early twentieth century, while young, single working women went to dances and promenaded with their friends, meet-

8. See, for example, Elizabeth Roberts, *Women and families: An oral history, 1940–1970* (Oxford: Blackwell, 1995), 99–100.

9. Claire Langhamer, *Women's leisure in England 1920–60* (Manchester and New York: Manchester University Press, 2000), 2

10. Andrew Davies, "Leisure in the 'classic slum,'" in *Workers' worlds: Cultures and communities in Manchester and Salford, 1880–1939,* Andrew Davies and Steven Fielding, eds. (Manchester and New York: Manchester University Press, 1992), 107. See also Andrew Davies, *Leisure, gender and poverty: Working-class culture in Salford and Manchester, 1900–1939* (Buckingham and Philadelphia: Open University Press, 1992); John K. Walton, *Lancashire: A Social History, 1558–1939* (Manchester University Press, 1987), 297–300.

ing single young men on "monkey parades," married working-class women engaged in few formal leisure activities outside the home.[11] This was related to financial resources: poorer families—particularly those with many young children at the low point of the poverty cycle—could less afford purchased entertainment, such as music hall tickets and seaside daytrips or holidays, than more prosperous families.[12] Furthermore, despite rising wages, interruptions of employment affected working-class financial decisions, limiting recreational spending.[13] As household managers, married women paid the bills and distributed "pocket money" to wage-earning husbands and children. In many cases, there was little left for women to spend on themselves—particularly for entertainment, although this generalization also affected necessities, such as food, furniture, and clothing.[14]

The effort necessary to manage the household, do the housework, care for men and children, and (sometimes) work outside the home both limited women's leisure time and rendered porous the boundaries between labor and other activities. Furthermore, the reputation for constant work and devotion to duty enhanced a woman's status. For these reasons, working-class women's recreation was normatively intertwined with their work. As indicated in chapter 2, their conversations with neighbors on the street, over backyard walls and washing lines, in corner shops, traveling to and from work, and in factories cemented relationships and supported mutual aid; chatting was also an important form of leisure for working-class women. Mrs. Boyle, born in 1936, who lived in a poor working-class Preston neighborhood, remembered:

> Well, I were never one for going out, but we could never afford, could we, for one thing? B[ob] [husband] used to go for a drink. Like I say, we got into that house on Allen Street, and I always had Marie and Jean to keep me company, always, you know. . . . Oh yes, and we always, if it was summer, they always sat on my step . . . with a brew, you know. And two of us smoked, me and Marie, there was always fag ends from where we had smoked, we always had to sweep up the morning after. Jean didn't smoke. Oh yes, we sat on the step while half past ten. But so did every-

11. For discussion of the courting ritual referred to as a "monkey walk," "monkey run," or "monkey parade," see Davies, *Leisure, gender and poverty*, 102–8; David Fowler, "Teenage consumers? Young wage-earners and leisure in Manchester, 1919–1939," in *Workers' worlds: Cultures and communities in Manchester and Salford, 1880–1939*, Andrew Davies and Steven Fielding, eds. (Manchester and New York: Manchester University Press, 1992), 148; Langhamer, *Women's leisure*, 119.

12. See, for example, John K. Walton, *The British seaside: Holidays and resorts in the twentieth century* (Manchester and New York: Manchester University Press, 2000), 15, 51–72.

13. John Benson, *The rise of consumer society in Britain, 1880–1980* (London and New York: Longman, 1994), 14, 26; Walton, *Lancashire: A Social History*, 283–84, 325–54.

14. See, for example, Laura Oren, "The welfare of women in laboring families: England, 1860–1950," in Mary Hartman and Lois W. Banner, eds., *Clio's consciousness raised: New perspectives on the history of women* (New York: Harper Torchbooks, 1974), 226–44.

body then, didn't they, old ladies used to be sat out in their chairs, you know, or their little stools. And everybody used to be sat out at the doors usually, you used to hear everybody coming home from the pubs and that, you know, and we used to say, "Pubs are loose and we are going in." So we knew then that it was time to go in. Then B[ob] was coming home after having a drink and that. . . . I didn't drink a lot then. An odd time I've gone out, I've gone to my mum and my dad and had a game of bingo at the club and then I've come home, yes. But, no, I didn't used to like drink a lot, no. Never were into drinking. I weren't one for going out anyway, but you know I wouldn't leave the kids with anybody.[15]

This account illustrates several characteristics of working-class women's leisure: its collective, informal, sex-segregated nature; its difference from that of men; its operation within the limits of male domination; and its association with respectability. Even into the 1950s and '60s, good working-class married women did not drink much, except perhaps at Christmas-time. They mainly associated socially with other married women and family members. And they did not leave their children in other people's care in order to go out and enjoy themselves.

HEALTHY READING: *WOMAN'S WEEKLY*

Oral history informants remembered their mothers engaging in little leisure activity, even within the home. Reading was considered within this category. Mrs. Ackerman, born in 1904, said, "Mum never read a book, she never had time. I think she was so tired at night that she was glad to get to bed."[16] Similarly, Mr. Best, born in 1897, remembered: "The only time m'mother used to read was Sunday afternoon. She was always working, looking after the family but Sundays, no work on Sundays, nothing had to be done. You hadn't even to sew a button on. . . . After Sunday dinner mother used to get these little books like *Home Chat* and she'd read those and *St. Mark's Church Magazine* . . . and Mother used to love the *War Cry* [a Salvation Army magazine]."[17]

As these examples indicate, reading at home was a respectable, inexpensive, and comparatively flexible recreational activity for working-class married women. After the 1870 Education Act, literacy levels rose. Few oral history informants remembered mothers who were unable to read.[18] Some informants recalled mothers reading books or regularly patronizing a public library. These activities were especially respectable and associated

15. Mrs. B11P, 56. See also Roberts, *A woman's place*, 188–89.
16. Mrs. A2B, 20. See also Mrs. C2B, 8.
17. Mr. B1B, 88. See also Mr. R1L, 37.
18. See, for example, Mrs. P1P, 40; Mr. P1B, 29.

with upward-mobility aspirations. For example, Mr. Carson, born in 1902 in Lancaster, said of his mother:

> She was in domestic service and of course I assume she had access to books of the household and she acquired quite a general knowledge that way, and she could retain it because she had a wonderful memory. . . . For what she was, she was really an intelligent woman. She could talk on almost any topic and she'd read a lot and kept herself up-to-date with papers, right up till she couldn't bother any more, it was too much trouble. She always got a daily paper and the *Observer,* of course, which was the best paper in the town, much better than the [*Lancaster*] *Guardian.*[19]

However, informants also recalled disadvantages to reading books. New ones were expensive and, as indicated in chapter 4, library books were thought to transmit contagious diseases. Mr. Kirby, born in Barrow in 1921, said, "My mother was probably averse to borrowing books from the library that other people had had. And that sort of thing, you know. . . . In the old days they thought you would get some disease off them, or something I think."[20] Furthermore, books were long; some informants remembered that reading books was considered a waste of time.[21]

It was more usual for women to read magazines and newspapers, which were also popular with other family members.[22] Indeed, reading of proliferating periodical genres was both gender- and age-related. Children tended to purchase comics; teens got age- and interest-related magazines; women bought women's magazines and romance serials; and newspapers, although read by all family members, were most strongly associated with men. Mr. Trickett, born in 1921, remembered, "My mum didn't read an awful lot, she liked a magazine because she used to get *Woman.*" His father read newspapers:

> We got the *Daily Express,* partly because his dad had got the *Daily Express* before him, not from politics, I don't think. And he got the *Sunday Express* and the *Daily Mail.* I think we might have got the *Barrow News,* and he also read very regularly the *Thompson Weekly News,* a Scottish paper. We used to get it from a neighbor and then we got it ourselves, you know, for quite a while, with Black Bob and all the rest. Oh yes, my mother got passed on a *People's Friend,* so that was another Scottish influence. . . . My sister used to get the *School Friend* and I got the *School*

19. Mr. C1L, 15.
20. Mr. K1B, 27.
21. See, for example, Mrs. A3B, 36.
22. See, for example, Mr. A2B, 96; Mr. D2P, 59; Mrs. H5L, 31; Mrs. H6L, 36; Mr. H7L, 28; Mrs. L3L, 24; Mr. R1L, 37; Mrs. R4B, 28.

Friend, and we got a kiddy one called *Play Box,* or something, and then we moved on to the *Topper.*[23]

Magazines were especially important recreational materials for married women—a fact indicated by the booming market. Cynthia White dates the escalation in the number of magazines published for women from the last twenty years of the nineteenth century, saying, "Excluding family journals and all-fiction periodicals, both of which had a feminine bias, not less than 48 new titles entered the field between 1880 and 1900."[24] According to Ros Ballaster and her coauthors:

> By 1900 most of the characteristic elements of the late-twentieth-century women's magazine were already being used in different combinations in *Home Chat, Woman, Woman at Home, The Gentlewoman* and other magazines of the period. There were the short stories and serials (almost always romantic), the articles on housekeeping, childcare and family relationships, the recipes, the fashion-plates and pull-out dress patterns, the letters pages addressing "personal" problems, dress, appearance or medical matters, the illustrated articles about the famous and royal, the competitions, the gossip columns, the advertisements for aids to beauty and home.[25]

The early years of the twentieth century witnessed periodical publishers reaching farther down the social scale than ever before, targeting the non-servant-keeping housewife and the factory worker.[26] Margaret Beetham observes, "The most important journalistic development of the 1890s in terms of women's reading was the cheap, that is the penny, domestic weekly. By 1910 it had established that dominance in the market which it was to retain unbroken for the rest of the twentieth century. Simultaneously cheap and 'respectable,' these magazines used the well-established formula of the genre to revitalize the tradition of the English domestic woman's journal which stretched back to Beeton in mid-century."[27] An important reason for the increase in the number of women's magazines in the early years of the study period was the targeting of women as consumers. Advertisers and publishers became mutually dependent; both reached out to working-class

---

23. Mr. T4B, 49–50.

24. Cynthia L. White, *Women's magazines 1693–1968* (London: Michael Joseph, 1970), 58.

25. Ros Ballaster, Margaret Beetham, Elizabeth Frazer, and Sandra Hebron, *Women's worlds: Ideology, femininity and the woman's magazine* (Houndmills and London: Macmillan Education, 1991), 118.

26. White, *Women's magazines,* 70.

27. Margaret Beetham, *A magazine of her own? Domesticity and desire in the woman's magazine, 1800–1914* (London and New York: Routledge, 1996), 190.

women as the main purchasers of consumer goods for their households.[28]

These magazines reached both their buyers and a much larger group of readers, since a single magazine tended to be passed around the family and neighborhood. Contents of magazines informed women's conversations. For example, Mrs. Peterson, born in 1899, said, "I used to get the *Woman's Companion* and there used to be stories in it all about babies. . . . The woman across the street got the *Woman's Companion* and we would be at the door sometimes discussing the stories."[29]

The oral evidence indicates that working-class women enjoyed the variety of features in magazines. Mrs. Owen, born in 1916, said:

I bought magazines and read them there. My husband was in the library.

Interviewer: What magazines did you enjoy, when she [daughter] was younger, say?

Informant: Oh, I've forgotten. Was it *Peg's Papers?* Oh, I've forgotten now, I couldn't remember. I'd also forgotten I used to get the *Woman* or the *Realm*, all those, but I can't remember.

Interviewer: What did you like especially about women's magazines?

Informant: I used to like the cookery and the agony page, love story, that was all.[30]

Mrs. Horton, born in 1903 in Lancaster, remembered, "I always bought *Red Letter.*" When asked, "What was that?" she replied, "One serial and one or two short stories like *Woman's Weekly* is now. One or two stories complete and then there would be one or two that was serials."[31] Women read magazines sometimes in spite of male disapproval. Mrs. Howard, born in 1931, commented: "You know, there was a magazine out called *Red Letter, Silver Star,* no they weren't allowed in the house. . . . Do you know he [father] wouldn't even buy the *News of the World,* because scandal was in it. *News of the World* was the paper that you just daren't look at, and my mother, I remember she used to get one or two magazines and hide them. And she used to say, 'Shift that *Red Star,*' or 'Mind that. Wait a minute, I'll have to hide this before your dad comes in.' Because he would just tear them up and throw them on the fire."[32] In this account, the romances Mrs. Howard's father found silly or immoral were thought respectable by her mother and may even have been associated with the same femaleness as was the infor-

---

28. See, for example, Benson, *Rise of consumer society,* 28; White, *Women's magazines,* 65–66.

29. Mrs. P1P, 40.

30. Mrs. O1B, 46.

31. Mrs. H3L, 47. The *Red Letter* series was a numbered series of short romantic novels, hundreds of which were published in the 1920s and '30s. Like similar series, such as *Silver Star,* these pamphlets sold "for coppers," according to Mrs. A2B, 110.

32. Mrs. H5L, 31.

mation about and evidence of menstruation, which also had to be hidden from men. It is arguable that women's magazines helped to both construct and represent women's changing identities and roles as the study period progressed.[33]

One constant aspect of those identities and roles was the woman's "natural" association with health-related decision making and caregiving. Women's magazines reflected and helped to shape health-related beliefs and behaviors through advertisements, stories, and advice columns.[34] To explore the health content of a magazine available to and read by working-class women in Barrow, Lancaster, and Preston, we will examine the pages of *Woman's Weekly,* a magazine first published by Newnes in 1911, when it sold for one penny per issue, and which remains among the most popular women's magazines in Britain.[35] From the beginning, the magazine contained advice columns, knitting and sewing patterns, short stories and serials, and the inevitable advertisements; it clearly targeted as its audience respectable young unmarried women (employed and unemployed), as well as wives, homemakers, mothers, and older women. Several oral history informants remembered reading *Woman's Weekly* themselves or women relatives regularly purchasing it.[36]

In its first issue the magazine's editor addressed readers thus:

> First of all, I should like to tell you the dominant note throughout is that of "usefulness." You will find that page after page is crammed with information and help that will assist women in their daily lives as no other journal has attempted before. Our one desire is to please the average woman. I say frankly that the women of Mayfair and the lady who lives in the castle are not catered for in this paper. But the woman who lives in the villa or the cottage, in a large house or a small house— the woman who rules the destinies of the home, is going to be helped in her life, her work, and her recreation by this journal.[37]

33. This is an argument made by Penny Tinkler in *Constructing girlhood: Popular magazines for girls growing up in England, 1920–1950* (London: Taylor and Francis, 1995), and Ballister et al., in *Women's worlds.*

34. See, for example, White, *Women's magazines,* 102.

35. Beetham, *A magazine of her own,* 203. According to Ballister et al., *Women's worlds,* "In 1988, *Woman's Weekly* had a circulation of 1,325,742—largest of the weeklies reviewed for this book" (179). I reviewed issues of the magazine at five-year intervals (1911, 1916, 1921, etc., to 1970) to observe change and continuity in the ways health-related matters were presented. While other women's magazines (*Woman's Own, Woman*) would also have offered appropriate source material, as a cheap weekly published for much of the study period that had a large working-class circulation, *Woman's Weekly* seemed the most appropriate for the purposes of my project. *Woman's Weekly* is still published, targeting mainly women readers over age 50. See, for example, Joan Barrell and Brian Braithwaite, *The business of women's magazines* (London: Kogan Page, 1979), 143–44.

36. See, for example, Mrs. H3L, 47; Mr. P5B, 36; Mrs. R4B, 28.

37. *Woman's Weekly* 1:1 (1911): 2.

In its 36 pages, this issue contained ten advertisements with health-related content (for baby and infant foods (4), hair improvement and removal (2), a series of books on women's life stages (defined by fertility and reproduction, menstruation and menopause), a weight-loss product, a headache treatment, and a cure for skin blemishes). It also included an advice column on infant feeding written by "our own Medical Adviser"; a column on "How to become a Nurse," by Miss E. Margaret Fox, Matron of the Prince of Wales's Hospital, London; and a serial story about a horrid newly rich widow with one little boy: "Her child had his nurse, his servants, his toys, and a doctor to attend him periodically. What more could he want? One thing, and one thing only, and that Leonora Templecore had not to give him—true motherly love."[38] The contents of this issue emphasized the mother's special responsibility for her children's health and supported her independence in caring for them—even when severe health problems, such as convulsions, occurred. In just one situation, that of serious illness due to teething, did the writer suggest consulting a doctor—in this case, to have the infant's gums lanced.[39] The only references to official medical authority were in advertisements: to a nurse, who provided a testimonial for "The great Antipon treatment" for weight loss, and to "medical men" for St. Ivel Lactic Cheese, "which eliminate[s] the poisons that other foods create, and thus keep[s] the system in splendid condition."[40] The issue contributed to an image of motherhood that was both natural and learned but always central to women's identity. The column "How to become a Nurse" emphasized the centrality of caregiving to women's nature: "The wish to relieve suffering is happily a Divine instinct planted in every womanly heart; and when a kindly sympathetic girl has perhaps for the first time had an opportunity of helping the doctor in an emergency and been praised for her presence of mind, or has successfully nursed a friend through an attack of illness, and been gratefully thanked for her services, it is quite natural that the pleasant experience should make her think there is no occupation in life so desirable as that of caring for the sick."

In this piece, while the doctor's presence in a medical emergency is presumed, trained nursing is defined not in terms of being his second-in-command but as "a reliable, useful means of making a living, so that whether I marry or remain single, I may always be of real use to other people."[41] By contrast, "The Experiences of a Hospital Nurse," published in 1916, focused on proper etiquette between doctors and nurses and the physician's superior authoritative role.[42]

Early issues of *Woman's Weekly* emphasized a domestic ideology and a

38. Ibid., 6.
39. Ibid., 5.
40. Ibid., 15, inside back cover.
41. Ibid., 35.
42. *Woman's Weekly* 9:239 (1916): 621.

traditional version of femininity that the magazine intended to enhance
by providing a little expert or modern advice. For example, from the start
most issues contained advertisements for manufactured sanitary towels
(which few working-class women used until 20 years later); this suggests
both a modern orientation and a traditional just-between-us-girls effort (by
virtue of publication in a magazine for women) to keep information about
menstruation from men.[43] There were also regular reminders of the dangers of "germs," new enemies for traditional homemakers to be aware of
and combat. In December 1911, one article warned mothers about "germ-
laden milk," while the column "Pantry Points" reminded readers, "One
must not forget that much dirt—and often the most deadly sort too—is
of the invisible kind, which cannot be detected by even the most sharp-
sighted housewife."[44] New scientific information was sometimes combined
with old-fashioned domestic crafts. A 1919 issue included a pattern for a
cover to "Keep out the flies. You must keep the flies out of milk and other
foods as you don't know from what dirty place they have just flown. You
want a cover that will keep out foreigners, but at the same time let in the
air, so here is the very thing. Take a piece of net or old lace and cut into a
circle," which was then edged with beads to hold the cover over the cup,
jar, or bowl.[45]

By the same token, old-fashioned ideas, relationships, and practices
were sometimes validated by professional experts. In a 1919 advice feature,
"A Page for the Children," the author described coltsfoot as "a very common thing given to children for coughs before so many patent medicines
came into use," while in the same year a new advice column by Florence
Stacpoole, "For Mother and Home," answered the question, "I am advised
by a friend to leave off my three-months-old baby's binder. I mean the flannel abdominal swathe. I have my doubts as to whether this advice is wise.
Do you think it is?" with the following response:

> Indeed it is *not.* It is most dangerous advice. . . . Read this quotation
> from Dr. O'Hea's little book, *The Rearing of Children.* "An adult has
> under the skin of the abdomen a layer of fat, and this fat is a bad
> conductor of heat. Deeper still, under the muscles of this part, there
> is a fatty apron which hangs down over the coils of the intestines, or
> bowels, like a protecting shield. Those layers of fat prevent the cold
> from 'striking through,' as the popular saying is, to the delicate organs
> of the abdomen; or more correctly speaking, prevents too great a loss

43. Many issues also contain advertisements for abortifacients under vague titles such as
"Ladies! Safeguard your health!"; "What every woman ought to know"; and "Catherine Kearsley's
original Widow Welch's female pills. Prompt and reliable for ladies." See, for example, *Woman's
Weekly* 9:219 (1916): inside back cover; *Woman's Weekly* 47:209 (1935): 30.
    44. *Woman's Weekly* 1:5 (1911): 146; *Woman's Weekly* 1:6 (1911): 175.
    45. *Woman's Weekly* 16:401 (1919): 14.

of heat from those organs. A baby is poorly provided with abdominal fat, compared with an adult. The deeper layer of fat in the abdomen of a baby is badly developed and hence there is a greater susceptibility to cold. Many attacks of diarrhea are set up in this way."[46]

Both the qualified, published physician-expert and the traditional female health authority figure (the older woman adviser) approved use of an infant garment that was on its way to the biomedical scrap heap. The doctor's argument for the binder, however, was couched in modern scientific language.

Similarly, in a 1916 series, "Mrs. Barker's Second Baby," the district nurse, Mrs. Merrydew, both a representative of modern trained nursing and a throwback to the female neighborhood health authority, gave advice on a comprehensive range of issues to a young pregnant woman whose husband was in military service at the Front. (Among other things, the nurse told Mrs. Barker that "rickets is sometimes one of the consequences of nursing too long.") Mrs. Merrydew adopted an authoritative, patronizing demeanor toward Mrs. Barker, on one occasion expressing shock that the young woman had started to take in washing to augment her income: "'You threw all those sheets and tablecloths over those lines yourself?' 'Yes, of course I did,' said Mrs. Barker proudly. 'Well, sister,' said the nurse impressively, 'Many a one has done the same when in your condition, and has rued the day—all her life after. It is a most unsafe thing to do, and is a frequent cause of internal mischief—perhaps permanent mischief.'" Mrs. Merrydew and Mrs. Barker's mother, Mrs. Bramble, attended the young woman during the final days of her pregnancy, collaborating, for example, on care of a decayed tooth, for which (on the authority of "all the best doctors") the mother recommended extraction and Mrs. Merrydew advised getting a powder from the chemist, meanwhile suggesting a home remedy (rinsing the mouth with warm water and baking soda). The district nurse combined this scattergun approach with a mixture of scientific and traditional wisdom, saying: "I wish I had known earlier about the tooth going. I would have recommended you to take a little phosphate of lime. You see, Mrs. Barker, what is often forgotten is that there is a great drain of lime from the mother's system before her baby is born, and this leads to tooth decay and toothache. It has given rise to the old saying, 'For every child a tooth.'" Mrs. Merrydew and Mrs. Bramble eventually delivered the baby safely at home (without a doctor), keeping from Mrs. Barker the news that her husband was missing in action on the grounds that "bad news sud-

46. *Woman's Weekly* 15:379 (1919): 81; *Woman's Weekly* 16:401 (1919): 16. In an earlier column (1/11/19), Ms. Stacpoole advised that the baby wear the binder "until all the first teeth are cut; or it may be replaced rather earlier by a pair of legless drawers—not open ones, but closed up—so as to keep an even warmth round the intestines. The too early removal of this, or the 'binder' may do serious harm" (20).

denly told to a newly-made mother has often cost her her life. The shock
may throw her into a fever, or bring on some serious complication. . . . A
healthy young woman like Mrs. Barker will soon be able to nurse her baby,
if we can but keep her mind tranquil." Happily, at the end of the story Mr.
Barker arrived home safe and sound.[47] This formula of fictional characters
with whom readers could identify; health advice blending common sense,
traditional home-based care, and scientific authority; and a dramatic timely
plot provides a useful illustration of the strength of women's magazines in
delivering health content.

Woman's Weekly's health advice was sometimes politically contextual-
ized—particularly in wartime. For example, on January 1, 1916, the new
agony aunt, Mrs. Marryat, addressed her readers with this "New Year's Message": "Never before in our country's history has the life of a baby been so
valuable as it is now. Our babies of today are the citizens of the future; they
are the Empire-makers of the years ahead. If we are to have any Empire at
all, if we are to keep our enemies at bay in the years to come, we must have
strong and brave men and healthy, vigorous women as the future fathers
and mothers of our English race."[48] Similarly, later that month an advertisement for Hall's Wine asserted:

> Only the healthy count today. It is the duty of Every Englishman and
> Englishwoman to safeguard Health. These sudden new duties, these
> drastic changes from old routine, these swift and heavy calls upon our
> strength are apt to show very clearly how much below the best health-
> standard many of us are. Tens of thousands of us have managed to "get
> along all right," but now we keenly realize we were getting on without a
> scrap of health-reserve, and now is the time that an unfailing tonic and
> restorative like Hall's Wine is of such enormous service.[49]

Both columns and advertisements validated their messages with the authority of physicians and trained nurses. For example, Angier's Emulsion, a
cough remedy, was "strongly recommended by the medical profession, not
only for colds, coughs, whooping cough, bronchitis, and all lung affections,
but also for scrofula, rickets, malnutrition and wasting diseases generally."[50]
Dr. Ridge's Patent Cooked Food was "praised by doctors, nurses, and thousands of mothers."[51] Cecile's Cookery Column on "Tempting Dishes for the
Invalid," which included raw beef tea, baked fish, tripe, barley water, and
steamed mutton chop, advised, "If allowed by the doctor, a finely chopped

47. *Woman's Weekly* 9:227 (1916): 282; *Woman's Weekly* 9:228 (1916): 313; *Woman's Weekly* 9:231 (1916): 398; *Woman's Weekly* 9:235 (1916): 507.

48. *Woman's Weekly* 9:218, 1.

49. *Woman's Weekly* 9:221 (1916): 110.

50. *Woman's Weekly* 1:7 (1911): inside front cover.

51. *Woman's Weekly* 9:221 (1916): 103.

boiled onion can be added to the tripe. Once must remember that, as a rule, only a very light seasoning of pepper and salt is allowed for an invalid; in this also the doctor's orders must be followed implicitly."[52] Advertisements also supported trends in official medical and public health advice. For example, a 1930 ad for Ovaltine targeted new mothers and advocated breast-feeding:

> Happy Babies are Breast-Fed. During the weeks before baby arrives there is one service of love even more important than the tiny garments so carefully chosen. . . . *Make sure that you will be able to feed baby yourself.* So much depends upon this. Maternal milk is germ-free and of correct composition. No substitute is equal to it for safeguarding the child against nutritional diseases, such as rickets, and building a sure foundation for future health. Doctors, nurses and mothers daily testify to the remarkable qualities of Ovaltine for promoting a rich supply of maternal milk. This delicious beverage also maintains the mother's strength while nursing and ensures a quick return to normal health. . . . One cup of Ovaltine supplies more nourishment than three eggs.[53]

The magazine also endorsed the developing image of the physician as infallible. A 1916 column, "Every Doctor a Detective," informed the reader, "Do you know that if you were to walk straight into a doctor's consulting-room and seat yourself in the chair, he could probably tell just what was amiss without your having given him a single symptom of your malady?"[54] In addition, columnists advised readers about appropriate patient behavior. For example, one columnist did not believe "in allowing children who have had measles or any other infectious illness, to get up until the doctor gives leave [or] in calling a doctor and then disobeying his orders."[55] This trend perhaps reached its zenith in Anne Campbell's 1940 poem, "The Doctor":

> How can we thank the doctor?
> Where is the shining phrase
> That will reward the doctor
> For lengthening our days?
> We come through the gloomy country
> Of half life and half death
> And think of the weary doctor
> Who gave us back our breath.
> His hands are the strong and healing

52. *Woman's Weekly* 9:232 (1916): 427.
53. *Woman's Weekly* 37:948 (1930): 23. Italics in the original.
54. *Woman's Weekly* 9:218 (1916): 18.
55. *Woman's Weekly* 9:229 (1916): 340.

Hands of a surgeon born.
His brain, with machine precision,
Plans for the sick and worn.
Something of God through his fingers
Surges to make us blest.
Our healing is of the spirit.
We lean on his soul for rest.
How can we thank the doctor?
Money and words are vain.
Only God can reward him
Who gives us our life again![56]

In addition to creating and projecting idealized images of physicians, *Woman's Weekly* writers supported medical interventions that were sometimes resisted by patients and their families. A 1919 "For Mother and Home" column answered the question, "Do you consider that pulmonary tuberculosis can really be permanently cured, if slight, by entering a sanatorium?" with the response, "Yes: it often can be cured if taken in time. And sanatorium treatment—or treatment at home on the same lines, if this can be had—is often very successful, and should always be tried." Later that year the same advisor wrote: "Mrs. R. P.—When you are inclined to doubt the value of vaccination as a protection from smallpox, I advise you to consider the case of the Gloucester epidemic in 1896. In that outbreak of smallpox, only 26 vaccinated children under 10 years old took the disease, and of those only one died; of unvaccinated children 680 took smallpox, and of these *two hundred and seventy-nine* died. In all epidemics much the same thing happens."[57]

It is noteworthy that the pedigrees of advice columnists became increasingly official as time went on; unlike Mrs. Marryat and Mrs. Merrydew, they were qualified, not by their age and experience, but by training and occupational status. In 1926 the author of a new column, "What They Ask Matron," was purportedly the "Matron of a big welfare center, whose homely advice brings solace to dozens of mothers every week."[58] Her recommendations, although still containing a good deal of folksy common sense, also included more references to professional medical and public health services. In an early column, "the Matron" wrote: "It would certainly be worthwhile to find out if 'Artificial Sunlight' is what would suit your baby. Only doctors can take the responsibility of advising a course of exposures, because it is a special study, and close observation has to be kept. I have the good fortune at our Welfare Centre to see the results from one of the kinds of lamps that are used for treatments. The marked improve-

56. *Woman's Weekly* 57:1,471 (1940): 55.
57. *Woman's Weekly* 15:382 (1919): 141; *Woman's Weekly* 15:390 (1919): 312. Italics in the original.
58. *Woman's Weekly* 29:740 (1926): 25.

ment in the general well-being of the babies well rewards the mothers who give up the necessary length of time to attend."[59] She also advised women suffering from morning sickness to see "a doctor or qualified nurse, such as you find at a welfare center" and told mothers whose children showed signs of measles, "If you have not already sent for the doctor, do not delay any longer. He will guide you in preventing the complications that cause the risks in this infectious illness."[60] The Matron supported the authority of physicians and public health clinics as well as encouraging mothers to use these biomedical resources.

However, this column also continued the magazine's tendency to respect readers' traditional backgrounds and perspectives, at the same time providing "modern" information in a comprehensible way. For instance, in 1926 a reader asked, "Can you tell me whether camphor put into a little bag and worn round the neck is any protection against infection? My mother used to do this for us and as there is scarlet fever at my little boy's school I thought I would try it. I am giving him cod-liver oil and malt, which he likes." The Matron replied, "You can rest assured that the little bag containing camphor which your boy wears can do no harm because camphor is a mild antiseptic and by smelling the bag it may help to keep his nose free from infection." She also said that it might repel fleas. Nonetheless, she was most enthusiastic about administration of cod-liver oil and malt extract "that will help to maintain him a sound standard of health during the winter."[61]

Stories published in *Woman's Weekly* reinforced and dramatized the positive images of medical personnel and institutions, at the same time encouraging cooperation and dependence on the part of laypeople. Standard themes involved hospital environments, beautiful young female nurses, good-looking dedicated physicians or surgeons (mostly male), and sick children who often needed adoption.[62] For example, Henry and Sylvia Lieferant's 1930 story, "Doctor Lady," included a "new woman" general practitioner, a crusty surgeon, and a cute child patient, and helped to humanize medicine and hospitals.[63] The January 6, 1940, issue inaugurated two new serials with medical themes: "Hands of Healing: Behind the Scenes in a Hospital for Suffering Animals," which sported a picture

59. *Woman's Weekly* 29:742 (1926): 81.

60. *Woman's Weekly* 29:744 (1926): 165; *Woman's Weekly* 29:746 (1926): 263.

61. *Woman's Weekly* 29:742 (1926): 147.

62. See, for example, Laura Kingscote, "Dr. Mac: Or handsome is that handsome does," *Woman's Weekly* 1:2 (1911): 55–56; Henry T. Johnson, "Joey's visitors: Telling how Cupid used a lonely little boy to make three people happy," *Woman's Weekly* 9:231 (1916): 374–76; "The doctor's secretary," *Woman's Weekly* 47:1,209 (1935): 21; Teresa Hyde Phillips, "Private case," *Woman's Weekly* 47:1,211 (1935): 115–47; Dorothy Quentin, "Traveler's Star," first episode, *Woman's Weekly* 67:1,731 (1945): 11ff; Norah Smaridge, "A very nice arrangement," *Woman's Weekly* 67:1,736 (1945): 144–46; *Woman's Weekly* 67:1,741 (1945); Anne Vernon, "The girl he left," 318–21.

63. *Woman's Weekly* 37:952 (1930).

of a beautiful nurse wearing a full veil headdress with two handsome dogs, and "Love is for Ever: The Story of An Assistant Matron," which dealt with drugs, misunderstanding, and romance between a wise doctor and a true-hearted boarding school matron.[64] A 1945 serial, "Time Will Tell" began:

> Living in the hospital was Clunie's first experience of life in a community. For her it was exciting, when she was alone in her little bedroom, to know that downstairs all manner of dramatic happenings were taking place. Today, perhaps, a new life was coming into the world. Last night for hours, doctors and nurses had fought a battle with death over the broken body of a young airman and had won. Tomorrow, the unwrapping of a bandage would give the answer as to whether an operation had given a girl the sight she had lost in childhood, or that she must remain in darkness.[65]

Like Clunie, the story's readers observed an increasingly familiar account of metaphorical battle and victory, peopled by increasingly stereotyped characters. Such stories in women's magazines glamorized medicine in general and nursing in particular, probably helping with nurse recruitment at a time of rising hospital utilization and (due to low pay and status) chronic shortage of nurses.[66]

New stereotypes of doctors and nurses also appeared in popular songs published in *Woman's Weekly*. For example, reflecting a common wartime experience, in June 1919, a ditty entitled "I don't want to get well" contained the following lyrics:

> I don't want to get well, I don't want to get well,
> I'm in love with a beautiful nurse.
> Early every morning, night and noon,
> The cutest little girlie comes and feeds me with a spoon;
> I don't want to get well, I don't want to get well,
> I'm glad they shot me on the fighting line—fine!
> The Doctor says that I'm in bad condition,
> But Oh, Oh, Oh, I've got so much ambition,
> I don't want to get well, I don't want to get well,
> For I'm having a wonderful time.

While these lyrics constructed and drew on the long-lived portrayal of the nurse as an object of sexual fantasy and fun (consider *M*A*S*H*'s Marga-

64. *Woman's Weekly* 57:1,470 (1940): 11ff, 21.
65. *Woman's Weekly* 67:1,732 (1945): 45–46.
66. See, for example, Celia Davies, "A constant casualty: Nurse education in Britain and the USA to 1939," in Celia Davies, ed., *Rewriting nursing history* (London: Croom Helm, 1980), 102–22.

ret "Hot Lips" Houlihan or the nurse characters in the popular *Carry On* films), they also revealed the then newly normative image of the doctor and nurse at the patient's hospital bedside.

By the 1940s, *Woman's Weekly* was serving as an outlet for official health information, running full-page advertisement-like statements from the Ministry of Health and Central Council for Health Education. Borrowing from successful advice columns and ads, these statements embedded health information in a fictional scenario. For example, in January 1945, the inside back cover read:

> From a doctor's diary. This is based on a doctor's experience of cases of VD. It has been carefully edited so that the people concerned shall not be recognized. "Then it wasn't VD after all, Doctor?" I was able to tell this patient that she had not got VD. She was a woman of 36 who had formed a friendship with a man, and one night intimacy took place. Later, he told her he was being treated for gonorrhea. She was terrified and when she developed a discharge shortly afterwards, quite naturally believed she had caught gonorrhea from him. After some very anxious weeks, she at last made up her mind to visit a clinic. She had feared she might be seen going in or coming out. But clinics are usually in very inconspicuous places, often inside hospitals, so *that* risk hardly exists. After tests had been made, I was able to tell her there was no outward sign of VD. I saw her again a week later, and then after another three months. The tests were negative in each case. She had been very fortunate—she had not contracted the disease.[67]

Similarly, in the same year the Ministry of Food ran what might be called "info-ads" about healthy diet: on March 10, 1945 the topic was "Tempting the convalescent."

After World War II, the pages of *Woman's Weekly* reflected a national health culture that linked medicine with science. A 1948 advertisement for Evans Medical Supplies, which showed Petri dishes labeled "Examination of Diphtheria Bacilli," contained the text "When Sickness strikes and you call in the doctor, you enlist far more than one man's knowledge and ability. Behind the doctor are the scientist in the laboratory, the pharmacist in his dispensary . . . all are partners in the battle against disease. In the vital field of research and discovery, the name of Evans holds a distinguished

67. *Woman's Weekly* 67:1,733 (1945). Italics in the original. See also *Woman's Weekly* 67:1,743 (1945); *Woman's Weekly* 67:1,754 (1945): inside back cover, when the scenarios vary, but the message remains the same. See also *Woman's Weekly* 67:1,734; *Woman's Weekly* 67:1,738; *Woman's Weekly* 67:1,747 (1945): inside back cover, when the message advocated immunization against diphtheria. In 1950, the "Doctor's Diary" info-ads were being copied by a private vendor, who borrowed their authority for a "new vaccine for catarrh and bronchitis, Lantigen 'B.'" See *Woman's Weekly* 77:1,992 (1950): inside front cover.

place." As this copy attests, the advertisers also presumed general acceptance and expectation for an expanding range of health matters—from
selection of sanitary napkins to childbirth and care of the sick—to be managed by officially qualified workers in clinic and hospital settings. So, for
example, an advertisement for Dettol (a disinfectant) created the scenario
of a woman asking

> "Tell me, Doctor . . . How did women learn about Dettol?" In maternity
> hospitals, during and after childbirth, women observed that Dettol
> was used to guard them against infection. In clinics, from doctors and
> nurses, they learned how non-poisonous Dettol remained efficient even
> when greatly diluted. Then in their own homes they discovered how
> very agreeable this gentle, non-staining, deodorant antiseptic could be
> for intimate use. They decided that Dettol was made for women, and
> forthwith made Dettol their own. Dettol, the modern antiseptic.[68]

This advertisement, based on "Doctor's" authority, enhanced the reputation of a common household disinfectant by linking it to use in hospitals,
whose cleanliness was presumed to be above reproach. It even suggested
that women use this doctor-approved chemical as a douche—thereby cleaning their insides as well as their environments.

Regularly appearing features similarly indicated normative dependence
on and compliance with professional medicine and public health. The February 21, 1948, column, "The adventures of the Robin family," described a
familiar scenario:

> It was most unusual for Rosemary Robin to be late in getting up for
> breakfast. Her brother Roley could hardly believe his eyes when he saw
> her still in bed—and he was almost dressed. But when Rosemary told
> him that she was feeling funny and her throat hurt, Roley knew there
> must be something wrong. So did Mrs. Robin, when her little son came
> racing into the kitchen with the news. . . . [S]o she hurried upstairs and
> when she had seen her small daughter, she hurried to the telephone.
> Mrs. Robin called up Dr. Robbie Robin, who said he would come right
> over. Rosemary had probably caught the mumps, there were several
> cases about, and little Richard was in bed with it too. "I have advised
> Miss Owl to close her school for a time," said Dr. Robbie. When Roley
> heard this he could hardly hide his joy. But he did feel sorry for his
> sister. Roley had already had the mumps—and he knew it wouldn't be
> any fun for Rosemary.[69]

68. *Woman's Weekly* (2/7/48): inside back cover. A 1950s advertisement for Dettol shows
a midwife on a bicycle, riding through rainy dark streets, above the text, "That must be Nurse
Lucas on an urgent call. . . Mrs. Barrington, no doubt. . . In her bag Nurse Lucas—like almost
every other District Nurse and Midwife in Great Britain—carries a bottle of 'Dettol.'"

69. *Woman's Weekly* (2/21/48): 208. Despite the middle-class connotations of the Robin

At this point, *Woman's Weekly*'s depiction of illness, medicine, care, and treatment portrayed and reinforced a more homogenous national health culture than had existed in the magazine's early days before World War I. This new culture presumed public ignorance and helplessness regarding even routine illness, lay familiarity with and regular consultation of doctors, and physicians' authority over nonmedical matters and institutions.

RADIO DOCTORING

Emerging later than magazines as pervasive resources for working-class entertainment and edification were radio broadcasts. While Marconi's first successful experiments with "wireless telegraphy" were in 1896 and Britain's first legislation regulating this activity was passed in 1904, not until after the formation of the British Broadcasting Company (BBC) in 1922 did people other than radio hobbyists come into routine contact with "wireless" programming.[70] Early "crystal" radio sets were expensive and required assembly. Furthermore, the network was incomplete in the 1920s, mainly reaching major population centers. Things changed after about 1929, when transmission extended to most areas of the country and increasingly affordable mass-produced receivers began to dominate the industry. According to Gordon Bussey, 1931 was a turning point when the new "superhet" design quickly became the market leader: "In 1924, 12 would have bought no more than a single valve set and accessories, requiring constant attention to all its battery supplies, the problems of a full-scale outdoor aerial and the inconvenience of headphones; by 1934 the same sum would have given a choice of several first class mains operated receivers capable of picking up most European broadcasting with no external aerial, all at the 'flick of a switch.'"[71]

Radio differed from magazines in its dependence on a totally new, apparently magical technology and access to equipment requiring what for working-class households was a significant financial outlay. It was also different because the BBC, from the beginning conceptualized as a public service, did not defer to regional or working-class tastes but, to the contrary, attempted deliberately to shape and change them. According to Mark Pegg, "A common reason for criticizing the BBC in its formative period was its insularity. Critics argued that the Director General, Sir John Reith,

family's home telephone, this vignette's appearance in a regular feature for working-class readers suggests that calling the doctor for minor childhood ailments had become part of those readers' experience.

70. Mark Pegg, *Broadcasting and society 1918–1939* (London and Canberra: Croom Helm, 1983), 2. See also Asa Briggs, *The BBC: The first fifty years* (Oxford and New York: Oxford University Press, 1985). This volume is an abridgement of a detailed four-volume study of the BBC published by the author between 1961 and 1979.

71. Gordon Bussey, *Wireless, the crucial decade: History of the British wireless industry 1924–34* (London: Peter Peregrinus, 1990), 59, 65, 69, 76, 83.

then indisputably the personification of British broadcasting, represented an organization which relied entirely on independent judgments from its hierarchy to establish moral and cultural standards for programmes and produced programmes based upon artistic judgments that had little regard for the varied tastes of its audience."[72] Dominating the organization from 1922 until his resignation in 1938, Reith personified what many viewed as "Aunty Beeb's" middle-class emphasis on high culture, religion, and education, coupled with a paternalistic certainty that it knew what people needed and did not care what they wanted. Thus, unlike magazines targeting working-class readers, radio was not expected to provide popular entertainment. Nonetheless, members of all classes increasingly bought radios; while 1 percent of British households had radio licenses in 1922, 71 percent had them in 1939, when 8,893,582 licenses were issued.[73] Although there was some concern that the "wireless" threatened distinctive local cultures, there was also optimism that an appropriately managed medium could foster an educated, democratic polity, in direct contrast to contemporary European dictators' use of radio to shape popular adherence to fascist or Marxist ideologies. Radio also served as a vehicle for development of a more homogenous British national culture, with its own language ("BBC English"), tastes, and values.

The oral history evidence reveals that working-class residents of Barrow, Lancaster, and Preston followed national trends regarding radio-ownership and -listening. For example, Mrs. Shelby, born in 1898, said that in 1929, "Mr. S[helby] and two or three more built theirs and we had them in this cupboard. My husband said, 'I'm going to close this in because I don't want the doctor to know we have one.' It's a closed cupboard and I still have it. We used to listen to all these things. It was 'Shut up, be quiet,' it was awful. Our kiddies used to listen, and our Peggy and Betty said, 'We want to listen to "Hello Twins."' They used to listen to Uncle Mac. It was the 'Children's Hour.'"[74] Similarly, Mr. Langley, born in 1900, remembered:

> Round about 1928 or 29, when we were in Foundry Street. It must have been about 1930 and we had headphones then. There was no loudspeaker. It was Mr. Willetts and he dabbled in wireless and stuff, and he had one going and we could hear it sometimes. I said, "By gum, it is marvelous, this." He said, "I'll tell you what to do, Billy, I know what I want and I'll buy part of it each week." I said, "Well, that is the only way because I can't pay for it." He said, "Yes, things are tight." He was in the Social Security office, Means Test carry-on. If you'd a piano, you'd to sell it, and all this carry-on. How we got our first, we bought a little bit

72. Pegg, *Broadcasting and society*, 92–93.
73. Ibid., 7. In 1939, there were an estimated 12,503,000 households in Britain, containing a total of 47,762,000 people.
74. Mrs. S1L, 28. See also Mr. G6P, 26.

every week, a coil or something like that, and the last thing he bought was the head-phones. . . . He put it together and made it in a little box. He put it on and by gum we did enjoy it.[75]

As these examples suggest, in the late 1920s a radio was considered, like a piano, to be a luxury item. Mr. Shelby, presuming general practitioners charged on a sliding scale depending on patients' resource, speculated that the possession of a radio might inflate his doctor's bill, while Mr. Langley's friend, who was on public assistance, was worried the welfare officer might either force him to sell his radio or cut off the family's benefits because he owned one. And radio maintenance was a significant expense. Mr. Adderly, born in 1926 in Lancaster, remembered:

> Our first [household] appliance was an old battery, a radio, they had wet batteries and dry batteries, and we used to tune in to Athlone. I always remember that. The local station, the most popular station was Athlone, all right until the batteries went dry. Wet batteries used to last about a week, but the big battery, when that went, oh, that was a week's wage replacing that. . . . Then, to answer your question a bit further, when we were over at Skerton [beginning in 1937], we got a bit more modern radio, which was nothing elaborate, just a more modern electric set.[76]

While in the early days neighbors might listen to the radio as a group, by the 1930s this activity was largely confined to individual homes, although it was often still collective because household members listened together. Radio appealed, in particular, to homemakers because they could tune in at home and combine the activity with household tasks.[77] Therefore, it is likely that programs with health content, including advice and educational features and dramas or serials with medical themes, particularly influenced women. It is clear that from its earliest days both the BBC programming staff and interest groups including the Ministry of Health (established in 1920) and the British Medical Association understood that radio could be a vehicle for official health information.[78] Furthermore, the medical establishment vetted the topics that could be broadcast and the ways medical workers and institutions were presented. In addition, the BBC itself made decisions aligned with the positions of organized medicine regarding what was or was not "suitable" for broadcasting. For example, in 1948 it refused the Abortion Law Reform Association's request for a debate on

75. Mr. L2B, 13.
76. Mr. A4L, 13.
77. Pegg, *Broadcasting and society*, 197–98.
78. Karpf, *Doctoring the media*, 32–50.

the subject and dealt similarly with the topic of birth control.[79] For these reasons, the radio programs heard by the British public projected views concerning health and medicine that were congruent with the perspectives and interests of physicians. While these views arguably paralleled the attitudes, experiences, and politics of middle-class listeners, they also helped to create new perspectives and expectations among working-class audience members.

Radio delivered health messages differently than did women's magazines. Organized and run as a public service, BBC programming was not supported by advertisements. Its drama lacked the sensational romance of *Woman's Weekly*'s stories. However, as Ann Karpf points out, from its inception in the 1920s the national radio network was viewed as a powerful tool for disease prevention and health maintenance: "As early as 1927, Friday morning radio talks were given under the auspices of the Ministry of Health, on Health in Autumn, How to Keep Fit at Fifty, How to Avoid Infection. From their inception, they were seen as an unqualified success: the first quarter's broadcasts in 1929 garnered 20,000 letters from a listener population of approximately 10 million."[80] In the 1930s, broadcasters provided advice on diet and, at the end of the decade, inaugurated a daily exercise program.

Despite—or perhaps because of—the popularity of health-related programs, BBC management ventured timidly into this highly politicized arena. While ongoing concerns about national fitness and competitiveness drove interest in improving general health—particularly among working-class people—controversy about the root causes of illness (e.g., low wages and poor living and working environments versus the ignorance and negligence of poor people) threatened to further splinter listeners along social class and political party lines.[81] Furthermore, the Ministry of Health had its own agenda and reputation to protect and was quite determined to control both reporting about the population's health and any health-related advice offered to the mushrooming radio audience.[82] In addition, clinical and public health interests were jockeying for position with voters and policymakers as medical services were increasingly viewed as both necessities and public responsibilities. In consequence, the BBC's health programming avoided controversial topics and offered a highly individual view of fitness, while also helping to inflate the image and reputation of physicians.

Enter the Radio Doctor. Charles Hill, eventually titled Lord Hill of

79. Ibid., 163–64.

80. Ibid., 32–33.

81. See, for example, Charles Webster, "Healthy or hungry thirties?" *History Workshop* 13 (1982): 110–29; Virginia Berridge, Mark Harrison, and Paul Weindling, "The impact of war and depression, 1918 to 1948," in Charles Webster, ed., *Caring for health: History and diversity* (Milton Keynes: Open University Press, 1993).

82. Karpf, *Doctoring the media*, 35–42.

Luton, was born into a working-class London family, educated as a scholarship student, received his medical training from Cambridge and the London Hospital, and spent much of his career working for the British Medical Association (BMA), resigning his post as Secretary when he was elected as a Conservative Member of Parliament in 1950.[83] His first BBC broadcasts were a 1933 series of four programs presenting to the public results of the BMA's recently released "Nutrition Report." After contributing pieces sporadically during the 1930s, in 1941 Hill presented the daytime "Kitchen Front" series, sponsored by the Ministry of Food and targeting homemakers, which initially addressed wartime dietary issues. Hill remembered, "One morning, without previous warning, I heard the introductory words, 'Here is the Radio Doctor,' and thereafter the same formula was used each week."[84] As time went on, the series expanded to cover a broad spectrum of health issues, eventually attracting a listening audience of approximately fourteen million. In 1942 Hill inaugurated an evening program, "Doctors Agree," which expanded his audience to include more men and children. At this point he was both Secretary of the British Medical Association and Chairman of the Central Council of Health Education. Thus, the information he provided carried the authority of both organizations.[85] Furthermore, Hill was the official medical adviser to the BBC, helping to shape programming beyond his own. He continued broadcasting as the Radio Doctor until 1950.

Unlike the usual reserved and formal BBC presenter, Hill was chatty and colloquial. His folksy style was probably particularly attractive to working-class listeners, bridging the social distance between them and their own physicians. One example will illustrate this aspect of the Radio Doctor's programs. On December 26, 1949, for a broadcast called "Hallo Children," he said:

This is stomach speaking. Yes, I mean it, *your* stomach. In fact, I'm the shop-steward of the society of Suffering Stomachs. Stomachs don't often speak. As a rule I get on with my job without as much as a murmur or rumble. You don't even know that I am doing it. But I've got something to say this morning, at least to some of you. Yesterday—Christmas Day— you bullied me. . . . At breakfast, well, you are fairly well-behaved. Some of you got so excited that you didn't want much breakfast: I can't work when you're all of a dither. But then, in the middle of the morning, the trouble started again. Down the chute they came, sweet after sweet, nut after nut, biscuits, oranges. If there is anything that upsets me it's sweet things between meals.

83. Charles Hill, Lord Hill of Luton, *Both sides of the Hill* (London: Heinemann, 1964), 17–50.

84. Ibid., 106.

85. Karpf, *Doctoring the media*, 44–47.

The personified stomach's perspective on Christmas Day continued pre-
dictably; at the end the organ threatened that unless it received better
treatment, "I warn you, I shall make an example of some of you; it won't
be a stay-in strike either. Oh, no, it will be a put-out strike. Ups-a-daisy it
will come. Well, have a good Boxing Day, but the kinder you are to me the
better you'll enjoy it."[86] Hill extended the impact of his radio programs
by publishing a number of inexpensive short books on health topics for
general readers.[87]

Charles Hill, according to Ann Karpf,

> bridged the worlds of medicine and broadcasting, contributing simuta-
> neously to the democratization of medical knowledge and to the spread
> of the idea that doctors were uncontestable experts on health. Since he
> frequently broadcast with the authority of a doctor on subjects about
> which medicine had no special knowledge, his talks are also an early
> example of medicalization. . . . The Radio Doctor played a powerful
> mythical role in British culture, both at the time and subsequently. If
> the nation shared a doctor, it could also be said to share the same illness
> and treatment. Mass health interventions and broadcasts directed at
> the whole population implied that all were similarly wanting. After the
> raging public debates about malnutrition, unemployment, and poverty,
> the Radio Doctor reconstituted everyone as equal citizens and patients,
> equally affected by the difficulties of the war—adieu health differences
> by class, region, or gender.[88]

More authoritatively than magazine advice columnists, Charles Hill helped
to draw working-class people into a national health culture. It is therefore
ironic that he spearheaded professional medical opposition to the establishment of the National Health Service.[89]

Hill's preferred health care world was peopled by wise, independent,
prosperous physicians advising educated, self-controlled, provident, and
compliant patients. This world was mirrored in one hugely popular radio
drama series, "Mrs. Dale's Diary," launched in January 1948. The title

86. Hill, *Both sides*, 119–21.

87. See, for example, Charles Hill, *The Radio Doctor. Your body: How it works and how to keep
it working well* (London: Burke Publishing, 1944); Charles Hill, *Wednesday morning early or A little
of what you fancy, by the Radio Doctor* (London, New York, and Melbourne: Hutchinson and Co.;
no dates given, although suggestion is during WWII) [1944, NLM Catalog]; Charles Hill, *Good
health, children! By the Radio Doctor* (London: Sir Isaac Pitman and Sons, 1944); Charles Hill, *The
Radio Doctor. Bringing up your child* (London: Phoenix House, 1950).

88. Karpf, *Doctoring the media*, 47.

89. Hill, *Both sides*, 75–103. In another irony, with John Woodcock, Charles Hill published a
book, *The National Health Service* (London: Christopher Johnson, 1949), to explain "in language
as simple as accuracy permits the anatomy and physiology of the National Health Service as it is
at the outset of the service."

character was a middle-class doctor's wife, Mary, who with her husband, Jim, lived at Virginia Lodge in the Middlesex suburb of Parkwood Hill. Renamed "The Dales" during the 1960s and concluding in 1969, the BBC's first radio soap opera was aimed at a listening audience of housewives. Like the even more popular program "The Archers," which began in 1950 with input from the Ministry of Agriculture, "Mrs. Dale's Diary" consciously fostered Englishness viewed largely through a middle-class lens.[90] Like some post–World War II television "doctor shows," such as *Marcus Welby, M.D.*, "Mrs. Dale's Diary" both humanized physicians by locating them in private family lives and enhanced their reputations for being not only good technicians, but wise and good men. As a result, radio dramas with medical characters and themes enhanced the educational messages of didactic health programming, rendering formal medicine more familiar and appealing.

CONSTRUCTING MODERN MEDICINE: BOX-OFFICE FILMS

While—or somewhat earlier than—radio was changing the horizons of working-class domestic leisure, feature films transformed recreational opportunities outside the home. Particularly after the introduction of sound in the *Jazz Singer* in 1927, movies became the most popular form of commercial entertainment in Britain. According to Jeffrey Richards:

> The number of cinemas and the average attendance at them rose steadily throughout the decade. Annual admissions rose from 903 million in 1934, to 917 million in 1936, to 946 million in 1937, to 987 million in 1938, to 990 million in 1939, to 1,027 million in 1940. By 1939 the cinema industry itself estimated its average weekly admission figure at 23 million, though there were of course seasonal fluctuations. The number of cinemas also increased to meet the extra demand. There were an estimated 3,000 cinemas in operation in 1926. By 1935 there were 4,448 and by 1938 4,967.[91]

As was true of radio, there was early awareness of the potential influence of movies on audience members. According to the 1936 Moyne Committee Report on the working of the Cinematograph Films Act: "The cinematograph film is today one of the most widely used means for the amusement

90. See Wikipedia online entries for "Mrs. Dale's Diary" at http://en.wikipedia.org/wiki/Mrs._Dale%27s_Diary; and for "The Archers" at http://en.wikipedia.org/wiki/The_Archers#History. Oral history informants remembered listening to both of these programs. See, for example, Mr. G6P, 26; Mrs. H6L, 34; Mrs. O1B, 46; Mrs. W4L, 67.

91. Jeffrey Richards, *The age of the dream palace: Cinema and society in Britain 1930–1939* (London: Routledge and Kegan Paul, 1984), 11–12.

of the public at large. It is also undoubtedly a most important factor in the education of all classes of the community, in the spread of national culture and in presenting national ideas and customs to the world. Its potentialities moreover in shaping the idea of the very large numbers to whom it appeals are almost unlimited. The propaganda value of the film cannot be overemphasized."[92]

Although it would be overstating the case to argue a deliberate and concerted attempt on the part of producers, writers, and directors to insert medical propaganda into box-office movies, it is fair to observe the disproportionate number of medical plots and characters in what working-class people called "the pictures." Indeed, Michael Shortland comments that although films featuring medical personnel have many different types of plots—melodrama, suspense, comedy, etc.—"All the same, the language, idiom and rituals of medicine are still manifest in such films, albeit as a kind of residue. And it remains the case that one cannot find in the annals of Hollywood an equivalent mass of romances or thrillers involving say, members of the clergy or school teachers, though stories could be fashioned in equal numbers from their lives and labors."[93]

This "residue" of what might be called official health culture was not a naturally occurring byproduct of random storytelling. It was increasingly crafted in an atmosphere of vigilance regarding story lines or characters that might cast a negative light on biomedicine. According to Ann Karpf:

> In Britain in the 1930s, the state censor took care that the medical profession wasn't brought into disrepute: between 1934 and 1937, the British Board of Film Censors (to whom scripts had to be submitted for vetting in advance of production) banned nine proposals for films because they threatened the image of the medical profession. Shaw's "The Doctor's Dilemma" was among them. And a 1934 film about an agonizing visit to the dentist was banned for a time for "ridiculing the profession." But such controls were largely unnecessary, for film-makers had discovered the value of the doctor as hero.[94]

Even where an individual doctor was cast as a villain, or a medical institution was negatively portrayed, these situations were increasingly constructed as aberrant; both modern medicine and its trained professionals were pre-

---

92. Quoted in Anthony Aldgate and Jeffrey Richards, *Best of British: Cinema and society from 1930 to the present*, 2nd ed. (London and New York: I. B. Tauris, 1999), 1–2.

93. Shortland, *Medicine and film*, 7.

94. Karpf, *Doctoring the media*, 181. See also Richards, *Dream palace*, which makes clear that Britain did not have government-controlled censorship; however, the British Board of Film Censors was especially vigilant "because the cinema was *the* mass medium, regularly patronized by the working classes, and the working classes were deemed to be all too easily influenced" (89).

sumed to be normatively good.

Working-class residents of Barrow, Lancaster, and Preston regularly went to the movies.[95] According to Jeffrey Richards, a 1934 study estimated that there was one cinema seat for every nine persons in Lancashire, making it among the best-served areas in the country: there was a seat for every 14 people in London and the Home Counties. "But perhaps Rowson's most interesting conclusion is that 'about 43 per cent of all cinema admissions were at prices not exceeding 6d. each and about another 37 per cent paid not more than 10d. or, put another way, 80 per cent of cinema-goers went in the cheap seats. This suggests that the bulk of the cinema-goers were working-class, a conclusion supported by virtually all other surveys.'" Film attendance was age-related, with the young most likely to go and older married couples least likely to go. People with lower incomes and educational attainment went to the movies more often than the more prosperous and educated. People employed in light manufacturing went more often than those in other occupations. Women went more often than men.[96] Although there were gradations of both seats and theaters, from smoke-choked "flea-pits" to ornate "dream palaces," cinemas certainly provided welcome alternatives to cramped working-class homes and the often damp, chilly streets of working-class neighborhoods.[97]

Oral history informants remembered going frequently to the pictures, making it clear that, rather than targeting a specific film, they went regardless of what was showing. Mr. Most, born in Barrow in 1901, said, "I went to the cinema and I was there the first night that the old Electric opened. Two-pence it was to sit on the front row and I was there the first night of the Gaiety opening and also the Coliseum." His parents were also regular moviegoers. "A lot of it was habit. My father and mother had the two front seats behind the conductor booked every Thursday night for several years. They never missed going and always had these particular seats and went Thursday after Thursday regardless of what was on. That was like habit." He went on:

> We used to go perhaps every night, my wife and I. My mother-in-law was a rabid picture-goer, and she'd go twice a night if possible. This was in the twenties, going on to the thirties. She'd come out of the first house and go in the second house somewhere else. We were never like that, although once I kept a diary of what I'd seen, and I saw three hundred feature films in the year. . . . A lot of people would average twice a week. At that time there were several cinemas in Barrow, so you'd plenty of scope and they all changed twice a week. There were fourteen films

95. Roberts, *A woman's place*, 123–24; Roberts, *Women and families*, 62–63, 100.
96. Richards, *Dream palace*, 12–15.
97. See, for example, Mr. D2P, 25.

if you wanted to see them. . . . It got them out of theirselves and away from their troubles. There was plenty of trouble in the twenties and there was a lot of depression and unemployment.[98]

Although both men and women went to the movies, this new, inexpensive, respectable form of entertainment was particularly attractive to women. Mrs. Peterson, born in 1899 in Preston, recounted one reason cinema attendance appealed to young girls with limited financial resources: "The first costume [suit] that I had, it was from a second-hand shop in Avenham Lane. I would be well over 15. That was about 15/-d in them days and that was a lot of money. She [shop attendant] said, 'I have laid a little costume up for our Maggie. It will just suit her.' I thought, how wonderful, she does think a lot about me. But I were nearly in rags, you know. We would go to the pictures because nobody would see us in the dark. That was all we did, even when we were teenagers." She continued seeing films regularly after she married, indicating that this one commercial leisure activity figured significantly in her tense marriage and her management of the family's limited finances:

> Once a week I would go to the cinema.
> *Interviewer:* Did you go on your own?
> *Informant:* Yes. I daren't have any friends. I hadn't to have any neighbors in or anything. He were very jealous, my husband. I think it was the "dog in the manger." One time when cigarettes were two-pence a packet, I used to get paid on Friday night and I would pay everything out and I would put two-pence away or four-pence for the pictures. I would leave that as that was for the pictures for next Thursday. I daren't spend it. Oftener than not he has come on a Thursday night and he would ask for two-pence for a packet of fags. I would just have that four-pence for the pictures. He would say, "Why can't you go on a Friday night?" How could I go on a Friday night when there used to be doctor fellow coming, paper fellow coming, milk fellow and different ones coming? I had to be there.[99]

Mrs. Peterson had four children and alternated between working as a weaver and staying at home when they were small. Her husband was a low-paid outdoor laborer.

The pattern, conventional during the interwar years, of going to the cinema at least once a week and often seeing more than one film meant that working-class people routinely saw movies with medical themes.

98. Mr. M8B, 3, 8, 10. See also, for example, Mrs. A1L, 15; Mr. A2B, 47–48; Mrs. A2B, 56; Mrs. A3B, 13, 44; Mr. B1B, 63; Mr. C1L, 26; Mr. C3L, 4; Mrs. D2B, 10; Mr. H1L, 32; Mr. K1L, 40; Mr. M1L, 34; Mr. P1B, 45; Mrs. S2B, 19.

99. Mrs. P1P, 24, 46.

These films, more often than not, were American-made and consequently reflected a health care system and culture that were quite different from those experienced by British viewers. Because of their enormous popularity and ubiquity, these Hollywood movies likely not only helped to shape viewers' perspectives on health and medicine but also influenced the self-image and presentation of British medicine as it developed in the interwar and post–World War II years. British films with medical themes, such as *The Citadel* (1938), which juxtaposed an idealistic young doctor with the short-comings of the medical establishment, and *Vigil in the Night* (1940), which highlighted the underfunding and poor management of a provincial voluntary hospital during an epidemic, sometimes reflected tensions within the developing health care delivery system but also projected the same altruistic heroic image of doctors and nurses as did American products.

The zenith of film viewing in Britain came in the early 1950s. Thereafter, the audience moved home to watch proliferating numbers of "doctor shows" on the newest form of mass media, television.[100] There, myths and stereotypes privileging professional and institutional medicine predominated during the 1950s and '60s, continuing the images generated by feature films during the previous two decades. However, before the critical 1970s, these images tended to reinforce new working-class assumptions regarding biomedicine that reflected a more homogenous national health culture than had ever existed before.

While the Radio Doctor packaged biomedicine in commonsense advice for self-care and "Mrs. Dale's Diary" embedded the normative physician in "ordinary" community life, feature films with medical characters and themes more resembled the romances and melodramas of magazine stories. They tended to construct problems that were ultimately solved by intelligent, well-trained, morally sound doctors and nurses. Whether based on historical persons or events, such as *Florence Nightingale* (1915), *The Story of Louis Pasteur* (1936), *Dr. Ehrlich's Magic Bullet* (1940), *Madame Curie* (1943), and *Sister Kenny* (1946), or exemplifying medical personnel and environments, such as the *Dr. Kildare* series (beginning in 1938 with *Young Dr. Kildare*), *Men in White* (1934), *White Corridors* (1951), and *Magnificent Obsession* (1935 and 1954), movies invested medical encounters with drama and health care personnel with sanctity and heroism. Even critical films, such as *Arrowsmith* (1931), whose main character sacrificed his wife and a number of (Caribbean island) plague victims to his scientific research design, and *Not as a Stranger* (1955), in which a brilliant (and unfaithful) physician learned that empathy is as important as scientific knowledge, implied the premise that, notwithstanding individual human frailties, biomedicine is essentially

100. See, for example, Karpf, *Doctoring the media*, 180–206; Joseph Turow, *Playing doctor: Television, storytelling, and medical power* (Oxford and New York: Oxford University Press, 1989).

noble and effective.[101] And, as Ann Karpf points out, even where medical institutions are portrayed as evil, such as the state insane asylum in *The Snake Pit* (1948), the doctor is often good.[102]

The positive images of doctors and nurses themselves had a history in film, with a disproportionately large number of early movies, such as *The Doctor's Favorite Patient* (1903), *The Medicine Bottle* (1909), *The Doctor's Bride* (1909), and *The Love Auction* (1919), depicting weak or nefarious physician characters, while films released after 1920 were more likely to show the heroic side of professional medicine. This trend may be related to changes in medicine itself; for instance, in *The Prodigal Wife* (1918), "A woman abandons her surgeon husband because he is miserably poor and has no career prospects"—a scenario that had lost its meaning by the mid-twentieth century.[103] By contrast, in *Emergency Call* (1933), "A talented surgeon finds his hospital controlled by ambulance-chasing racketeers; after the death of a friend on the operating table as a result of a defective anesthetic, he mounts a crusade to clean up the hospital."[104] This change may also have been related to increasing pressure from organized medicine for films to cast biomedicine in a good light. Authorities agree that the American Medical Association brought significant influence to bear in Hollywood, while the British Board of Film banned or required changes in movies that criticized the profession.[105]

Whatever the interpretation, by the 1930s the familiar stereotypes of the brilliant, self-sacrificing doctor who is sometimes lacking in social skills and the beautiful, plucky nurse who usually ends up in his arms were fully fleshed out and launched. From the trenches of World War I to the African jungle, from London to Beverly Hills, from rural solo family practices to metropolitan high-rise research hospitals, nurses and doctors faced and beat challenges, garbed in the white that increasingly represented their germlessness, association with science, and devotion to a uniformed higher calling that distinguished them from ordinary mortals. This was not a conspiracy in the sense of an organized, concerted attempt at propaganda. However, it was good business for both filmmakers and professional medicine, harnessing the powerful dream machine to the dramatic scientific and therapeutic achievements of the mid-twentieth century. It also lent the luster of the fictional images and scenarios of the "pictures" to their local manifestations—the doctors, trained nurses, and hospitals that were becoming increasingly familiar to working-class patients and their family members.

---

101. Shortland, *Medicine and film*, 8.
102. Karpf, *Doctoring the media*, 182.
103. Shortland, *Medicine and film*, 18.
104. Ibid., 21.
105. Ibid., 8; Karpf, *Doctoring the media*, 181–82.

MASS MEDIA, "PROPAGANDA,"
AND PUBLIC HEALTH

Magazines, radio programs, and feature films delivered health information and medical images to a mass audience. The oral evidence shows that working-class people in Barrow, Lancaster, and Preston consumed these types of media. In addition, however, as public health authorities began to believe in the power of propaganda to influence attitudes and behavior—and particularly after the Ministry of Health (established in 1920) officially made health education a local responsibility—Medical Officers of Health started reporting their efforts in this area, which generally took the forms of posters, leaflets, lectures, exhibitions, and distribution of the Central Council for Health Education's magazine, *Better Health.* Target audiences included working-class mothers, schoolchildren, teachers, and local organizations. Topics ranged from infant care and personal hygiene to prevention and management of infectious diseases. For example, in 1922 Barrow's MOH reported: "A series of lectures were delivered by the Superintendent Nurse and the Health Visitors, and other ladies, at the various Centres during the year, dealing with every phase of maternity and child welfare and a special lecture on 'The Care of the Teeth,' was given by the Dental Officer (Mr. W. Harvie Kerr). It is believed, judging by the appreciation with which these lectures are received, that much is done thereby."[106] Such earnest endeavors were categorized in official reports as "Propaganda Work" and joined the one-to-one advice administered by health visitors in the ongoing attempt to influence what Lancaster's MOH described in 1921 as "ignorance on the part of the public of elementary hygienic principles, and a dormant or apathetic public sanitary conscience."[107]

Public health authorities worked with other organizations to reach a wider audience. Their lectures, posters, and pamphlets were supplemented by stories in local newspapers. In 1948 Barrow's MOH reported, "Good relations exist with the local Press which has always shown itself willing to cooperate in publishing any item to which it is considered the public attention should be drawn."[108] Health officials also worked with voluntary organizations focusing on specific issues. For example, in 1914 Preston's MOH wrote:

> Arrangements with the National Society for the Prevention of Consumption, resulted in the Tuberculosis Exhibition, which had been traveling the Country and had already been shown in many places, coming to the town. By means of exhibits of various kinds—such as

---

106. Barrow MOH Report, 1922, 344. See also, for example, Lancaster MOH Report, 1927, 53.

107. Lancaster MOH Report, 1921, 17.

108. Barrow MOH Report, 1948, 16.

models of sanitary and insanitary dwellings—striking pictures, and wall sheets of statistics, it endeavored to impress upon the public mind the fact that Tuberculosis, whilst causing so much sickness and mortality, was really a preventable disease, but also one which, if precautions were neglected, could, mainly through the sputum of the patient, readily be spread throughout a household. These points were further stated and emphasized in a series of Evening Lectures given by Medical men who kindly volunteered, and these lectures, like the Exhibition itself, were well attended.[109]

Medical Officers of Health recognized early the power of film to educate and influence audiences. In 1917 in Preston:

With a view to making the subject of Infant Welfare more widely known, and of arousing public interest, it was decided under the auspices of the National Baby Week Council to hold a Baby Week in the early part of July. This was a first effort in this direction, and consequently only on a small scale, whilst owing to the limited time available, the preparation was somewhat hurried. Proceedings commenced with the exhibition on Sunday, July 2nd, of the film, "Motherhood," at one of the Theatres. . . . At the same time a practical address was delivered by Mr. Alderman Smith, of the Bradford Corporation, a town which has deservedly earned a reputation for its initiative, and progressive action, in matters connected with Infant Welfare.[110]

Similarly, in 1920 the MOH reported: "The Preston Branch of the National Committee for Combating Venereal Diseases has continued its activities under the able chairmanship of Alderman Henry Cartmell. Educational films such as 'The End of the Road,' 'How Life Begins,' and 'The Shadow,' have been shown. Lectures by prominent speakers for mixed audiences and for the sexes separately have been enthusiastically received by the public."[111] By the early 1930s, Timothy Boon estimates, several million people saw such VD films every year.[112]

In addition to films produced by other organizations, public health authorities commissioned their own pictures. For example, the silent subtitled 1928 film "Tuberculosis Sanatorium at Ulverston" was made to inform the public about tuberculosis and, by allaying fears of sanatorium treat-

    109. Preston MOH Report, 1914, 8.
    110. Preston MOH Report, 1917, 9.
    111. Preston MOH Report, 1920, 63.
    112. Timothy Martyn Boon, "Films and the Contestation of Public Health in Interwar Britain," unpublished PhD dissertation, London University, 1999, 18.

ment, encourage compliance with prescribed sanatorium admission.[113] The movie portrays "the life of a patient at a Lancashire Sanatorium" from his diagnosis, through treatment at the High Carly Sanatorium, to his discharge as a healthy man. It provides a good deal of clinical detail, for example showing an x-ray with a clear right lung and two affected areas on the left lung, and explaining, "Bacteriological Tests are made at the Sanatorium of patient's sputum or spit in order to detect the presence or otherwise of the tubercle bacillus, that is, the germ which causes tuberculosis." In addition to demystifying the process of diagnosis, care and treatment, however, the film shows sunlit breezy rural scenes, with bedridden patients resting in the fresh air attended by white-uniformed nurses and doctors, and recuperating patients hiking, gardening, or playing games outside. Everyone is smiling, matter-of-fact, and (particularly the men) smoking. At the end of the movie, "After nine months' treatment our chosen patient has made an excellent recovery and is fit to return to employment. He is here seen bidding goodbye to the male patients, taking farewell of the Medical Superintendent, Matron, and staff." Such films, reaching a smaller audience than box-office features, nonetheless benefited from people's huge appetite for movies and their growing familiarity with information and images delivered in this way. Like the approximately 350 documentary films on public health topics produced in Britain in the interwar period, "Tuberculosis Sanatorium at Ulverston" exploited "the most powerful contemporary medium of persuasion . . . to enroll audiences in different interpretations of the public health"—in this case, institutional treatment for TB.[114]

CONCLUSION

If feature films, radio dramas, and magazine stories can be viewed as art imitating life, public health films, posters, and magazines turned this relationship around, using the conventions of entertainment media to educate and influence behavior. That this happened at all testifies to the influence of truly popular media on people's attitudes and actions—regarding health and medicine as well as other matters. Unlike traditional lectures, magazines, radio programs, and feature films were pleasurable to consume and delivered information in new and powerful ways.

This was all happening in the interwar period, when, as we have seen, working-class people in Barrow, Lancaster, and Preston began calling the doctor, going to the hospital, and using public health clinics more habitually than ever before. I think an important reason they changed their tra-

113. North West Film Archive, Film 163: "TB Sanatorium at Ulverston," 1926.
114. Boon, *Films*, 6.

ditional attitudes and behaviors is that the media they consumed rendered such behaviors normal, safe, and respectable. Furthermore, the images of doctors, nurses, medical interventions, and hospitals encapsulated in popular media presentations lent professional medicine a cultural authority it had not previously enjoyed among working-class people. The media educated working-class perceptions and interpretations of medicine and public health. It built a market for health care services and products that required only the establishment of the National Health Service to explode.

Chapter Eight

≈

"The best thing since wearing boots"

Working-Class Health Culture after 1948

INTRODUCTION:
DEPRESSION, WAR, AND PEACE

After World War II, traditional working-class health culture faded and a national culture regarding conceptualization and management of health and illness developed in Britain. This transition is associated with the introduction of the National Health Service in 1948. However, I argue that, like that legislation, alterations in working-class health behavior and beliefs were evolutionary rather than revolutionary, fostered by earlier social policies and programs, and nurtured by public education and the popular media. Changes that can clearly be observed after 1948 have roots particularly in the interwar years, which served as a watershed for the transformation of formal health care delivery and the hegemonic development of professional medicine's cultural authority among working-class people in Barrow, Lancaster, and Preston. They also stem from wartime policies and social developments that increased working-class utilization of official health services, undermined the previous multitiered delivery system, and encouraged the collective expectation that after the shared agony and challenge of war, a new Britain would shed some of its former inequalities—including those associated with health and medical care.

As we have seen, the 1920s and '30s witnessed significant expansion of formal health services in the study cities, including maternity and child welfare clinics, school medical and dental care, and provision of hospital beds for a widening range of conditions (e.g., tuberculosis, tonsillectomy, and childbirth) and individuals (e.g., children and pregnant women). At the same time, a growing number of wage earners were covered by National Health Insurance (NHI) for services from general practitioners (GPs), and

hospital prepayment "schemes" provided low-cost or free in- and outpatient care to rising numbers of working-class people, including women and children. Furthermore, admission to isolation hospitals, recommended and sometimes enforced by local health authorities, made hospitalization an increasingly familiar and expected experience for working-class children.

Accompanying proliferation of and easing access to formal health services was escalating pressure to use those services. In the era of social medicine and advocacy for health citizenship, some of this pressure was policy-driven and supported by public revenues; both school and local authority health care provision, initiated before World War I, expanded after 1918.[1] Schoolchildren were examined by doctors and nurses; sent to dentists, physicians, public health clinics, and open-air schools for treatment; and taught about germs, personal hygiene, and the importance of professional medical attention. Mothers of infants and ailing schoolchildren received mandated visits and recommendations from health visitors; those recommendations often included the instruction to consult the "family doctor." At the same time, infant welfare clinics wooed mothers by offering cheap or free milk and other supplies along with professional advice about child care. As we have seen, these services were not universally popular, but they did become routine aspects of working-class life in Barrow, Lancaster, and Preston.

More subtle pressure to use formal health services came from the popular media. Box-office films, which were especially popular with working-class audiences, glamorized white-uniformed doctors and nurses and endowed their endeavors with dramatic urgency and altruism. Radio programs broadcast advice based on current biomedical knowledge, "keep fit" routines, and medical dramas into millions of working-class homes. Through advertisements, advice columns, and stories, popular magazines targeting working-class readers straddled these approaches, offering both information from "experts" and entertainment glorifying professional medicine. And health-related organizations ranging from the British Medical Association and the Central Council for Health Education to the Empire Marketing Board and the British Social Hygiene Council used propaganda approaches borrowed from the popular media and advertising, including posters, magazine articles, films, and public events, to change working-class behavior and attitudes regarding health, illness, and medicine.

Paralleling the enthusiasm for "modern medicine" projected by such material was repudiation of "old wives' tales," which encompassed the

---

1. See, for example, Jane Lewis, *What price community medicine: The philosophy, practice and politics of public health since 1919* (Brighton, Sussex: Wheatsheaf Books, 1986); Dorothy Porter, "From social structure to social behavior in Britain after the Second World War," *Contemporary British History* 16:3 (2002): 58–80; Bernard Harris, *The health of the schoolchild: A history of the school medical service in England and Wales* (Buckingham and Philadelphia: Open University Press, 1995).

information and advice these tales contained as well as the tellers—the informal working-class health authorities whose knowledge and techniques were marginalized, invalidated, and ultimately demonized. Indeed, regardless of whether traditional health lore "worked," through the social class and professional power dynamics identified by Beverley Skeggs, by the mid-twentieth century this lore had become non-knowledge and its purveyors tinged with suspicion of dirt, vice, and illegal activities.[2] At the same time, information provided by medical experts—regardless of ongoing changes and contradictions in that information or, indeed, whether it proved to be right, wrong, effective, or dangerous—because of its association with science and professional authority became the only valid knowledge regarding a widening range of human activities and experiences.

Despite powerful pressure in the 1920s and '30s for working-class people to alter their traditional ways of preventing illness and managing birth, disability, and death, the oral evidence shows that those ways survived and were usual in most working-class households in Barrow, Lancaster, and Preston until World War II. "Doctor's medicine," although increasingly sought or experienced for reasons explored in chapter 3, remained either a luxury or an unpleasant necessity. Women, mainly without formal medical training, continued to manage health events in dwellings and neighborhoods using traditional knowledge and home- and over-the-counter remedies. How can we account for this survival?

One contributing factor was the economic downturn that followed World War I and lingered until the late 1930s. The cotton and shipbuilding industries of Preston and Barrow were particularly affected. According to Elizabeth Roberts, "Unemployment was a serious problem in the interwar years, especially in Barrow where 49 percent of the insured workers were unemployed in 1922, and in Preston, where 27 percent were unemployed in 1931."[3] Indeed, between 1921 and 1931, Barrow's population dropped by 16.2 percent as residents left to seek work elsewhere.[4] Even in Lancaster, where oilcloth, linoleum, and services provided a more stable employment base, hours and wages were cut, and unemployment rose.[5] Regardless, then, of the general improvement during this period in work-

2. For example, both Dr. Armstrong of Lancaster (born 1918) and Mrs. Jenkins (born in Barrow 1932) remembered babies' "wind" (gas) being relieved by cinder tea made of the ashes from the fire, despite their recognition that this technique, used by "Granny," was outdated. See chapter 6, n145. Chapter 5 explored the memories that oral history informants had of stereotypical criminal backstreet abortionists, who were perhaps the quintessentially demonized old wives. Regarding knowledge, social class, gender, and legitimacy of knowledge, see Beverley Skeggs, *Formations of class and gender* (London: Sage Publications, 1997), 19–20.

3. Elizabeth Roberts, *A woman's place: An oral history of working-class women 1890–1940* (Oxford: Basil Blackwell, 1984), 136. See also David Hunt, *A history of Preston* (Preston: Carnegie Publishing, in conjunction with Preston Borough Council, 1992), 232–33.

4. Roberts, *A woman's place*, 181.

5. See, for example, Lancaster MOH Report, 1925, 9–10.

ing-class lifestyles, housing, and health that has been observed by many scholars, the oral history evidence records memories of comparative want and widespread exercise of the traditional skill of making the best of very little.[6] Furthermore, it is clear that women, always both the health care and budget decision-makers and the least advantaged regarding resource distribution in working-class homes, experienced disproportionately high levels of need when work and wages declined.[7]

Economic insecurity fostered continued reliance on neighborhood mutual aid, which for many was a preferable alternative to the financial and medical support available through means-tested public assistance.[8] While, as chapter 2 indicates, neighbors and relatives did not always help each other, tradition favored this type of support, which was especially requested and given during times of ill-health. And informal assistance was both less expensive than care from a general practitioner and less stigmatized than medical attention provided *via* the Poor Law Guardians or later local welfare authorities. Even maternity and child health clinics were considered by some to be part of the same operation as the former Poor Law infirmaries; therefore, respectable working-class people avoided the stain of pauperization that clung to use of such facilities and preferred to depend on relatives, neighbors, and informal home care. While the more prosperous increasingly consulted physicians, went to hospitals, and took advice from public health professionals, poorer families continued to deal with health matters traditionally. Thus, the Depression arguably delayed the transformation of working-class health culture.

However, after 1939, with the dislocation of peacetime society coupled with enhanced governmental involvement in daily life—including health care provision—working-class utilization of formal health services grew. In the course of planning for civilian and military casualties, Britain's hospitals were nationalized and regionalized.[9] This brought to an end older categories of hospitals—voluntary, Poor Law, local authority—bringing them all under central governmental control, beginning expansion programs that would continue after the war, and eliminating barriers (such as required payment or the need for a "recommend" from an employer or governmental official) to working-class admission. Furthermore, policy-backed social services, from wartime nurseries to evacuation of children

6. See, for example, Ann Digby, *British welfare policy: Workhouse to workfare* (London and Boston: Faber and Faber, 1989), 53; Charles Webster, "Healthy or hungry thirties?" *History Workshop* 13 (1982): 110–29.

7. See, for example, Helen Jones, *Health and society in twentieth-century Britain* (London and New York: Longman, 1994), 58–87; Margery Spring Rice, *Working-class wives* (London: Penguin, 1939).

8. See, for example, Digby, *British welfare policy*, 51–52. See also Roberts, *A woman's place*, 181–82, 199–200.

9. Charles Webster, *The National Health Service: A political history*, 2nd ed. (Oxford: Oxford University Press, 2002. First published 1998), 17–19.

from areas under direct military threat, ratcheted up working-class contact with official health care providers and advice. As a shared enterprise and experience, World War II brought the social classes together as, perhaps, never before. World War II generated consensus that change was necessary and possible—in matters of health and medicine as well as other quality-of-life issues.

ESTABLISHMENT OF THE NATIONAL HEALTH SERVICE

Articulating a local expression of the national consensus regarding need for post–World War II reconstruction, in 1945 Barrow's Medical Officer of Health, A. R. Forrest, wrote: "One hopes that in the future post-war world that we shall see freedom from want, economic security for the family by full employment and adequate wages which will not require the mothers to work in industry, and better housing so that each family can have a decent home of their own in order to bring up their children."[10] Oral history informants echoed Forrest's hopes. Mr. Rollins, born in 1931 in Barrow, said his parents were very pleased with the new Labor government that came to power in 1945: "We are going to progress and everything is going to improve and everybody is going to be more or less equal."[11] The National Health Service (NHS), initiated in 1948, by offering medical and public health services based on the latest biomedical science free at the point of use, was expected to eliminate disparities in access, service provision, and health status among Britain's social classes.

As unexpectedly high initial utilization figures indicate, from its inception the NHS was popular with patients from all social backgrounds.[12] The popular stereotype of an avalanche of demand for dentures and spectacles is borne out by statistics. According to Charles Webster, "During the first eight months of the new service, the rate of demand for the general dental service ran at about eight million cases a year, which was twice the expected level. One-third of the patients treated required dentures." Similarly, in the same time period, "some five million people had their eyes tested and the public was supplied with no fewer than 8.3 million pairs of glasses."[13]

10. Barrow MOH Report, 1945, 12.
11. Mr. R3B, 50.
12. Webster, *The National Health Service*, 29–31.
13. Ibid., 48–49. According to Brian Watkin, "By 1953, nearly 7 million people, or one in six of the population, were wearing a full set of dentures, nearly 6 million pairs of which had been issued under the NHS" (*The National Health Service: The first phase. 1948–1974 and after* [London: George Allen and Unwin, 1978], 32–33). Similarly, the cost of optical services was more than 20 times the original estimate: "By 1953, about 19.5 million people had been supplied with 26.1 million pairs of spectacles" (33). However, once the initial need was filled, demand for spectacles and dentures declined.

Oral history informants and scholars agree that the early and continued high demand for medical services revealed, not working-class greed and improvidence, but needs that had hitherto gone unmet. Mr. Boswell, born in 1920 in Barrow, observed:

> People wanted their teeth out . . . and wanted a set of dentures, they just could not afford to buy them, so they had aching teeth. . . . Or somebody was ill, send for the doctor, you would get a bill. So they would go down to the chemist and make a bottle up or something like that, you know, and of course the result was that people snuffed it. They had diseases that could have been cured, but they went on too far, so the population was beset with illnesses. . . . And they could not afford to get them treated, so it was the best thing since wearing boots when that [the NHS] came on.[14]

Helen Jones argues that the NHS benefited working-class women in particular. "The full extent of women's ill health had never before been revealed. One woman doctor who qualified on the day the NHS came into operation recalled women queuing with thyroid deficiency, gynecological problems, painful varicose veins, or with menopausal difficulties. The biggest increase in visits to the GP came from the elderly and from women aged up to thirty-five."[15]

In addition to addressing unmet needs, the NHS undermined previous class- and financially based differences in the ways general practitioners treated private and "panel" patients. Margot Jeffreys grew up in a small town near London. Her middle-class family consulted a GP who "lived in an elegant house in the High Street. As private, paying, patients . . . we went in through the front door and waited to see him in a well-furnished sitting room. . . . Our doctor also had panel patients. They were mainly working-class men, entitled to consult him by virtue of their compulsory NHI payments. They used a side entrance to his house, and waited to see him on benches along a passageway."[16] As indicated in chapter 3, oral history informants remembered friendly society ("club") and NHI panel patients receiving less respect and possibly a lower quality of care from GPs than private patients.[17] Recounting her mother's memories of consulting the doctor before the NHS, Mrs. Harrison, born in Preston in 1945, said, "Dr. Simpson . . . was a mean Scotsman. He used to make you wash your

14. Mr. B4B, 30. See also Mrs. B2B, 54; Mr. K1B, 13; Mr. P6B, 31; Mrs. P6B, 121; Mr. S7L, 74.

15. Jones, *Health and society,* 123–24.

16. Margot Jeffreys, "General practitioners and the other caring professions," *General practice under the National Health Service 1948–1997,* Irvine Loudon, John Horder and Charles Webster, eds. (London: Clarendon Press, 1998), 129.

17. See, for example, Mr. M1B, 17; Mr. F2B, 7–8.

bandages and those sorts of things then." When asked what her mother thought of the National Health Service, Mrs. Harrison responded, "Bevan was her hero, certainly. Yes, she thought it was wonderful, you know, after experiencing the meanness of doctors like Simpson and others, the discretionary treatment."[18] By contrast with the past, because most private patients elected to join NHS panels in 1948, such distinctions faded in the postwar period when "going to the doctor" or requesting a home visit became a universal working-class experience for the first time.[19]

The National Health Service also eliminated the stigma attached to requesting or receiving care paid for by public assistance. As we have seen, only the very poor who lacked adequate support from relatives and neighbors sought or accepted admission to a workhouse infirmary or treatment from a doctor compensated by the Poor Law guardians. Such pauperization risked individual and family reputations, as well as generating shame over personal inability to meet the normative role expectations of working and meeting one's needs and those of close family members. The vestiges of the Poor Law were swept away by the advent of what some have termed the "classic welfare state" of the 1940s.[20] Health care provided by the NHS was universal, not means-tested, and funded by general taxation. Mr. Morton, born in 1927 in Barrow, said his family thought the NHS was "First class. They had worked hard for it."[21] Mr. Kirby, born in Barrow in 1921, remembered, "People thought, 'Well, at least we can afford to be ill now,' whereas before they tended not to go to the doctor's unless they had to because they had to pay, that was the simple thinking behind it. If you were paying a contribution towards it, you felt as though it was an insurance, really."[22] Citizens accessed NHS services by right, and increasingly were judged more harshly for *not* using than for using them.

After 1948, working-class willingness to consult general practitioners and use hospitals for in- and outpatient treatment grew, while reliance on traditional ways of dealing with health and illness declined. Mr. Lodge, born in 1919 in Preston, commented:

> You see, before the war, if you went to a doctor, you had to pay. You had to pay for that treatment, there was no free medicine. Now, when the Beveridge plan came in, it was free, so naturally you relied more or less on the doctors, than your own remedies. Mind you, it came sometimes, when you wouldn't be bothered going, you'd say, "Oh, I'll do what my mother did." Same as if I couldn't sleep at night for coughing, I'd boil

18. Mrs. H9P, 38–39.

19. Ian Tait and Susanna Graham-Jones, "General practice, its patients, and the public," in *General practice*, Loudon et al., eds. (London: Clarendon Press, 1998), 227–28.

20. See, for example, Digby, *British welfare policy*, 6.

21. Mr. M13B, 59.

22. Mr. K1B, 13.

some milk and get a spoonful of treacle and put it in and stir it round, and drink it, that would ease it, and you'd sleep all night, you see. Things like that.[23]

Mrs. Owen's only daughter was born in 1940. While continuing her close relationship with her own mother, who lived nearby, Mrs. Owen transferred her reliance in medical matters to her GP. She said, "If something happened to her [the child], I used to take her to the doctor's and get the *proper* thing." She tolerated her mother's home remedies, allowing "Mum to goose grease her if she had a bad chest. I used to say, 'That child's got a bad chest,' and out would come the jar of goose grease. An earthenware jar with a piece of brown paper with a rubber ring round, and she would come down and rub her back and front. In the end, I took her [daughter] to the doctor, and he gave me some antibiotics, and it cleared up in no time."[24] These accounts illustrate the extensive overlapping of traditional and "modern" health cultures, which straddled the introduction of the National Health Service. They also remind us that, as was true in the early twentieth century, working-class people were selective about the formal services they sought and accepted after 1948, and did not operate as an undifferentiated cohort. There were continuing differences between the "rough" and the "respectable," the more and less prosperous, the old and the young. As Virginia Berridge observes, relatives (particularly mothers and daughters) continued to support each other in times of ill-health, and certain forms of traditional behavior, including self-medication, continued.[25] Nonetheless, the oral history evidence reveals an important shift in normative attitudes and behavior.

Elizabeth Roberts argues that after World War II, "There was a strong feeling that professional services were better than those provided by well-meaning amateurs. Mothers of babies and small children particularly sought professional help. Increasingly, the advice of doctors and health visitors was preferred to that of older women in the family or neighborhood."[26] As Mrs. Owen suggested, people who had experienced traditional domestic and community management of illness as children made different choices within their adult households. When asked where he and his wife obtained medical advice for their own children, Mr. Norton, born in 1931 in Lancaster, said "the doctor":

23. Mrs. L3P, 35.
24. Mrs. O1B, 58.
25. Virginia Berridge, *Health and society in Britain since 1939* (Cambridge: Cambridge University Press, 1999). Berridge's discussion also suggests geographical differences in working-class health culture.
26. Roberts, *Women and families,* 12.

If Mum had called, we would ask, but basically, no, we talked to the doctor.

Interviewer: Why was there this change?

Informant: Because, I think, the world had changed, the responsibility levels had changed, knowledge had changed. The doctors had got a lot more knowledge and were a lot more available.[27]

Other informants reported a similar change—higher levels of consultation of doctors combined with reduced confidence in informal health authorities.

This shift paralleled dramatic changes in the effectiveness of medical intervention. It is arguable that the development and growth of public health services before 1948 stemmed in part from comparative clinical helplessness, when prevention was regarded as the more powerful alternative. After 1948, with development of a growing range of successful interventions—from antibacterial and psychoactive drugs to increasingly ambitious surgeries and use of new technologies—despite institutionalization of social medicine, the policy focus shifted to treatment, with a special emphasis on medical specialists and the hospitals in which they were based.[28] The hospitals and specialist consultants, and, to a lesser degree, the primary care services involving "independent contractors" (general practitioners, dentists, opticians, and pharmacists), attracted the lion's share of public attention and resources. Although local-authority public health services continued and successfully administered immunization, midwifery, home visiting, social work, and family planning services, their status and influence declined from the high point of the 1930s. When working-class informants talked about "modern medicine," they were more likely to mention clinical interventions than prevention and to refer to "doctors," who were gatekeepers for the miraculous cures of the brave new postwar world.

After 1948, most health care moved from homes to offices, clinics, or hospitals. Although GPs continued to make house calls and until the 1970s a declining but significant percentage of Barrow, Lancaster, and Preston births occurred at home, the balance shifted in favor of institutional attention—whether for well care, diagnosis, monitoring (of a pregnancy or chronic condition), intervention, or nursing. This transition accompanied a change in the power dynamics of the relationship between patients and their families, on the one hand, and professional care providers, on the other. When most treatment and care took place in the home, although the GP, MOH, health visitor, qualified midwife, or district nurse might carry

27. Mr. N2L, 58.

28. Webster, *The National Health Service*, 39. Regarding institutionalization of social medicine, see Dorothy Porter, "From social structure to social behavior."

the weight of social class, professional, or official authority, patients and family members had significant control of the situation. They admitted or denied entry to the care provider, took or did not take medical advice, and followed or did not follow "orders." The home environment was as much a part of the care provider's culture as it was part of the patient's; providers expected to work in private homes with patients and their families to achieve a variety of goals, including compliance, cure or amelioration of the condition occasioning the visit, and (sometimes) payment for services rendered.

By contrast, in offices, clinics, and hospitals, medical professionals were firmly in charge of interactions with patients, who were expected to defer to official authorities and comply with institutional rules. These rules quickly undermined traditional roles and relationships during times of ill-health: for example, mothers had access to hospitalized children only at the ward sister's discretion, and fathers were not allowed to hold their newborn infants. Institutional environments contributed to the mushrooming cultural authority of professional medicine, which became spatially distant from sufferers' home and neighborhood environments, and figuratively distant from lay knowledge and understanding.[29] As health care moved to institutions, homes and laypeople became both unfit to provide it and increasingly dependant on occupational experts. Nonetheless, because of continuing social class distance from medical professionals, in the post–World War II era, working-class people were more deferent and less able to assert their own needs or question medical authority than their middle- and upper-class counterparts.

With hindsight, it is clear that inequalities in health and access to health services persisted after the introduction of the NHS.[30] Furthermore, while life expectancy improved and death rates declined in the generation after 1948, these advances were slower than in the years before World War II and lagged behind those of many other European countries.[31] This evidence indicates that the NHS did not accomplish the utopian goals its advocates set for it. However, it did complete the long process of cementing working-class "buy-in" to biomedicine and the formal health care delivery system. Because its services were universal and, with the exception of small fees charged for some services beginning in 1951, free at the point of use, the NHS converted professional treatment from a luxury (or quasi-punitive requirement) to a necessary, routine element of daily life. As a result of its philosophical and cultural distance from welfare, the NHS reduced barri-

29. See, for example, Paul Starr, *The social transformation of American medicine* (New York: Basic Books, 1982), 14.

30. See, for example, *The Black Report: The health divide* (New York: Penguin, 1988); John Whitelegg, *Inequalities in health care: Problems of access and provision* (Rettford, Nottinghamshire: Straw Barnes, 1982); Jones, *Health and society*, 125–27.

31. David Widgery, *Health in danger* (London: Macmillan, 1979), 33–35.

ers to use of affordable medical services. Working-class women, continuing in their roles as family health care decision-makers, became enthusiastic patrons of the National Health Service, within a generation dropping their traditional positions as diagnosticians, makers and administrators of remedies, skilled nurses, and officiators at birth- and deathbeds.

MODERN LIFE, RESPECTABILITY, AND WORKING-CLASS HEALTH CULTURE

After World War II, social class remained an important component of identity, opportunity, health, and longevity in Britain.[32] Class distinctions survive; people still identify themselves as working-class, however difficult it may be to define what that means.[33] However, I will argue here that postwar changes in working-class standards of living, neighborhoods, access to a publicly provided social safety net, and consumption of popular media significantly influenced the ways people thought about and dealt with health and illness, contributing to decline of traditional working-class ways of managing ill-health and development of a national health culture.

Perhaps the most important contribution to working-class living standards was the transformation of housing that escalated with construction of local authority council houses and demolition of "slums" after World War I, and continued after World War II.[34] For example, in 1964 Preston's Medical Officer of Health reported that over 6,000 unfit houses had been eliminated in the postwar period.[35] New housing updated standards and expectations regarding amenities, including private indoor sources of cold and hot water; private indoor toilets; plumbed-in baths; and domestic electricity and gas supplies for lighting, heating, and appliances. Council housing incorporated and projected these new standards, making them affordable for a growing number of working-class people. According to Alison Ravetz, "At its peak around 1975 council housing supplied nearly a third of the nation's housing stock and (since it was primarily for families with children) the homes of something more than a third of the population."[36] Built on the outskirts of towns, council estates were intended to

32. See, for example, Andrew Rosen, *The transformation of British life 1950–2000: A social history* (Manchester and New York: Manchester University Press, 2003), 5.

33. See, for example, Elizabeth Roberts, *Women and families: An oral history, 1940–1970* (Oxford: Blackwell, 1995), 237.

34. I use the word "escalated" because, as indicated in chapter 2, reform of working-class housing arguably began with construction of "bye-law" housing in the late nineteenth century. See, for example, John Burnett, *A social history of housing 1815–1985*, 2nd ed. (London and New York: Methuen, 1986. First published in 1978), 217–330; Alison Ravetz, *Council housing and culture: The history of a social experiment* (London and New York: Routledge, 2001).

35. Preston MOH Report, 1964, 6.

36. Ravetz, *Council housing*, 2.

facilitate working-class moral and physical health by substituting light, space, and modern appointments for the poor sanitation, darkness, and crowding thought to breed disease and vice in old inner-city neighborhoods. Private home construction paralleled development of council housing, expanding owner occupation among all social classes. John Burnett points out, "In 1945 only 26 percent of all houses in England and Wales were owner-occupied; by 1966, the proportion was 47 per cent, and in 1983 63 per cent."[37]

Changes in housing paralleled changes in employment and income. After the war, working-class employment began its long shift from manufacturing to services. This change reduced the concentration of working-class wage earners in factories—often located within walking distance from where the workers lived—thus undermining the generations-old link between workplace, neighborhood, and household. Preston was particularly affected, with the cotton textile industry, after a brief postwar revival, shuddering to a halt by the late 1960s when "its era as a mill town was over."[38] Lancaster's more diversified factories, which boomed for twenty years after the war, began to contract and close in the late 1960s, while Barrow's workforce continued to be disproportionately employed by Vickers's shipyards throughout the study period.[39] The shift toward nonfactory jobs did not damage working-class incomes overall. Indeed, nationwide the incomes of manual workers rose considerably during the twentieth century—over 400 percent between 1900 and 1981.[40] Thus, in the second half of the twentieth century, working-class people could afford better housing and pay for the transportation required to commute longer distances to work.

With the dismembering of old neighborhoods by "slum clearance," factory closures, council estate construction, and family mobility, traditional neighborhood relationships broke down. Many oral history informants remembered positive aspects of moving to better dwellings. For example, Mrs. Boyle was born in 1936 in a two-up-two-down rented house in Preston. When she was 16, the family moved to a council house on Preston's Larches Estate, "which were like a palace then really, to us. Because it had three bedrooms, a back garden, a front garden, a hallway, a big kitchen, a washhouse, a big living room. Bathroom. We thought it were great."[41] Similarly, Mrs. Hunter, born in Preston in 1931, said:

37. Burnett, *Social history of housing,* 282.

38. David Hunt, *A history of Preston* (Preston: Carnegie Publishing, in conjunction with Preston Borough Council, 1992), 250.

39. Steven Constantine and Alan Warde, "Challenge and change in the twentieth century," in *A history of Lancaster 1893–1993,* Andrew White, ed. (Keele: Ryburn Publishing, Keele University Press, 1993), 199–244, 229–31.

40. John Benson, *The rise of consumer society in Britain, 1880–1980* (London and New York: Longman, 1994), 26.

41. Mrs. B11P, 7. See also Mr. G6P, 2; Mrs. Y1L, 5, 7.

My first house I remember was a council house, which we apparently moved into when I was about one. . . . Well to me it was great, far superior to the houses of my friends, because they had the old-fashioned houses. One particular friend didn't even have electricity, she went to bed with a candle. But we had three bedrooms and hot and cold water. We had a bathroom downstairs which was rather unusual and I don't think we really liked. A little garden at the front and a big one at the back.

Interviewer: And at that point how big a family were you?

Informant: Just my mum and dad, and elder brother and myself.

The family had moved from a house that had been condemned.[42]

However, informants also recalled negative aspects of moving to council housing. Although the houses themselves were indisputably better than antiquated, bug-infested terraced homes, people missed the social closeness of traditional neighborhoods. In the 1950s and early '60s, Mr. and Mrs. Boyle lived in a small house on a run-down Preston Street. Mr. Boyle said of his wife, "No, if you asked her could she go back to when we were first married, to when we were in that two-up and two-down in Allen Street, bugs dropping off the ceiling and one thing and another, she would go back to that tomorrow." When the interviewer asked Mrs. Boyle, "Would you?" she replied, "Yes, to the neighbors." She went on to recall mutual aid in her traditional neighborhood:

> But like if you was ill or anything like that, you know they would come and help you, and it were good. They would take one another's children to school for you, my mother would end up taking us to the park, but we would end up taking about twelve of us. Everybody joined in, do you know what I mean? Not like today, although we used to fight and fall out, but don't get me wrong, because kids won't be kids unless they did, but you could play together and nobody seemed any better than anybody, you know, nobody were upper-class. But nobody thought themselves any better than anybody, you know.[43]

Normative mutual aid was a casualty of the dissolution of older neighborhoods. With higher wages and the social safety net created by the post-1948 welfare state, the help of neighbors was neither needed nor trusted; instead, increasingly prosperous working-class women "kept themselves to themselves" and depended on professionals for expert assistance.[44]

Therefore, there was declining emphasis on family respectability to

42. Mrs. H3P, 1.
43. Mrs. B11P, 14–15. See also Mr. M7P, 19.
44. See, for example, Judy Giles, *Women, identity and private life in Britain, 1900–50* (New York: St. Martin's Press, 1995), 101.

maintain access to neighborhood mutual aid. This does not mean that reputation no longer mattered to working-class people after World War II. However, its components and goals changed form. Before World War II, respectability was based in part on housekeeping standards—donkey-stoned front steps, gleaming white lace curtains, black-leaded ranges. With limited resources, working-class people's ability to keep a respectable home depended on their capacity to improvise creatively, to "make do and mend," and to "make a penny do a pound's work."[45] With growing prosperity, these capabilities became comparatively less important than using new purchasing power and "do-it-yourself" skills to represent family respectability through home appearance and contents.

From the 1950s, working-class people could afford a proliferating range of domestic consumer goods. Andrew Rosen reminds us that "in 1956 only 8 per cent of British households had refrigerators and as recently as the 1960s the majority of British households did not possess telephones or cars and only slightly more than half had washing machines."[46] Thus, there was plenty of scope for consumption, consumer objects were expensive and desirable, and they arguably became the currency of new measures for family reputations. Mr. Goodwin's comments about the Preston council estate he grew up in during the 1950s and '60s are illustrative:

> Even though it was a corporation, council estate, it was nice. Everybody knew each other, the kids were all, you knew all the kids. It was a nice street, it was. And everybody kept the gardens nice, these days the council estates seem to have let things go, but there everybody kept—and they had a pride with their gardens. Well, we had to look after and mow the lawns and things like that. Yes, everything was in nice condition, yes.
>
> *Interviewer:* Do you remember the neighbors popping in to see your mum or her popping in to see them?
> *Informant:* Usually with talking over the fence, I don't think they popped in.[47]

The well-kept garden, the three-piece suite (sofa and two armchairs), and (ultimately) the automobile, together with the endless housework that homemakers performed with additional consumer goods (and status symbols) such as the Hoover (still a generic term for vacuum cleaner in Britain) and twin-tub washing machine, increasingly signified family providence, hard work, and independence. After the war, working-class respectability was commodified.

45. See, for example, Roberts, *A woman's place*, 128–29, 150–51.
46. Andrew Rosen, *The transformation of British life 1950–2000: A social history* (Manchester and New York: Manchester University Press, 2003), 14.
47. Mr. G6P, 5.

Similarly, while keeping children clean and well-dressed remained a mark of family and maternal respectability, these endeavors were assisted and represented by purchase of goods including expensive prams, clothing, shoes, and toys. Responsible childcare was also signified by dependence on experts—doctors, health visitors, teachers, and others—to guide development, identify and forestall problems, and enhance parents' (read "mothers'") knowledge and skills.

Since the goals of working-class respectability no longer included accessing mutual aid, what had they become? This question is difficult to answer. Perhaps the need to maintain standards before the neighbors was vestigial, with no real current objective except to distinguish one's family as "respectable," as opposed to the stigmatized "rough" other. Perhaps the new commodified respectability was constructed by the same middle-class social reformers who designed council estates, child welfare clinics, and state comprehensive schools to re-engineer a working class in their own image—and, thus, the primary goal of respectability was pleasing those same experts. Alternatively, perhaps postwar changes in components and functions of working-class respectability, like changes in health culture, were part of the larger processes of deindustrialization, the blurring of class distinctions, and the development of a national culture.

This process was aided by universal primary and secondary education, which after 1947 required attendance up to age 15. Working-class children spent increasing time in classrooms where they were taught approved lessons about personal hygiene, sex, and homemaking. They also took science courses informed by developments in biomedicine. They were given milk, meals, emulsion, and physical training to support their health and prevent disease. Classroom teachers, school doctors, and nurses inspected them, identified physical and mental "deficiencies," and referred them for treatment. Above all, teachers and medical professionals encountered at school represented expertise, authority, and modernity, in direct contrast to the comparative old-fashioned ignorance of students' parents. School encouraged adoption of officially endorsed health behavior—whether it be hand-washing, acceptance of diagnostic x-rays and immunization, or consultation of physicians. Public education is probably an important reason that oral history informants born after about 1920 tended to remember experiencing traditional informal home-based care as children but using formal institutionally based care in their adult households.

Another influential factor in this transition was universal exposure to an expanding range of popular media. Chapter 7 explored working-class consumption of magazines, radio programs, and films with content that glamorized and encouraged people to use professional institutional medicine. In the postwar era, this consumption continued, enhanced by the advent of television, which provided both informational and fictional programming about health, illness, hospitals, and medical personnel. Ann Karpf

observes that TV medical documentaries portrayed doctors as "scientific wizards with formidable technical skills," while medical dramas emphasized physicians' surgical flair, razor-sharp intelligence, and "superlative aptitude for handling emotions." Programs such as *Emergency Ward 10* (1957–67) helped relieve popular anxieties about hospital treatment, while in the late 1960s *Marcus Welby, M.D.* exemplified the idealized family doctor dwelling in both British and American mythology.[48] An "exotic curiosity" in 1950, within the next half-century the television became "a normal part of virtually every household," and "doctor shows" helped shape national health culture.[49]

That culture was characterized by automatic normative consultation of professional health care providers for virtually all matters related to health and illness and internalization of the "cultural authority" of the physician:

> Patients consult physicians not just for advice, but first of all to find out whether they are "really" sick and what their symptoms mean. "What have I got, Doc?" they ask. "Is it serious?" Cultural authority, in this context, is antecedent to action. The authority to interpret signs and symptoms, to diagnose health or illness, to name diseases, and to offer prognoses is the foundation of any social authority the physician can assume. By shaping the patients' understanding of their own experience, physicians create the conditions under which their advice seems appropriate.[50]

By 1970, the end date of this study, routine dependence on professional medicine extended beyond experienced symptoms to symptom-free ills, such as hypertension or the early stages of many cancers, which required knowledge and technology. This dependence also involved ingesting (or administering to children) large amounts of prescribed medication, routine attendance at health care facilities, and hospital admission for an ever-expanding range of ills and therapies. For members of all social classes—particularly for working-class women—this dependence also involved relinquishing personal knowledge of, discretion regarding, or participation in the medical care of self or loved ones. By 1970 the ideal patient was the compliant patient illustrated in the comments of Mr. Thornbarrow, born in 1949: "No, we knew the doctors very well, we had had the family doctor from the early forties, and no, we didn't have any home cures. . . . It was one of them families where what the doctor said, that was it. You know,

48. Ann Karpf, *Doctoring the media: The reporting of health and medicine* (London: Routledge, 1988), 183, 187–88. See also Joseph Turow, *Playing doctor: Television, storytelling, and medical power* (Oxford and New York: Oxford University Press, 1989).

49. In 2000, 99 percent of British households had a color television set. Rosen, *Transformation of British life,* 14.

50. Starr, *Social transformation,* 14.

it wasn't open for negotiation."[51] And, although 1970 arguably marked a turning point, when middle-class patients in particular began to be critical of professional medicine and to demand greater participation in health care decision-making, processes, and environments, working-class patients continued, in general, to be dependent on and deferent to medical authority.

This transition involves both gains and losses. It is difficult to argue a downside to the eradication of smallpox and polio and the improvement of longevity and quality of life resulting from widespread access to bypass surgery for circulatory diseases and insulin treatment for diabetes. It would be churlish to attack the dedication and altruism of the medical practitioners who deal and have dealt with working-class health problems and people with imagination and good humor. However, it is fair to observe that dependence on medical expertise has undermined the traditional role and confidence of working-class women as health care authorities in their homes and neighborhoods, as well as invalidating their knowledge. With increasing costs of and decreasing resources for formal health care services at the beginning of the twenty-first century, it is ironic that people of all social classes are now being urged to be more active participants in prevention and treatment of illness, as well as to care for the ailing at home. Thus, perhaps we are in the midst of a new transformation of health culture.

IMPLICATIONS

This book has been a case study, firmly located in a particular time and place, of a phenomenon that has occurred in all industrialized nations and is now happening worldwide. While it is about Barrow, Lancaster, and Preston, it belongs more firmly to the history of public health and medicine than it does to local history. However, its local evidence reminds us that the shift from traditional to biomedical conceptualization and management of health and ill-health happens at different times in different places and differently among women, men, and members of different social classes. Although this study has not dealt with issues of race and ethnicity, these identifiers also affect transitions in health culture.

In most circumstances, these transitions are stimulated and enforced from the top down. Reformers know what should be done and are prepared to make people change for their own good. In the process, reformers tend to identify the evil with the victim and to be comparatively blind and tone-deaf to the wider environmental, political, and cultural circumstances of the people they are trying to help. Current global struggles with AIDS, malaria, overpopulation, malnutrition, and other killers are powerful reminders that elite knowledge and strategies rarely result in progress

51. Mr. T4B, 78. See also Mrs. M12B, 71; Mrs. P3L, 49–50; Mrs. S3B, 71.

or happiness unless sufferers are engaged and invested in solutions. Furthermore, the desired conversion of populations to modern western medicine carries the twin burdens of loss of lay ability to prevent and manage ill-health, on the one hand, and demand that political elites and medical professionals meet proliferating health care needs, on the other.

Working-class experience in Barrow, Lancaster, and Preston also reminds us that health culture touches almost every aspect of life—from housing, diet, and play to dress, sex, and death. As a result of their own heritage and the types of source materials they employ, the histories of public health and medicine have tended to be ghettoized within their associated professions and institutions. This isolation has conferred ownership of these histories on professional medicine and public health and ignored the expertise and agency of the people whose health and illnesses have, after all, been the foci of both endeavors.

This book has not been about doctor-bashing, although some readers may experience it in that way. Indeed, physicians have been comparatively peripheral to this study—as sufferers and patients often are in histories of medicine and public health. It is not that professional medicine is unimportant in the history of health and illness but that it is just one of many factors involved in the universal experiences of suffering, healing, prevention, and caregiving. By looking through another lens of the telescope, this study attempts to provide alternative perspectives about these matters.

Appendix

Oral History Informants

The following information was drawn from "biography cards" kept regarding each of the 239 oral history informants whose evidence was used for this book and from appendices of Elizabeth Roberts's *A woman's place: An oral history of working-class women 1890–1940* (Oxford: Basil Blackwell, 1984, 207–13) and *Women and families: An oral history, 1940–1970* (Oxford: Basil Blackwell, 1995, 241–48). Entries appearing below use italics for informants' families of birth and ordinary text for their adult experiences. Entries are categorized by informants' cities of residence. Since interviews varied in length, depth, and subject matter, information about informants' backgrounds is inconsistent. Some of the younger informants are children of people whom Roberts interviewed in the 1970s. Several informants (two chemists and two physicians) were interviewed because of their special roles in and perspectives regarding working-class neighborhoods.

Barrow

Mrs. A1B (Mrs. Anderson), b. 1872. *Oldest informant. Father, blacksmith in Vickers shipyard. Eldest of 10 children.* Domestic servant and cook. Married, 4 children.

Mr. A2B (Mr. Ackerman), b. 1904. *Father a prosperous pawnbroker. Second of 4 children (1 died).* Worked as a carpenter and became a leading Socialist politician in Barrow. Married. 1 child.

Mrs. A2B (Mrs. Ackerman), b. 1904. *Father a boilermaker's assistant. Mother, from Ireland, domestic servant before marriage; afterwards cleaner, laundress, and nurse. Very poor family. Eldest of 4 children.* Domestic servant and shop assistant. Married, 1 child.

Mrs. A3B (Mrs. Addison), b. 1892. *Father, laborer. Mother ran a shop before marriage; afterwards took in washing and went out cleaning. Eldest of 9 children (2 died).* Domestic servant and cook. Married. 6 children (3 died).

Mr. B1B (Mr. Best), b. 1897. *Father, coachman. Mother, domestic servant. Youngest of 13 children (2 died).* Baker in the Barrow workhouse. Married. 2 children.

Mr. B2B (Mr. Burrell), b. 1931. *Father, gun-fitter and munitions manager in Vickers. Mother, homemaker. Youngest of 7 children.* Fitter, merchant seaman. Married. 3 children.

Mrs. B2B (Mrs. Burrell), b. 1931. *Father, welder for Vickers. Mother, homemaker. Elder of 2 children.* Chemist's assistant before and after marriage; later did part-time shop and clerical work. Married. 3 children.

Mr. B3B (Mr. Barlow), b. 1915. *Father, plumber. Mother, weaver and shopkeeper. Younger of 2 children.* Did office and clerical work before World War II; later, teacher. Married. 3 children.

Mrs. B3B (Mrs. Barlow), b. 1928. *Father plater in Vickers, who was frequently unemployed and died in a shipyard accident in 1935. Mother, teacher before marriage and when widowed; also kept a lodging house. Only child.* Teacher. Married, 3 children.

Mr. B4B (Mr. Boswell), b. 1920. *Father, merchant seaman who also worked for Vickers as a fitter. Mother, munitions worker during World War I and homemaker after marriage. Second of 7 children.* Fitter. Married, 3 children.

Mr. C1B (Mr. Clarke), b. 1900. *Father, carpenter. Mother laborer in boot factory in Northern Ireland before marriage. Homemaker. One of 4 children.* Worked for Vickers. Married.

Mrs. C1B (Mrs. Clarke), b. 1900. *Father, raftsman on timber pond. Mother, domestic service before marriage. Homemaker. One of 8 children.* Did shop work before marriage.

Mrs. C2B (Mrs. Chase), b. 1887. *Irish immigrant family. Father, moulder. Mother, homemaker. Youngest of 8 children.* Married, 3 children.

Miss C3B (Miss Carter), b. 1958. *Father, chemist. Mother, part-time work as telephonist and shop assistant. Eldest of 4 children.* As adult, informant did hotel work and worked for community program assisting elderly people. Frequently unemployed and on public assistance.

Mrs. D1B (Mrs. Drake), b. 1899. *Father, sailor and laborer. Mother, farm servant before marriage. One of 9 children (1 died).* Domestic servant, munitions worker, cleaner. Married, 1 child.

Mrs. D2B (Mrs. Dalkey), b. 1896. *Father, shipwright who left job due to ill health. Later did office work. Mother, homemaker. Youngest of 21 children (12 died).* Shop assistant. Married, 2 children.

Mr. E1B (Mr. Eaton), b. 1902. *Father, ship painter killed in 1905. Mother deserted family around 1911. One of 2 children. Brought up by grandparents and stepfather: spent some time in the workhouse.* Office work, farm labor, gardening, and laboring in steel works.

Mr. F2B (Mr. Finch), b. 1900. *Father, tailor and postman. Mother, servant at 10 Downing Street before marriage. Homemaker. One of 3 children.* Railway clerk. Unmarried.

Mrs. G1B (Mrs. Garvey), b. 1888. *Father, fitter and turner. Mother, homemaker. One of 16 children (5 died).* Before marriage, ran domestic register. Later, homemaker. Married, 2 children.

Mrs. H1B (Mrs. Hancock), b. 1893. *Father, boilermaker and laborer on railway and dredgers. Mother, lady's maid before marriage. Homemaker. One of 4 children.*

Domestic, munitions, and shop work. Married, 1 child.

Mr. H1B (Mr. Hancock), b. 1894. *Father, fruit and vegetable seller. Mother, house-keeper for aunt before marriage. Worked in family shop after marriage. One of 5 children.* Wheelwright and joiner. Married, 1 child.

Mr. H2B (Mr. Hunt), b. 1888. *Father, shop manager and baker. Mother helped in family shop. Youngest of 4 children.* Moulder. Married, no children.

Mrs. H2B (Mrs. Hunt), b. 1885. *Father, railway carter. Mother, domestic servant before marriage; took in lodgers and sewed after marriage. Youngest of 4 children.* Dressmaker. Married, no children.

Mrs. H3B (Mrs. Hampton), b. 1887. *Father, clerk. Mother, teacher before marriage; kept embroidery shop after marriage. Eldest of 6 children.* Worked as clerk and untrained teacher. Married, no children.

Mrs. H6B (Mrs. Hetherington), b. 1948. . *Father, joiner. Mother, clerk for railway before marriage. After marriage, kept lodgers and did evening shiftwork at factory. Eldest of 3 children (1 died).* University lecturer. Married (lecturer); adopted 2 children.

Mrs. J1B (Mrs. Jenkins), b. 1932. *Father, railway laborer. Mother, cleaner, laundry worker, and bus conductress. Elder of 2 children.* Domestic servant, shop assistant, and bookkeeper; after marriage, worked as clerk. Married (joiner), 3 children.

Mr. K1B (Mr. Kirby), b. 1921. *Father, joiner in family business. Mother, shop assistant before marriage; homemaker. Only child.* Apprenticed as joiner; after work injury, worked as clerk for local council. Married (nurse), 1 child.

Mr. L2B (Mr. Langley), b. 1900. *Father, railway worker.* Initially lamp boy, later shunter on the railway. Married, 2 children.

Mrs. L2B (Mrs. Langley), b. 1900. *Father, laborer. Mother, barmaid and munitions worker. One of 6 children.* Confectioner and barmaid. Married, 2 children.

Mrs. L3B (Mrs. Lewthwaite), b. 1920. *Father, long periods of unemployment before becoming storeman in Vickers in late 1930s. Mother, domestic servant before marriage; cleaner afterwards. One of 2 children.* Worked as servant, shop assistant, munitions worker until birth of only child. Married.

Mr. L4B (Mr. Latham), b. 1931. *Father, chemist. Mother, tracer in Vickers before marriage; helped in family shop after marriage. Only child.* Informant went to university but failed degree course. Career in city government. Married, no children.

Mr. L5B (Mr. Lucas), b. 1950. *Father, blast-furnaceman; Mother, laundry-worker and seamstress (after marriage). One of three children.* Worked as draftsman and merchant seaman. Married, 1 adopted child.

Mrs. L5B (Mrs. Lucas), b. 1943. *Father, draftsman. Mother, shop assistant before marriage. One of three children.* Teacher. 1 adopted child.

Mr. M1B (Mr. Martin), b. 1892. *Father, railway laborer. Mother, domestic service before marriage. 5th of 12 children (2 died). Very poor family.* Worked for the Co-op shops. Married.

Mrs. M1B (Mrs. Martin), b. 1898. *Father, boilermaker at steelworks. Mother, domestic service before marriage. Youngest of 5 children (1 died).* Homemaker. Family prosperity and social aspirations ruined by Depression.

Mr. M2B (Mr. Middleton), b. 1898. *Father, sailor who died when informant was 3. Informant raised by mother, uncle, and grandfather.* Worked for Vickers.

Mrs. M3B (Mrs. Musgrove), b. 1886. *Parents from Ireland. Father, shipwright. Mother,*

cook before marriage; later ran a parlor shop. One of 10 children (5 died). Pupil teacher, Suffragette, active in Girl Guides and church. Married, no children.

Mr. M5B (Mr. Mitton), b. 1892. *Father, miner. Mother died when informant was a child.* Informant came to Barrow as munitions worker from Canada in 1915.

Mrs. M6B (Mrs. Mallingham), b. 1896. *Father, laborer from Scotland. Mother, dressmaker. One of 16 children (13 died).* Professional musician. Married, 1 child.

Mr. M6B (Mr. Mallingham), b. 1892. *Grew up in Tyneside. One of 12 children. Munitions worker during World War I; leader of unemployed during 1920s.* Married, 1 child.

Mr. M7B (Mr. Maines), b. 1897. *Father kept fish and chip shop. Mother worked in the jute works before marriage and in the family shop after marriage. Fourth of 12 children (2 died).* Apprenticed as a draftsman.

Mr. M8B (Mr. Most), b. 1901. *Father, commercial traveler and shop assistant. Mother, homemaker.* Rent collector. Married, 1 child.

Mrs. M10B (Mrs. Marsh), b. 1908. *Father, foreman in brass finishing shop, Vickers. Mother, dressmaker before marriage. One of 4 children.* Secretary in Vickers. Married, 1 child.

Mrs. M11B (Mrs. Marley), b. 1914. *Father killed in World War I. Mother, confectioner before marriage and Blackpool landlady after marriage. Only child.* Market trader. Married (plasterer, sailor, and clerk of works), 2 children.

Mr. M12 B (Mr. Morris), b. 1933. *Father, joiner. Mother, musician. Only child.* Worked in accounts office. Married, 2 children.

Mrs. M12B (Mrs. Morris), b. 1936. *Father, skilled factory work. Mother, tailor. One of 4 children.* Accounting machine operator. Married, 2 children.

Mr. M13B (Mr. Morton), b. 1927. *Father, fitter for railway and Vickers. Mother, mill work before and for first two years of marriage. Fourth of 6 children.* Fitter at Vickers. Secretary, Engineering Union. Married, 1 child.

Mr. M14B (Mr. Matthews), b. 1931. *Father, miner from South Wales. Mother, homemaker. Sixth of 7 children. Very poor family. Informant had rickets as a child.* Laborer. Never married.

Mrs. 01B (Mrs. Owen), b. 1916. *Father died in 1921. Stepfather, crane-driver. Mother, cook before marriage. Part-time cook and cleaner after marriage. One of 6 children (3 died).* Shop assistant before marriage (factory worker). One child.

Mr. P1B (Mr. Perkins), b. 1900. *Father, laborer. Mother, factory work before marriage. Fourth of 6 children.* Fitter and turner at Vickers. Married, 3 children.

Mrs. P2B (Mrs. Pinkerton), b. 1902. *Father, boilermaker; frequently unemployed. Mother, cook before marriage; cleaner in shipyard when widowed.* Office girl in Town Hall.

Mrs. P3B (Mrs. Parton), b. 1873. *Father, sea captain and dock-worker. Mother died when informant was a young child. Informant never went to school.* Domestic servant.

Mr. P4B (Mr. Place), b. 1899. *Father, blacksmith in Vickers. Mother (Spanish), shop assistant before marriage. Third of 5 children.*

Mr. P5B (Mr. Priestley), b. 1950. *Father, fitter. Mother, office worker. One of 2 children.* Fitter. Married, 5 children.

Mrs. P5B (Mrs. Priestley), b. 1950. *Father, skilled factory work. Mother, part-time shop assistant. One of 3 children.* Married, 5 children.

Mr. P6B (Mr. Peel), b. 1909. *Father, joiner, policeman, time clerk at Vickers. Mother, nurse before marriage. Homemaker. Youngest of 11 children.* Welder at Vickers.

Married twice (first wife died). 2 children.

Mrs. P6B (Mrs. Peel), b. 1921. *Father, postal worker. Mother, worked in pub before marriage; ran boarding house after widowed. One of 2 children.* Shop assistant, publican; married 3 times (divorced philandering first husband; second husband died). 4 children.

Mr. Q1B (Mr. Quayle), b. 1897. *Father died before informant was born. Younger of 2 children.* Apprenticed as Co-op grocer.

Mrs. R1B (Mrs. Ralston), b. 1889. *Father, captain of his own coastal vessel. Later, berthing master at harbor. Mother, weaver in jute works before marriage. Second of 6 children.* Worked at jute works before mother's death. Married, 2 children.

Mr. R3B (Mr. Rollins), b. 1931. *Father, skilled railway worker. Elder of 2 children.* Rose through ranks in Co-op shops. Married (Co-op worker), 2 children.

Mrs. R4B (Mrs. Ruthven), b. 1936. *Father, draftsman, later manager in Vickers. Mother, secretary before marriage. Only child.* Teacher. Married (teacher), 2 children.

Mr. S1B (Mr. Sage), b. 1896. *Father, stonemason. One of 5 children.* Skilled worker and union official.

Mrs. S2B (Mrs. Smith), b. 1895. *Father, laborer. Mother, took in sewing and went out nursing. One of 10 children.* Tailor. Married, 4 children.

Mrs. S3B (Mrs. Sykes), b. 1927. *Father, electrician's mate. Mother, shop assistant before marriage. One of 3 children.* Shop assistant and clerk before birth of first child. Married (skilled worker), 2 children.

Mr. S4B (Mr. Sullivan), b. 1922. *Father, railway laborer. Mother, butcher's assistant before marriage. One of 3 children.* Warehouseman and insurance agent; various jobs at Vickers. Married, no children.

Mr. T1B (Mr. Tomlinson), b. 1884. *Father, skilled work at Vickers and shopkeeper. Mother, matron in boarding school and shopkeeper. One of 5 children.* Worked for National Telephone Company.

Miss T2B (Miss Thistle), b. 1888. *Father, manager of corn mill (died, 1900). Mother, teacher before marriage; cook after widowed. One of 13 children (1 died).* Domestic servant.

Mrs. T3B (Mrs. Tinley), b. 1910. *Father, driller in Vickers. Mother went out cleaning after marriage. Elder of 2 children.* Worked in chemist's shop.

Mr. T4B (Mr. Thornbarrow), b. 1949. *Father, butcher before 1960. Then storeman in Vickers. Mother trained as nurse and helped in butcher shop. Only child.* Civil Servant. Married (librarian), no children.

Mrs. T4B (Mrs. Thornbarrow), b. 1948. *Father, shipwright. Mother, part-time shop assistant. One of 2 children.* Librarian. Married, no children.

Mr. T5B (Mr. Trickett), b. 1923. *Father, street vendor, often unemployed, deserted family in 1930. Mother took in washing and went out cleaning. One of 4 children (1 died).* Laborer in brewery, merchant seaman, laborer in Vickers. Married, no children.

Mrs. W1B (Mrs. Wilson), b. 1900. *Father, moulder. Mother worked at box factory before marriage. One of 10 children (2 died).* Servant, later shop assistant. Married, 1 child.

Mrs. W2B (Mrs. White), b. 1889. *Father, shipwright. Mother, work in family shops. One of 15 children (5 died).* Weaver in jute mills before marriage. Married, 1 child.

Mrs. W3B (Mrs. West), b. 1884. *Father, miner from Cornwall. Second of 6 children.* Domestic servant before marriage. 2 children.

Mr. W4B (Mr. Wallace), b. 1923. *Father, skilled work in cotton mill. Only child.* Lived in Barrow, 1952–70. Engineer, Naval Base; later lecturer at Technical College. Wife worked in tax office before marriage. 4 children.

Mrs. W5B (Mrs. Wheaton), b. 1933. *Father, fitter in Vickers. Younger of 2 children.* Clerk in Town Hall. Married (Water Board official). 2 children.

Mrs. W6B (Mrs. Walker), b. 1936. *Father, Co-op shop assistant and manager. Mother, domestic work before marriage. One of 2 children.* Typist before birth of first child. Married (gardener, meter collector), 2 children.

Mr. W7B (Mr. Watkinson), b. 1945. *Father, machinist in Vickers. Mother, midwife. Younger of 2 children.* Butcher's boy, fitter at Vickers, policeman after 1968. Married (nurse trainee), 2 children.

Lancaster

Mrs. A1L (Mrs. Allen), b. 1908. *Father, laborer. Mother, weaver. One of 2 children.* Weaver. Married, no children.

Mr. A2L (Mr. Ash), b. 1905. *Father, skilled worker. Mother, domestic service before marriage. Died when informant was 12. Eldest of 4 children (2 died).* Heating and ventilating engineer. Married, 1 child.

Mrs. A2L (Mrs. Ash), b. 1907. *Father, gardener. Mother, mill worker before marriage. One of 2 children.* Confectioner. Married, 1 child.

Mrs. A3L (Mrs. Atkin), b. 1944. *Father kept fish and chip shop and worked as foreman for the River Board. Mother did mill work, then farm work. Second of 3 children.* Nursery Assistant. Married (mechanical engineer, Williamson's; draftsman, Storey's), 2 children.

Mr. A4L (Mr. Adderley), b. 1926. *Father, laborer. Mother, usherette before marriage; munitions worker during World War II; sewing at home. One of 8 children.* Farm worker, military service, factory work (severely injured), sales rep for Hoover, publican. Married, 3 children.

Mrs. A4L (Mrs. Adderley), b. 1932. *Father, farm worker. Mother, mill worker before marriage. One of 2 children.* Shop assistant and clerk before marriage; after marriage, shop assistant and pub landlady. 3 children.

Dr. A5L (Dr. Armstrong), b. 1918. *Father, clerk with Scottish Oils (subsidiary of British Petroleum). Mother, homemaker.* General Practitioner who began practice in Lancaster in 1948.

Mrs. B1L (Mrs. Ball), b. 1888. *Father, mill laborer. Mother, weaver before and after marriage. One of 5 children.* Weaver. Married, 4 children.

Mr. B2L (Mr. Barnes), b. 1907. *Stepfather, railway laborer. Mother, domestic servant before marriage; went out cleaning after marriage. One of 4 children.* Mule-spinner in cotton mill.

Mr. C1L (Mr. Carson), b. 1902. *Father, fireman at mill. Also made money by gambling. Mother, cook before and occasionally after marriage. One of 3 children.* Engineer at Storey's.

Miss C2L (Miss Coyle), b. 1903. *Father, skilled work and labor activist. Mother, caretaker and sewing before marriage. One of 4 children.* Weaver.

Mr. C3L (Mr. Carrington), b. 1898. *Father, professional soldier. Youngest of 6 children.* Clerk at Storey's.

Mr. C4L (Mr. Cross), b. 1914. *Father, gardener; soldier, World War I; Co-op collector; periods of unemployment. Mother, weaver before and after marriage; went out cleaning. Only child.* Office worker at Williamsons. Married, 1 child.

Mr. C6L (Mr. Chambers), b. 1896? *Father, chemist.* Chemist with a large working-class clientele. Wife (who contributed to interview) helped in chemist's shop.

Mrs. C7L (Mrs. Critchley), b. 1926. *Father, laborer. Mother, weaver before and after marriage. One of 5 children.* Post office worker until 18 months after marriage (to policeman). 3 children.

Mrs. C8L (Mrs. Center), b. 1942. *Mother, mill worker before and after marriage.* Mill work before and after marriage; part-time cleaner. Married (mechanic), 2 children.

Mr. F1L (Mr. Fleming), b. 1917. *Orphaned young. Raised by uncle (newsagent). Eldest of 3.* Butcher. Married, 6 children.

Mrs. F1L (Mrs. Fleming), b. 1921. *Father, railway worker. Mother, domestic service before marriage. One of 4 children.* Baker, munitions worker, part-time cleaning. Married, 6 children.

Mr. F2L (Mr. Farrell), b. 1946. *Father, butcher. Mother, domestic work. One of six children.* Mechanic. Married, 3 children.

Mr. G1L (Mr. Grand), b. 1904. *Father, laborer in Williamson's. Mother, domestic service before marriage; took in washing and went out cleaning afterwards. One of 5 children.* Laborer, then professional soldier. Married, 1 child.

Mr. G2L (Mr. Gordon), b. 1879. *Father, clerk. Mother, domestic service before marriage; homemaker. Youngest of 6 children.* Joiner, who started a successful business.

Mr. G3L (Mr. Graves), b. 1937. *Father, laborer. Mother, domestic service before marriage. Later, went out cleaning and took in lodgers. One of 5 children.* Storekeeper. Married (shop assistant), 2 children.

Mr. H1L (Mr. Hardine), b. 1904. *Father, bricklayer. Mother, seamstress before marriage. Both from Ireland. Very poor family that moved 21 times, mainly in Skerton area of Lancaster. One of 2 children.* Errand boy, later bricklayer. Married, no children.

Mrs. H2 L (Mrs. Harte), b. 1889. *Father, laborer. Mother, weaver before marriage; took in lodgers afterwards. One of 11 children (3 died).* Weaver, then domestic service. Married, 3 children.

Mr. H3L (Mr. Horton), b. 1904. *Father, blacksmith, caretaker, mill handyman. Lived for a time in Canada. Mother, weaver. Second of 4 children.* Skilled and unskilled mill work. Married, 3 children.

Mrs. H3L (Mrs. Horton), b. 1903. *Father, weaver who died in 1919. Mother, domestic service before marriage; childminding, laundry, and sewing afterwards. Eighth of 10 children (3 died).* Shop work, domestic service, and mill work. Married, 3 children.

Miss H4L (Miss Herndon), b. 1883. *Father, color mixer in textile mill. Mother, weaver before and after marriage. Only child.* Weaver.

Mrs. H5L (Mrs. Howard), b. 1931. *Father, bus conductor and shop assistant. Mother, shop assistant before marriage, part-time war work (clerk), hospital work. One of 7 children.* Office and factory work until birth of first child. Married (painter and decorator), 3 children. Divorced in early 1970s.

Mrs. H6L (Mrs. Hocking), b. 1933. *Father, tailor, deserted family after World War II. Mother, proof-reader after husband left. One of 2 children.* Key-punch operator, telephonist. Homemaker after marriage (to electrician and sales rep), 3 children.

Mr. H7L (Mr. Hinchcliffe), b. 1947. *Parents divorced when he was a child. Mother married three times. Mother, mill worker before marriage; went out cleaning after marriage. Informant closer to grandmother (with whom he lived) than mother. Only child.* Plumber. Never married.

Mr. H10L (Mr. Hope), b. 1915. Lancaster chemist who began work in 1930.

Mr. I1L (Mr. Ives), b. 1902. *Father, railway fireman, boilerman at Williamson's, munitions work during World War I. Mother, dressmaker before marriage. One of 3 children.* Apprenticed as cabinetmaker at Waring and Gillow.

Mr. I2L (Mr. Ingham), b. 1930. *Father, bookmaker and café proprietor. Mother, teacher before marriage. One of 7 children,.* Electrician. Married and divorced (shorthand typist), 1 child.

Mr. J1L (Mr. James), b. 1903. *Father, warehouseman at Storey's. Mother, dressmaker before marriage; took in sewing after marriage. Younger of 2 children.*

Mr. K1L (Mr. King), b. 1907. *Father, baker. Mother, weaver, cook, and munitions worker (World War I) before marriage; later took in lodgers. One of 4 children.* Baker. Married, 2 children.

Mr. L1L (Mr. Lane), b. 1896. *Father, docker in Salford. Second of 9 children.* Informant settled in Lancaster in 1921. Soldier, later laborer, active in left wing and trade union politics. Married, 2 children.

Mrs. L2L (Mrs. Leighton), b. 1941. *Father, dental technician. Mother, shop assistant before marriage and after children started school. One of 3 children.* Office work before and after marriage (to electrician). 2 children.

Mrs. L3L (Mrs. Lonsdale), b. 1947. *Father, unknown. Mother, factory worker. Middle of 3 children (1 given up for adoption).* Factory work before and after marriage (to electrician). Divorced and remarried. 2 children.

Mr. M1L (Mr. Madison), b. 1910. *Stepfather, mill laborer. (Father deserted family during World War I.) Mother, seamstress before marriage; later sold pies made at home. One of 7 children (all step-siblings.)* Warehouseman. Married, 8 children.

Mr. M3L (Mr. Melling), b. 1906. *Father, joiner. Mother, domestic service before marriage. One of 3 children.* Joiner. Married, 2 children.

Mrs. M3L (Mrs. Melling), b. 1917. *Father, fitter and laborer. Mother died young (as did stepmother). Informant kept house for the family afterwards. Sixth of 8 children.* Married, 2 children.

Miss M4L (Miss Meade), b. 1902. *Father, shop manager. Mother, shop assistant, then buyer. Only child.* Shop assistant, then kept house for mother.

Mrs. M5L (Mrs. Milton), b. 1914. *Father, street trader when not ill. Died in 1924. Mother took in washing. Youngest of 6 or 8 children.* Weaver. Married, no children.

Mr. M8L (Mr. Moudy), b. 1926. *Father, laborer at Williamson's. Youngest of 8 children.* Office worker before military service. Later owned and operated bakers and confectioner's shop.

Mr. M9L (Mr. Miller), b. 1924. *Father, skilled factory worker. Mother, spinner before birth of first child. Second of 4 children.* Skilled factory worker. Married, no children.

Mr. M10L (Mr. Monkham), b. 1948. *Father, laborer. Mother, mill worker before marriage, part-time cleaning after children at school. Fifth of 8 children.* Office and shop worker before he became a nurse. Married (office worker), 2 children.

Mrs. N1L (Mrs. Nance), b. 1899. *Father, painter and decorator who was often unemployed and regularly deserted the family. Mother, slubber (twisting wool for spinning) before marriage; later took in washing. One of at least 9 children.* Slubber. Married, 8 children.

Mr. N2L (Mr. Norton), b. 1931. *Father, bargeman for railway. Committed suicide in 1943. Mother, homemaker and informal neighborhood health authority. One of 2 children.* Joiner, laborer, plasterer, policeman, printer. Married (fish and chip shop worker), 4 children.

Mr. N3L (Mr. Needham), b. 1921. *Father, window cleaner. Mother, mill work before marriage; café work after marriage. One of 6 children.* Laborer before and after war service. Married, 4 children.

Mrs. N3L (Mrs. Needham), b. 1919. *Father, laborer who was disabled (gassed) during World War I service. Mother, mill work before marriage. Some home laundry afterwards.* Factory work. First child born out of wedlock in workhouse. Married, 4 children.

Mrs. N4L (Mrs. Norton, elder), b. 1909. *Father, tailor born in Ireland. Guarded German prisoners during World War I.* Domestic service before marriage. Married, 2 children.

Mr. P1L (Mr. Parke), b. 1894. *Father, clerk. Mother, homemaker. One of 3 children.* Engineer. Married, 1 child.

Mrs. P1L (Mrs. Parke), b. 1898. *Father, factory foreman. Mother, homemaker. One of 5 children (1 died).* Weaver and clerk at textile mill. Married, 1 child.

Mr. P2L (Mr. Pratt), b. 1899. *Father, laborer at Williamson's. Mother, confectioner before marriage. She died in 1912. One of 9 children.* Laborer. Married, 2 children.

Mrs. P3L (Mrs. Paulson), b. 1948. *Father, laborer. Mother, factory worker before and after marriage; later went out cleaning. One of 2 children.* Office work before and after marriage (to cook). Divorced. One child.

Mr. R1L (Mr. Ritter), b. 1894. *Father, driver who died in 1897. Mother took in washing. Third of 6 children (1 died). Informant and 3 siblings grew up in Ripley Hospital (orphanage).* Builder.

Mr. R2L (Mr. Rowse), b. 1903. *Father, coachman and chauffeur. Mother, domestic servant and housekeeper. Only child.* Apprenticed as motor mechanic and drove for a laundry.

Mr. R3L (Mr. Rust), b. 1890. *Father, wood carver and turner. Mother, nurse before marriage. One of two children.* Cabinet maker. Married, 6 children.

Mrs. S1L (Mrs. Shelby), b. 1898. *Father, tinsmith. Mother, weaver before marriage. Died in childbirth. Informant raised by grandparents.* One of 2 children. Shop assistant. Married, 3 children.

Miss S2L (Miss Sellers), b. 1894. *Father, baker.* Weaver, mainly in Halifax. Came to Lancaster in 1921. Active trade unionist.

Mr. S3L (Mr. Sanderson), b. 1884. *Father, carter. Youngest of 13 children.* Apprenticed as blacksmith. Married.

Mrs. S3L (Mrs. Sanderson), b. 1892. *Father, mill laborer. Mother, weaver before mar-*

riage; childminder and laundress after marriage. Tenter and winder at mill. Married.

Mrs. S4L (Mrs. Scales), b. 1896. *Father, gravedigger. Mother, washerwoman before and after marriage. Eighth of 9 children.* Weaver. Married, 1 child.

Mrs. S5L (Mrs. Struck), b. 1897. *Father, foreman at Williamson's. Mother, dressmaker before and after marriage. One of 2 children. Prosperous upwardly mobile family until father deserted them in the 1920s.* Apprenticed as dressmaker, then worked at home.

Mrs. S6L (Mrs. Swallow), b. 1948. *Father, laborer. After marriage, mother did evening factory shift, then nursing. Sixth of 9 children.* Nurse and social worker. Married (engineer), 2 children.

Mr. S7L (Mr. Simpkins), b. 1932. *Father, newspaper seller, Died, 1938. Mother, homemaker who depended on public assistance after husband's death. Middle of 5 children (1 died).* Weaver, widow cleaner, hypnotist. Married and divorced (clerk). Second wife, a nurse. 3 children.

Mr. T1L (Mr. Turner), b. 1888. *Father, electric wirer. Mother, farm hand before marriage, washerwoman after. One of 7 children (1 died).* Painter. Married, 2 children.

Mrs. T2L (Mrs. Turnbull), b. 1932. *Father died before her birth. Stepfather, laborer. Mother, skilled mill work before and after marriage. Eldest (with twin) of 4 children.* Weaver. After marriage (soldier and laborer), home help and nursing. 4 children.

Mr. V1L (Mr. Vales), b. 1908. *Father, nurse in Moor (mental) Hospital. Mother, domestic service before marriage. Eldest of 4 children (1 died).* Joiner. Married, 2 children.

Mrs. W1L (Mrs. Wilkinson), b. 1881. *One of 12 children (4 died).* Came to Lancaster in 1895. Married in 1900 and, with her husband, kept Scotforth (south edge of Lancaster) Post Office and grocer's shop for many years.

Mrs. W2L (Mrs. Winder), b. 1910. *Father, grocer, later clerk. Mother, domestic service before marriage; took in sewing afterwards. One of 3 children.* Shop assistant. Married, 3 children.

Mr. W3L (Mr. Watkins), b. 1911. *Father, clerk at Williamson's. Mother ran family shop.* Joiner.

Mrs. W4L (Mrs. Wallington), b. 1923. *Father, painter and art shopkeeper. Mother, helped in family shop and later had her own grocery shop. During World War II, sewed for Waring and Gillow. Elder of 2 daughters.* Shop assistant, war work, secretary. In 1960, opened mixed grocery shop in the front room of her house. Married, 3 children (1 died).

Mr. W5L (Mr. Whiteside), b. 1940. *Father, fishmonger. Mother, domestic service before marriage; went out cleaning afterward. One of six children.* Factory worer. Married, 1 child.

Mrs. W5L (Mrs. Whiteside), b. 1943. *No details about parents.* After marriage, part-time cleaner and clerk. Married, 1 child.

Mr. W6L (Mr. Warwick), b. 1931. *Father, factory laborer who served in World War II. Mother, part-time mill work. Eldest of 3 children.* Electrician. Married, 2 children.

Mrs. W6L (Mrs. Warwick), b. 1937. *Father, merchant seaman. Mother, shop assistant before marriage. Sewed uniforms and packed food parcels during World War II.*

Youngest of 3 children. Shop assistant and bookkeeper before marriage. After marriage did shop work and evening work as domestic in hospital. Married, 2 children.

Mrs. Y1L (Mrs. Yardley), b. 1927. *Father, laborer before and after war service. Mother, munitions work during World War II. One of 7 children.* Factory work before and after marriage (soldier, laborer); part-time cleaning. 2 children.

Preston

Mrs. A1P (Mrs. Arnold), b. 1910. *Father, patternmaker. Mother, winder before marriage; part-time childminder afterwards. One of 5 children.* Weaver. Married (printer), no children.

Mrs. A2P (Mrs. Anston), b. 1900. *Father, domestic servant and caretaker. Mother, domestic servant. One of 10 children (8 died).* Winder, dressmaker, bookkeeper's clerk. Married, 4 children (2 died).

Miss A3P (Miss Alder), b. 1899. *Father, weaver. Mother, weaver; later childminder and washerwoman. One of 3 children (1 died).* Weaver.

Mrs. B1P (Mrs. Becker), b. 1900. *Father, skilled factory work. Mother died young. Father married 3 times, so informant had 3 half-sisters, 3 brothers and sisters, and 13 stepbrothers and sisters (9 died).* Weaver before and after marriage. Married, 4 children.

Mrs. B2P (Mrs. Black), b. 1916. *Father, laborer. Mother, skilled mill work before and after marriage. One of 2 children (1 died).* Weaver. Married, 2 children (1 died).

Miss B3P (Miss Bramley), b. 1900. *Father, baker. Mother, ring spinner; helped in family bakery shop after 1913. One of 9 children (3 died).* Weaver.

Mr. B4P (Mr. Barstow), b. 1896. *Father, factory work. Mother, poultry dresser. One of 10 children.* Bleacher. Married, no children.

Mrs. B5P (Mrs. Burton), b. 1898. *Father, docker. Mother took in washing. One of 8 children.* Weaver, laborer in shoe polish factory, and cleaner. Married, 2 children.

Mr. B8P (Mr. Brown), b. 1896. *Father, mule spinner. Married twice. One of 6 siblings and step-siblings.* Mule spinner. Married (weaver), 3 children.

Mr. B9P (Mr. Barrington), b. 1927. *Father, waiter. Mother, weaver before and after marriage. One of 2 children.* University lecturer.

Mrs. B10P (Mrs. Brayshaw), b. 1947. *Father, lorry driver and office work. Mother, bookkeeper. One of 3 children (1 stillborn).* Teacher. Married (teacher), 2 children.

Mr. B11P (Mr. Boyle), b. 1937. *Father, laborer. Stepfather, laborer. Mother, cleaner and factory worker. Lived with non-relatives for several years due to family poverty. One of 12 children (4 died).* Laborer, frequently unemployed. Married, 5 children.

Mrs. B11P (Mrs. Boyle), b. 1936. *Father, riveter on docks, then factory work. Mother, factory work before marriage; when youngest child was 3, factory cleaner. Second of 6 children.* Factory work before first child was born; later, childminding and sewing at home. Married, 5 children.

Mr. C1P (Mr. Cranston), b. 1884. *Father, railway worker from Isle of Man. Mother, weaver before marriage. One of 6 children (2 died).* Weaver. Married (weaver), no children.

Mrs. C2P (Mrs. Champion), b. 1899. *Father, tailor. Mother, tailor's machinist before*

marriage; afterwards, took in sewing. One of 3 children. Weaver. Married (farmer), 2 children.

Mrs. C3P (Mrs. Crest), b. 1897. *Born out of wedlock. Mother, weaver. Only child.* Shop assistant and commercial traveler. Married (craftsman), 1 child (died).

Miss C4P (Miss Cheswick), b. 1879. *Father, Manchester doctor.* Teaching nun, Preston, beginning in 1912.

Mr. C7P (Mr. Clay), b. 1892, Liverpool. Shopkeeper and insurance agent in Preston, 1920–1940. Married (part-time handicraft teacher), 3 children.

Mr. C8P (Mr. Christy), b. 1928. *Father (Mr. C7P), shopkeeper, insurance agent, war service, clerk. Mother, part-time teacher. One of 3 children.* Chemist. Married (laboratory assistant), 3 children.

Mrs. C8P (Mrs. Christy), b. 1939. *Father, laboratory assistant (unemployed after 1955). Mother, factory work before marriage; later, part-time domestic work. One of 5 children.* Laboratory technician. Married (analytical chemist), 3 children.

Mrs. D1P (Mrs. Dent), b. 1908. *Father, laborer. Mother, weaver; later, washerwoman. Only child.* Shop assistant; factory work. Married (husband died after one year of marriage), 1 child.

Mr. D2P (Mr. Danner), b. 1910. *Father, soldier from London. Mother, domestic service before marriage; took in sewing and cleaned afterward. One of 9 children (2 died).* Cabinetmaker and clerk. Married (teacher), 3 children.

Mrs. D3P (Mrs. Dorrington), b. 1905 in Wigan. *Father, miner; stepfather, paper deliverer and knocker-up from Preston. Mother, tailor before marriage; later, worked on munitions and took in lodgers. One of 2 children.* Factory work; after marriage, kept pubs with husband. 6 children.

Mr. E1P (Mr. Eckley), b. 1895. *Father, pub keeper and fish hawker. Died when informant was very young. Mother, mill work before marriage; kept pub later. Also died when informant was a child. One of 4 children.* Weaver, spinner, World War I service, hotel porter. Married (weaver before birth of first child), 2 children.

Mrs. E2P (Mrs. Emery), b. 1937. *Father, factory work. Mother, weaver before informant was born. Only child.* Factory and mill-worker before and after marriage (laborer). 2 children.

Mr. F1P (Mr. Ford), b. 1906. *Father, miner in Cumbria. Munitions worker, World War I. Poultry dresser in Preston. Mother, domestic service before marriage; took in washing afterwards. One of 5 children.* Electrician; unemployed 1926–8. Married (weaver), 1 child.

Mr. F2P (Mr. Flowers), b. 1909. *Father, soldier; later docker. Mother died at informant's birth. Informant raised by aunt and uncle. One of 2 children (1 died).* Various jobs, beginning as errand-boy and ending as area manager for large firm. Married, 2 children.

Mr. G1P (Mr. Grove), b. 1903. *Father, mill work. Mother, weaver. One of 8 children (2 died).* Weaver. Married (weaver), 5 children (1 died).

Mr. G2P (Mr. Gridley), b. 1903. *Father, blacksmith. Mother, mill worker before marriage. One of 4 children.* Blacksmith. Married, 2 children.

Mr. G3P (Mr. Glover), b. 1913. *Father, engineer. Mother, weaver before marriage; childminder afterwards. One of 4 children (1 died).* Mill worker. Married (weaver), 2 children.

Mr. G4P (Mr. Gardner), b. 1895. *Father, publican. Mother, weaver; later helped in pub. One of 4 children (1 died).* Weaver, later tackler (skilled mill work). Married

(weaver), 1 child.

Mrs. G5P (Mrs. Gerard), b. 1958. *Father, laborer. Mother, mill worker before marriage; later, childminding and sewing at home. One of 5 children.* Factory work before marriage (work study engineer, shopkeeper); cleaner afterwards. 3 children.

Mr. G6P (Mr. Goodwin), b. 1945. *Father, warehouse manager of cotton mill made redundant at age 54. Then factory laborer. Mother, weaver before marriage; afterwards, school dinner lady. Fourth of 5 children (1 died).* Clerk, printer. Unmarried.

Mr. G7P (Mr. Goodwin), b. 1941. Brother of Mr. G6P. *Third of 5 children (1 died).* Engineer. Married, 2 children.

Mrs. G7P (Mrs. Goodwin), b. 1944. *Father, Co-op shop assistant and manager. Mother, Co-op shop assistant; worked for Milk Marketing Board during World War II. Younger of 2 children.* Comptometer operator until birth of first child. Married, 2 children.

Mrs. H1P (Mrs. Hampton), b. 1911. *Father, publican. Mother helped in pub. One of 15 children (5 died.)* Weaver. Married, 3 children.

Mrs. H2P (Mrs. Howe), b., 1898. *Father, spinner and mule minder. Mother, weaver (until husband promoted). One of 3 children.* Weaver. Married (blacksmith and soldier), 1 child.

Mr. H3P (Mr. Hunter), b. 1928. *Father, factory worker, soldier, and professional football referee. Mother, factory work before marriage. Only child.* Teacher. Married (secretary), 1 child.

Mrs. H3P (Mrs. Hunter), b. 1931. Daughter of Mrs. B5P. *Father, laborer. Mother, weaver before marriage. Afterward, laborer in shoe polish factory and cleaner. One of 2 children (1 died).* Married, 1 child.

Mrs. H4P (Mrs. Havelock), b. 1903. *Father, fitter; frequently unemployed. Mother, weaver before marriage; afterward, intermittently weaver, cleaner, laundress. One of 10 children (2 died).* Weaver, domestic service. Married (laborer), 2 adopted children.

Mr. H6P (Mr. Hughes), b. 1896. *Father, blacksmith. Mother, weaver before marriage; helped on market stall afterwards. One of 6 children (2 died).* Weaver, soldier (World War I), miner. Married (weaver), 4 children (1 died).

Mrs. H7P (Mrs. Huddleston), b. 1916. *Father, railing maker and engine driver. Mother, mill worker. One of 6 children (3 died).* Weaver. Married (soldier), no children.

Mrs. H8P (Mrs. Hill), b. 1903. *Father, clogger. Mother, mill worker before marriage; childminder afterwards. One of 12 children (4 died).* Weaver. Married, 1 child.

Mrs. H9P (Mrs. Harrison), b. 1945. *Father, market gardener and laborer. Mother, weaver before marriage; afterwards, helped in market garden and shop assistant. One of 2 children.* Teacher, Married (teacher), no children.

Mrs. J1P (Mrs. Jelks), b. 1911. *Father, factory worker from London. After marriage, worked in wife's family's post office. Mother, ran post office. One of 4 children.* Post office work. Married (sailor, later helped in post office), 2 children.

Dr. K1P (Dr. Kuppersmith), b. 1900. General Practitioner in very poor area of Preston between 1928 and 1978.

Mr. K2P (Mr. Kennedy), b. 1930. *Father, docker. Mother, domestic service after marriage. Munitions work, 1939–67. Middle of 3 children.* Trawlerman, docker. Married (spinner before marriage; later part-time mail-order warehouse work), 6 children.

Mrs. K2P (Mrs. Kennedy), b. 1936. *Father, docker; soldier during World War II. Mother, weaver; munitions work during World War I. One of 8 children.* Spinner before marriage. Factory work from mid-1970s. Married, 6 children.

Mr. L1P (Mr. Lincoln), b. 1894. *Father, carter; casual work after injured. Family on poor relief; father broke stones at the workhouse. One of 12 children (1 died).* Weaver, soldier (World War I), loom-sweeper, munitions work (World War II). Married (weaver), 2 children.

Mrs. L1P (Mrs. Lincoln), b. 1900. *Father, carter. Mother took in washing, did midwifery and laying out after marriage. One of 10 children (1 died).* Weaver. Married, 2 children.

Mr. L3P (Mr. Lodge), b. 1919. *Father, mill worker. Mother, weaver and cleaner. One of 2 children.* War service, laborer, docker. Married, 4 children.

Mrs. L3P (Mrs. Lodge), b. 1922. *Mother, carder, part-time bookie's runner. One of 2 children.* Worked in lamp factory and went out cleaning. Married, 4 children.

Mrs. M1P (Mrs. Masterson), b. 1913. *Father, fitter and turner, died 1922. Mother, weaver before marriage; some childminding afterwards. One of 6 children (1 died).* Mill work. Married (airman killed in 1944), 2 children (1 died).

Mr. M2P (Mr. Malvern), b. 1901. *Father, crane driver at docks. Mother, weaver. One of 4 children.* Furniture builder, docker. Married, 2 children.

Mrs. M3P (Mrs. Maxwell), b. 1898. *Father, dock-worker. Mother, dressmaker before marriage; afterwards, went out cleaning. One of 7 children (4 died).* Weaver and factory worker; after marriage, went out cleaning. Married (weaver, soldier, warehouseman, factory worker, frequently unemployed 1926–32), 5 children.

Mrs. M6P (Mrs. Meadows), b. 1904. *Father, docker. Mother, weaver. One of 5 children (1 died).* Weaver. Married, no children.

Mr. M7P (Mr. Muldoon), born in Ireland, 1922. *Father, farmer. Mother helped on farm. One of 10 children.* Came to Preston at age 18. Docker. Married (school cleaner), 3 children.

Mrs. O1P (Mrs. Oxley), b. 1902. *Father, weaver. Mother, dressmaker. One of 11 children (2 died).* Weaver, piano teacher. Married (shop assistant), 4 children.

Mrs. P1P (Mrs. Peterson), b. 1899. *Father, blacksmith who left family when informant was very young. Mother, unskilled mill worker before marriage; hawker afterwards. One of 5 children (1 died).* Weaver and part-time cleaner. Married (laborer), 6 children (2 died).

Mrs. P2P (Mrs. Preston), b. 1907. *Father, skilled mill worker. Mother, weaver before marriage; shop-keeper afterwards. One of 6 children (2 died).* Weaver, factory worker, shop-keeper. Married (helped in family shop), 1 child.

Mr. R1P (Mr. Rowlandson), b. 1944. *Father, Co-op shop assistant, later manager. Mother, weaver before marriage; part-time cleaner and factory work afterwards. Only child.* Engineer. Married, 1 child.

Mrs. R1P (Mrs. Rowlandson), b. 1945. *Father, riveter. Mother, cook before marriage; childminder afterwards. One of 3 children.* Factory worker until birth of daughter. Married.

Mr. R3P (Mr. Read), b. 1931. *Father, caretaker for church and Sunday School. Mother, dressmaker at home. Elder of 2 children.* Factory worker, driver. Married, 3 children (1 died).

Mrs. R3P (Mrs. Read), b. 1927. *Father, laborer. Mother, weaver before marriage. One of*

4 children (1 died). Baker; weaver until first child was born. Married, 3 children (1 died).

Mr. S1P (Mr. Short), b. 1900. *Father, carter. Mother, domestic service before marriage; went out cleaning afterwards. One of 4 children.* Weaver, railwayman, soldier, laborer. Married (weaver), no children.

Mrs. S2P (Mrs. Strong), b. 1897. *Father, farmer (Ireland).* Farm servant. Married (laborer), 1 child.

Mrs. S3P (Mrs. Shirley), b. 1892. *Father, mill worker. Mother, weaver until there were too many children. One of at least 8 children (at least 2 died).* Ring spinner, Married (soldier killed in World War I 4 weeks after marriage). No children.

Mr. S4P (Mr. Southwort), b. 1915. *Father, patternmaker. Mother, machinist and teacher before marriage. One of 2 children (1 died).* Teacher. Married, 3 children.

Mrs. S5P (Mrs. Steele), b. 1898. *Father, blacksmith. Mother, ring spinner until third child was born. One of 10 children (2 died).* Weaver. Married (plasterer), no children.

Mrs. S7P (Mrs. Simpson), b. 1914. *Father, mill worker. Mother, weaver. One of 2 children.* Tailor. Married, 1 child.

Mr. S9P (Mr. Stephenson), b. 1925. *Youngest of 12 children. Orphaned young. Brought up by aunt and uncle. Uncle worked in family business.* Merchant seaman, engineer. Married (factory worker), 4 children.

Mr. T1P (Mr. Townley), b. 1897. *Father, docker. Mother, mill worker before marriage; later, kept a sweet shop. One of 17 children (4 died).* Weaver, loom sweeper, soldier, tram conductor, laborer; frequently unemployed. Married 3 times, 3 children (1 illegitimate, 2 died).

Mr. T2P (Mr. Thomas), b. 1903. *Father, laborer, soldier. Mother, weaver. One of 7 children (4 died).* Mill work, munitions work, railway driver. Married (factory worker), 1 child.

Mr. T3P (Mr. Tasker), b. 1886. *Father, farm laborer. Mother, mill work before marriage; washerwoman afterwards. One of 7 children (3 died).* Spinner, shuttlemaker, insurance collector. Married (spinner), 3 children (1 died).

Miss T4P (Miss Thompson), b. 1912. *Father, mill laborer. Mother, weaver. One of 5 children (1 died).* Weaver. No children.

Mrs. T5P (Mrs. Turner), b. 1905. *Father, skilled mill worker. Mother, weaver before marriage. Seventh of 10 children (1 died).* Weaver. Married, 2 children.

Mrs. W1P (Mrs. Warton), b. 1899. *Father, stoker in gas works. Mother, weaver before marriage. Died in 1906. One of 9 children (1 died).* Weaver, ring spinner. Married (factory worker, soldier, caretaker), 2 children.

Mrs. W4P (Mrs. Washburn), b. 1900. *Father, bricklayer who died when informant was one year old. Mother, barmaid before marriage; after widowed, kept a shop and took in lodgers. One of 10 children (2 died).* Weaver. Married (driver, deliveryman), 1 child.

Mr. W6P (Mr. Woods), b. 1887. *Father, itinerant preacher and baptizer, who died in 1891. Stepfather, soldier, farmer, dockworker, fireman. Mother, domestic servant; after marriage, kept a small shop.* Nurseryman. Unmarried, no children.

Mr. W7P (Mr. Whitaker), b. 1940. *Father, soldier. Mother, mill and munitions work. One of 2 children (1 died). Raised by grandparents.* Factory work. Married (factory worker and civil servant), no children.

Mr. W8P (Mr. Wheeler), b. 1949. *Son of Polish immigrants. Father, factory worker and*

self-employed photographer. Mother, factory worker. Elder of 2 children. Apprenticed as fitter. Married, no children.

Mr. Y1P (Mr. Young), b. 1948. *Father, mill worker. Mother, nurse and mill worker. Youngest of 3 children.* Began university. Computer programmer, laborer, frequently unemployed. Unmarried, no children.

Mrs. Y2P (Mrs. Young), b. 1915. Mother of Mr. Y1P. *Father, mill worker, served in World War I. Mother, weaver. One of 5 children. This informant spent much of her childhood in New England before returning to Preston in her early teens.* Mill worker, trained nurse. Married (construction worker), 3 children.

Bibliography

_≈

Primary Sources

Transcripts of 239 life history interviews conducted between 1974 and 1989 with working-class residents of Barrow, Lancaster, and Preston by Elizabeth Roberts (Administrator and later Director of the Centre for North-West Regional Studies, Lancaster University, United Kingdom) and Lucinda McCray Beier. Tapes and transcripts of these interviews are housed by the Elizabeth Roberts Oral History Archive, Lancaster University, United Kingdom. Footnote references to transcripts appear by the informant's code number and transcript page number. Barrow informants are indicated by the suffix "B," Lancaster informants by the suffix "L," and Preston informants by the suffix "P." Informants were promised confidentiality; thus, aliases are used in the text. Some of these aliases are the same as those appearing in Roberts's books, *A woman's place: An oral history of working-class women 1890–1940* (Oxford: Basil Blackwell, 1984) and *Women and families: An oral history, 1940–1970* (Oxford: Basil Blackwell, 1995). Others were created for this volume.

Reports of the Medical Officers of Health for Barrow (1883–1970), Lancaster (1907–1970), and Preston (1889–1970). These reports were given a variety of titles by the officials who wrote them. In footnotes, they are referred to as "[City Name] MOH Report, [Year of Report], [Page Number]."

Additional Primary Sources

The Black Report: The health divide. New York: Penguin, 1988.

Davis, M. B. *Hygiene and health education for colleges of education.* Eleven editions published by Longmans between 1932 and 1967.

Dickens, Charles. *Martin Chuzzlewit.* Harmondsworth: Penguin, 1968. First published in 1843–44.

Health in schools and workshops. London: Ward, Lock, & Co., 1888.

Hill, Charles, Lord Hill of Luton. *Both sides of the Hill.* London: Heinemann, 1964.

————. *Good health, children! By the Radio Doctor.* London: Sir Isaac Pitman and Sons, 1944.

————. *The Radio Doctor, Bringing up your child.* London: Phoenix House, 1950.

————. *The Radio Doctor. Your body: How it works and how to keep it working well.* London: Burke Publishing Co., 1944.

————. *Wednesday morning early or A little of what you fancy, by the Radio Doctor.* London, New York, and Melbourne: Hutchinson and Co. (no dates given, although suggestion is during WWII) [1944, National Library of Medicine Catalog].

Newsholme, Arthur. *School hygiene: The laws of health in relation to school life.* Boston: D. C. Heath and Co., 1904.

"The Royal Infirmary, Preston." (1936). Film #104, North West Film Archive.

Spring Rice, Margery, *Working-class wives: Their health and conditions.* 2nd. ed. London: Virago, 1981. First published in 1939.

"Tuberculosis Sanatorium at Ulverston." 1926. Film #163, North West Film Archive.

The Women's Co-operative Guild. *Maternity: Letters from working-women.* New York and London: Garland Publishing, Inc., 1980. Reprint of the 1915 ed. published by G. Bell.

Woman's Weekly. Selected issues 1911–70.

Secondary Sources

Abel, Emily K. *Hearts of wisdom: American women caring for kin.* Cambridge, MA: Harvard University Press, 2000.

Abel-Smith, Brian. *A History of the nursing profession.* London: Heinemann, 1960.

————. *The hospitals 1800–1948: A study in social administration in England and Wales.* Cambridge, MA: Harvard University Press, 1964.

Aldgate, Anthony and Jeffrey Richards. *Best of British: Cinema and society from 1930 to the present.* 2nd ed. London and New York: I. B. Tauris, 1999.

Anderson, Michael. *Family structure in nineteenth century Lancashire.* Cambridge: Cambridge University Press, 1971.

Anderson, Stuart. "'I remember it well': Oral history in the history of pharmacy." *Social History of Medicine* 10:2 (1997): 331–43.

———— and Virginia Berridge. "Opium in 20th-century Britain: Pharmacists, regulation and the people." *Addiction* 95:1 (2000): 23–36.

———— and Virginia Berridge. "The role of the community pharmacist in health and welfare, 1911–1986." In Joanna Bornat, Robert Perks, Paul Thompson, and Jan Walmsley, eds., *Oral history, health and welfare.* London and New York: Routledge, 2000. 48–74.

Armstrong, David. *Political anatomy of the body: Medical knowledge in Britain in the twentieth century.* Cambridge: Cambridge University Press, 1983.

Arnold, David. *Colonizing the body: State medicine and epidemic disease in nineteenth-century India.* Berkeley: University of California Press, 1993.

Ballaster, Ros, Margaret Beetham, Elizabeth Frazer, and Sandra Hebron. *Women's worlds: Ideology, femininity and the woman's magazine.* Houndmills and London: Macmillan Education, 1991.

Barrell, Joan and Brian Braithwaite. *The business of women's magazines.* London: Kogan Page, 1979.

Beetham, Margaret. *A magazine of her own? Domesticity and desire in the woman's magazine, 1800–1914.* London and New York: Routledge, 1996.

Behlmer, George K. *Friends of the family: The English home and its guardians, 1850–1940.* Stanford: Stanford University Press, 1998.

Beier, Lucinda McCray. "Contagion, policy, class, gender, and mid-twentieth-century Lancashire working-class health culture." *Hygiea International* 2:1 (2001): 7–24.

———. "Experience and experiment: Robert Hooke, illness and medicine." In Michael Hunter and Simon Schaffer, eds., *Robert Hooke: New studies.* Woodbridge, Suffolk: The Boydell Press, 1989. 235–52.

———. "Expertise and control: Childbearing in three twentieth-century working-class Lancashire communities." *Bulletin of the History of Medicine* 78:2 (2004): 379–409.

———. "The good death in seventeenth-century England." In Ralph Houlbrooke, ed., *Death, ritual and bereavement.* London: Routledge, 1989. 43–61.

———. "'I used to take her to the doctor's and get the *proper* thing': Twentieth-century health care choices in Lancashire working-class communities." In Michael H. Shirley and Todd E. A. Larson, eds., *Splendidly Victorian: Essays in nineteenth- and twentieth-century British history in honor of Walter L. Arnstein.* Aldershot: Ashgate Press, 2001. 331–41.

———. "In sickness and in health: The Josselins' experience." In Roy Porter, ed. *Patients and practitioners: Lay perceptions of medicine in pre-industrial society.* Cambridge: Cambridge University Press, 1985. 101–28.

———. "My twelve years in the UK health system." *Health Affairs* 19:3 (2000): 185–90.

———. "Seventeenth-century English surgery: The casebook of Joseph Binns." In Christopher Lawrence, ed., *Medical theory, surgical practice: Studies in the history of surgery.* London: Routledge, 1992. 48–84.

———. *Sufferers and healers: The experience of illness in seventeenth-century England.* Routledge and Kegan Paul, 1987.

———. "'We were green as grass: Learning about sex and reproduction in three working-class Lancashire communities, 1900–1970." *Social History of Medicine* 16:3 (2003): 461–80.

Benson, John. *The rise of consumer society in Britain 1880–1980.* London and New York: Longman, 1994.

Berridge, Virginia. *Health and society in Britain since 1939.* Cambridge: Cambridge University Press, 1999.

———, Mark Harrison, and Paul Weindling. "The impact of war and depression, 1918 to 1948." In Charles Webster, ed., *Caring for health: History and diversity.* Milton Keynes: Open University Press, 1993.

Blacktop, John G. *In times of need: The history and origin of the Royal Lancaster Infirmary.* No publisher, no date. Available at the Lancaster Public Library.

Boon, Timothy Martyn. "Films and the contestation of public health in interwar Britain." Unpublished PhD Dissertation. London University, 1999.

Bornat, Joanna, Robert Perks, Paul Thompson, and Jan Walmsley, eds. *Oral history, health and welfare.* London and New York: Routledge, 2000.

Bourke, Joanna. *Working-class cultures in Britain 1890–1960: Gender, class and ethnicity.* London and New York: Routledge, 1994.

Bradshaw, Ann. *The Nurse Apprentice, 1860–1977.* Aldersthot: Ashgate, 2001.

Briggs, Asa. *The BBC: The first fifty years.* Oxford and New York: Oxford University Press, 1985.

Brookes, Barbara. *Abortion in England 1900–1967.* London, New York, and Sydney: Croom Helm, 1988.

Bryder, Linda. *Below the magic mountain: A social history of tuberculosis in twentieth-century Britain.* Oxford and New York: Clarendon Press, 1988.

Burnett, John. *A social history of housing 1815–1985.* 2nd ed. London and New York: Methuen, 1986. First published in 1978.

Bussey, Gordon. *Wireless, the crucial decade: History of the British wireless industry 1924–34.* London: Peter Peregrinus, 1990.

Cartwright, Ann. *Parents and family planning services.* New York: Atherton Press, 1970.

Chinn, Carl. *Poverty amidst prosperity: The urban poor in England, 1834–1914.* Manchester and New York: Manchester University Press, 1995.

Chippendale, John H., Andrew L. Paton, and Sandy Clark. *100 years of the Dalton Square Practice.* Lancaster: Privately published, 2003.

Constantine, Steven and Alan Warde. "Challenge and change in the twentieth century." In Andrew White, ed., *A history of Lancaster 1193–1993.* Keele, Staffordshire: Ryburn Publishing, Keele University Press, 1993. 199–243.

Cooter, Roger, ed. *In the name of the child: Health and welfare, 1880–1940.* London and New York: Routledge, 1992.

Cooter, Roger and Bill Luckin, eds. *Accidents in history: Injuries, fatalities and social relations.* Amsterdan and Atlanta, GA: Rodopi, 1997.

Cornwell, Jocelyn. *Hard-earned lives: Accounts of health and illness from East London.* London: Tavistock, 1984.

Creighton, Charles. *History of epidemics in Britain.* Cambridge: Cambridge University Press, 1891.

Davies, Andrew. *Leisure, gender and poverty: Working-class culture in Salford and Manchester, 1900–1939.* Buckingham and Philadelphia: Open University Press, 1992.

———. "Leisure in the 'classic slum.'" In Andrew Davies and Steven Fielding, eds., *Workers' worlds: Cultures and communities in Manchester and Salford, 1880–1939.* Manchester and New York: Manchester University Press, 1992. 102–32.

Davies, Celia, ed. *Rewriting nursing history.* London: Croom Helm, 1980.

Davies, Celia. "The health visitor as mother's friend: A woman's place in public health, 1900–14." *Social History of Medicine* 1:1 (1988): 39–59.

———. "The sociology of professions and the profession of gender." *Sociology* 30:4 (1996): 661–78.

Davin, Anna. "Imperialism and motherhood." *History Workshop* 5 (1978): 9–65.

Digby, Ann. *British welfare policy: Workhouse to workfare.* London and Boston: Faber and Faber, 1989.

———. *The evolution of British general practice 1850–1948.* Oxford: Oxford University Press, 1999.

Dingwall, Robert, Anne Marie Rafferty, and Charles Webster. *A social history of nursing.* London: Routledge, 1988.

Donnison, Jean. *Midwives and medical men: A history of inter-professional rivalries and women's rights.* New York: Schocken, 1977.

Donzelot, Jacques. *The policing of families.* New York: Pantheon Books, 1979.

Durbach, Nadja. *Bodily matters: The anti-vaccination movement in England, 1853–1907.* Durham: Duke University Press, 2005.

———. "'They might as well brand us': Working-class resistance to compulsory vaccination in Victorian England." *Social History of Medicine* 13:1 (2000): 45–62.

Dwork, Deborah. *War is good for babies and other young children: A history of the infant and child welfare movement in England 1898–1918.* London and New York: Tavistock Publications, 1987.

Dyhouse, Carole. *Girls growing up in late Victorian and Edwardian England.* London: Routledge and Kegan Paul, 1981.

———. "Working-class mothers and infant mortality in England, 1895–1914." *Journal of Social History* 12:2 (1978): 248–67.

Englander, David. *Landlord and tenant in urban Britain 1838–1918.* Oxford: Clarendon Press, 1983.

Evans, David. "Tackling the 'hideous scourge': The creation of the venereal disease treatment centres in early twentieth-century Britain." *Social History of Medicine* 5:3 (1992): 413–33.

Evenden, Doreen. *The midwives of seventeenth-century London.* Cambridge: Cambridge University Press, 2000.

Fisher, Kate. "'She was quite satisfied with the arrangements I made': Gender and birth control in Britain 1920–1950." *Past and Present* 169 (2000): 161–93.

Forsyth, Gordon and Robert F. L. Logan. *The demand for medical care: A study of the case-load in the Barrow and Furness Group of Hospitals.* London, New York, and Toronto: Published for the Nuffield Provincial Hospital Trust by the Oxford University Press, 1960.

Foucault, Michel. *Discipline and punish: The birth of the prison.* New York: Vintage Books, 1979.

———. *The history of sexuality.* New York: Vintage, 1978.

Fowler, David. "Teenage consumers? Young wage-earners and leisure in Manchester, 1919–1939." In Andrew Davies and Steven Fielding, eds., *Workers' worlds: Cultures and communities in Manchester and Salford, 1880–1939.* Manchester and New York: Manchester University Press, 1992. 133–55.

Fox, Enid. "Powers of life and death: Aspects of maternal welfare in England and Wales between the wars." *Medical History* 35 (1991): 328–52.

Giles, Judy. *Women, identity and private life in Britain, 1900–50.* New York: St. Martin's Press, 1995.

Gittins, Diana. *Fair sex: Family size and structure in Britain, 1900–39.* New York: St. Martin's Press, 1982.

Gooderson, Philip J. *Lord Linoleum: Lord Ashton, Lancaster and the rise of the British oilcloth and linoleum industry.* Keele: Keele University Press, 1996.

Gramsci, Antonio. *Selections from the prison notebooks.* Quentin Hoare and Geoffrey Nowell Smith, eds. New York: International Publishers, 2003.

Grant, Mariel. *Propaganda and the role of the state in inter-war Britain.* Oxford: Clarendon Press, 1994.

Green, David G. *Working-class patients and the medical establishment: Self-help in Brit-*

ain from the mid-nineteenth century to 1948. New York: St. Martin's Press, 1985.

Griffiths, Trevor. *The Lancashire working classes c. 1880–1930.* Oxford: Clarendon Press, 2001.

Hall, Lesley A. *Sex, gender, and social change in Britain since 1880.* New York: St. Martin's Press, 2000.

———. "Venereal diseases and society in Britain, from the Contagious Diseases Acts to the National Health Service." In Roger Davidson and Lesley A. Hall, eds., *Sex, sin and suffering: Venereal disease and European society since 1870.* London and New York: Routledge, 2001. 120–36.

Hardy, Anne. *The epidemic streets: Infectious disease and the rise of preventive medicine, 1856–1900.* Oxford: Clarendon Press, 1993.

———. *Health and medicine in Britain since 1860.* Houndmills, Basingstoke, Hampshire: Palgrave, 2001.

———. "Tracheotomy versus intubation: Surgical intervention in diphtheria in Europe and the United States, 1825–1930." *Bulletin of the History of Medicine* 66 (1992): 536–59.

Harris, Bernard. *The health of the schoolchild: A history of the school medical service in England and Wales.* Buckingham and Philadelphia: Open University Press, 1995.

Hewitt, Margaret. *Wives and mothers in Victorian industry.* London: Rockliff, 1958.

Higgenbotham, Peter. "The Workhouse." http://users.ox.ac.uk/~peter/workhouse /index.html (accessed 12/5/05).

Hodgkinson, Ruth G. *The origins of the National Health Service: The medical services of the New Poor Law, 1834–1871.* Berkeley and Los Angeles: University of California Press, 1967.

Horden, Peregrine and Richard Smith, eds. *The locus of care: Families, communities, institutions, and the provision of welfare since antiquity.* London and New York: Routledge, 1998.

Humphries, Steve. *A secret world of sex: Forbidden fruit: the British experience 1900–1950.* London: Sidgwick and Jackson, 1988.

Hunt, David. *A history of Preston.* Preston: Carnegie Publishing, 1992.

Hurt, J. S. *Elementary schooling and the working classes 1860–1918.* London: Routledge and Kegan Paul, 1979.

Jackson, Louise. *Child sexual abuse in Victorian England.* London and New York: Routledge, 2000.

Jeffreys, Margot. "General practitioners and the other caring professions." In Irvine Loudon, John Horder, and Charles Webster, eds., *General practice under the National Health Service 1948–1997.* London: Clarendon Press, 1998. 128–45.

Jones, Greta. *Social hygiene in twentieth century Britain.* London: Croom Helm, 1986.

Jones, Helen. *Health and society in twentieth-century Britain.* London and New York: Longman, 1994.

Joyce, Patrick. *Visions of the people: Industrial England and the question of class, 1848–1914.* Cambridge: Cambridge University Press, 1991; paperback edition, 1994.

Karpf, Ann. *Doctoring the media: The reporting of health and medicine.* London: Routledge, 1988.

Kearns, Gerry and Charles W. J. Withers. "Introduction: Class, community, and the processes of urbanisation." In Gerry Kearns and Charles W. J. Withers, eds., *Urbanising Britain: Essays on class and community in the nineteenth century.* Cambridge: Cambridge University Press, 1991. 1–11.

Keown, John. *Abortion, doctors and the law: Some aspects of the legal regulation of abortion in England from 1803 to 1982.* Cambridge: Cambridge University Press, 1988.

Langhamer, Claire. *Women's leisure in England 1920–60.* Manchester and New York: Manchester University Press, 2000.

Laws, Sophie. *Issues of blood: The politics of menstruation.* Basingstoke: Macmillan, 1990.

Leap, Nicky and Billie Hunter, eds. *The midwife's tale: An oral history from handywoman to professional midwife.* London: Scarlet Press, 1993.

Leathard, Audrey. *The fight for family planning: The development of family planning services in Britain 1921–74.* London and Basingstoke: Macmillan, 1980.

Leavitt, Judith Walzer. *Brought to bed: Child-bearing in America, 1750–1950.* Oxford: Oxford University Press, 1986.

Lederer, Susan E. and Naomi Rogers. "Media." In Roger Cooter and John Pickstone, eds., *Medicine in the twentieth century.* Amsterdam: Harwood Academic Publishers, 2000. 487–502.

Levine-Clark, Marjorie. *Beyond the reproductive body: The politics of women's health and work in early Victorian England.* Columbus: The Ohio State University Press, 2004.

Lewis, Jane. *The politics of motherhood: Child and maternal welfare in England, 1900–1930.* London: Croom Helm, 1980.

———. *What price community medicine: The philosophy, practice and politics of public health since 1919.* Brighton, Sussex: Wheatsheaf Books, 1986.

Loudon, Irvine. "On maternal and infant mortality 1900–1960." *Social History of Medicine* 4:1 (1991): 29–74.

Marks, Lara. *Model mothers: Jewish mothers and maternity provision in East London, 1870–1939.* Oxford: Clarendon Press, 1994.

———. "Mothers, babies and hospitals: 'The London' and the provision of maternity care in East London, 1870–1939." In Valerie Fildes, Lara Marks, and Hilary Marland, eds., *Women and children first: International maternal and infant welfare 1870–1945.* London and New York: Routledge, 1992. 48–73.

Marland, Hilary and Anne Marie Rafferty, eds. *Midwives, society and childbirth: Debates and controversies in the modern period.* London and New York: Routledge, 1997.

Marshall, J. D. *Furness and the Industrial Revolution: An economic history of Furness (1711–1900) and the town of Barrow (1757–1897) with an epilogue.* Barrow-in-Furness: Barrow-in-Furness Library and Museum Committee, 1958.

Mayne, Alan. *The imagined slum: Newspaper representation in three cities 1870–1914.* Leicester, London, and New York: Leicester University Press, 1993.

McKeown, Thomas and R. G. Record. "Reasons for the decline of mortality in England and Wales during the nineteenth century." *Population Studies* 16:2 (1962): 94–122.

Meacham, Standish. *A life apart: The English working class 1890–1914.* London: Thames and Hudson, 1977.

Melosh, Barbara. *"The Physician's Hand": Work Culture and Conflict in American Nursing.* Philadelphia: Temple University Press, 1982.

Midwinter, E. C. *Social administration in Lancashire 1830–1860.* Manchester: Manchester University Press, 1969.

Mooney, Graham. "Public health versus private practice: The contested development of compulsory infectious disease notification in late-nineteenth-century Britain." *Bulletin of the History of Medicine* 73:2 (1999): 238–67.

Morgan, Nigel. *Deadly dwellings: Housing and health in a Lancashire cotton town. Preston from 1840 to 1914.* Preston: Mullion Books, 1993.

———. "Infant mortality, flies and horses in later-nineteenth-century towns: A case study of Preston." *Continuity and Change* 17:1 (2002): 97–132.

Mottram, Joan. "State control in local context: Public health and midwife regulation in Manchester, 1900–1914." In Hilary Marland and Anne Marie Rafferty, eds., *Midwives, society and childbirth: Debates and controversies in the modern period.* London and New York: Routledge, 1997. 134–52.

Neave, David. *Mutual aid in the Victorian countryside: Friendly societies in the rural East Riding 1830–1914.* Hull: Hull University Press, 1991.

Oakley, Ann. *The captured womb: A history of the medical care of pregnant women.* Oxford: Blackwell, 1984.

Oddy, Derek J. *From plain fare to fusion food: British diet from the 1890s to the 1990s.* Rochester, New York, and Woodbridge, Suffolk: Boydell Press, 2003.

Oren, Laura. "The welfare of women in laboring families: England, 1860–1950." In Mary Hartman and Lois W. Banner, eds., *Clio's consciousness raised: New perspectives on the history of women.* New York: Harper Torchbooks, 1974. 226–44.

Parker, David. "'A convenient dispensary': Elementary education and the influence of the school medical service 1907–39." *History of Education* 27:1 (1998): 59–83.

Passerini, Luisa. *Fascism in popular memory: The cultural experience of the Turin working class.* Trans. Robert Lumley and Jude Bloomfield. Cambridge: Cambridge University Press, 1988.

Pegg, Mark. *Broadcasting and society 1918–1939.* London and Canberra: Croom Helm, 1983.

Pelling, Margaret. *Cholera, fever and English medicine, 1825–1865.* Oxford and New York: Oxford University Press, 1978.

Pescosolido, Bernice A. and Jack K. Martin. "Cultural authority and the sovereignty of American medicine: The role of networks, class and community." *Journal of Health Politics, Policy and Law* 29:4–5 (2004): 735–56.

Peterson, M. Jeanne. *The medical profession in mid-Victorian London.* Berkeley: University of California Press, 1978.

Phillips, Howard and David Killingray, eds. *The Spanish influenza pandemic of 1918–19: New perspectives.* London and New York: Routledge, 2003.

Pickstone, John V. *Medicine and industrial society: A history of hospital development in Manchester and its region, 1752–1946.* Manchester: Manchester University Press, 1985.

Portelli, Alessandro. *The battle of Valle Giulia: Oral history and the art of dialogue.* Madison: University of Wisconsin Press, 1997.

Porter, Dorothy. "From social structure to social behavior in Britain after the

Second World War." *Contemporary British History* 16:3 (2002): 58–80.

———. *Health, civilization and the state: A history of public health from ancient to modern times*. London and New York: Routledge, 1999.

Porter, Roy. "The patient's view. Doing medical history from below." *Theory and Society* 14 (1985): 175–98.

Porter, Roy and Lesley Hall. *The facts of life: The creation of sexual knowledge in Britain, 1650–1950*. New Haven, CT: Yale University Pres, 1995.

Ravetz, Alison. *Council housing and culture: The history of a social experiment*. London: Routledge, 2001.

Reddy, William M. "The concept of class." In M. L. Bush, ed., *Social orders and social classes in Europe since 1500: Studies in social stratification*. London and New York: Longman, 1992. 13–25.

Reid, Alice. "The effects of the 1918–1919 influenza pandemic on infant and child health in Derbyshire." *Medical History* 49:1 (2005): 29–54.

Richards, Jeffrey. *The age of the dream palace: Cinema and society in Britain 1930–1939*. London: Routledge and Kegan Paul, 1984.

Riley, James C. *Sick, not dead: The health of British workingmen during the mortality decline*. Baltimore and London: Johns Hopkins University Press, 1997.

Roberts, Elizabeth. "The Lancashire way of death." In Ralph Houlbrooke, ed., *Death, ritual and bereavement*. London and New York: Routledge, 1989. 188–207.

———. "Oral history investigations of disease and its management by the Lancashire working class 1890–1939." In *Health, disease and medicine in Lancashire 1750–1950*. Occasional Publications, 2, Department of History, Science, and Technology, UMIST (1980). 33–51.

———. "The recipients' view of welfare." In Joanna Bornat, Robert Perks, Paul Thompson, and Jan Walmsley, eds., *Oral history, health and welfare*. London and New York: Routledge, 2000. 203–26.

———. *Women and families: An oral history, 1940–1970*. Oxford: Basil Blackwell, 1995.

———. *A woman's place: An oral history of working-class women 1890–1940*. Oxford: Basil Blackwell, 1984.

Roberts, Robert. *The classic slum: Salford life in the first quarter of the century*. Harmondsworth, Middlesex: Penguin, 1987. First published 1971.

Rosen, Andrew. *The transformation of British life 1950–2000: A social history*. Manchester and New York: Manchester University Press, 2003.

Rosen, George. *A history of public health*. Baltimore and London: Johns Hopkins University Press, 1993. First published 1958.

Ross, Ellen. *Love and toil: Motherhood in outcast London, 1870–1918*. New York and Oxford: Oxford University Press, 1993.

Royle, Edward. "Trends in post-war British social history." In James Obekevich and Peter Catterall, eds., *Understanding post-war British society*. London and New York: Routledge, 1994. 9–18.

Sandelowski, Margarete. *Devices and desires: Gender, technology and American nursing*. Chapel Hill: University of North Carolina Press, 2000.

Savage, Michael. *The dynamics of working-class politics: The labor movement in Preston, 1880–1940*. Cambridge: Cambridge University Press, 1987.

Seccombe, Wally. *Weathering the storm: Working-class families from the Industrial Revolution to the fertility decline.* London and New York: Verso, 1993.

Shorter, Edward. *A history of women's bodies.* Harmondsworth: Penguin, 1984.

Shortland, Michael. *Medicine and film: A checklist, survey and research resource.* Oxford: Wellcome Unit for the History of Medicine, 1989.

Showalter, Elaine and English. "Victorian Women and Menstruation." In Marsha Vicinus, ed., *Suffer and be still: Women in the Victorian age.* Bloomington and London: Indiana University Press, 1972. 38–44.

Skeggs, Beverley. *Formations of class and gender: Becoming respectable.* London: Sage Publications, 1997.

Smith, F. B. "The Contagious Diseases Acts reconsidered." *Social History of Medicine* 3:2 (1990): 197–215.

———. *The people's health 1830–1910.* New York: Holmes and Meier Publishers, 1979.

Soloway, Richard Allen. *Birth control and the population question in England, 1877–1930.* Chapel Hill and London: University of North Carolina Press, 1982.

Spring Rice, Margery. *Working-class wives.* 2nd ed. London: Virago, 1981. First published 1939.

Starr, Paul. *The social transformation of American medicine.* New York: Basic Books, 1982.

Stearns, Peter N. "Working-class women in Britain, 1890–1914." In Marsha Vicinus, ed., *Suffer and be still: Women in the Victorian age.* Bloomington and London: Indiana University Press, 1972. 100–120.

Stedman Jones, Gareth. *Languages of class: Studies in English working class history 1832–1982.* Cambridge: Cambridge University Press, 1983.

Stevens, Rosemary. *Medical practice in modern England: The impact of specialization and state medicine.* New Haven: Yale University Press, 1966.

Strange, Julie-Marie. "The assault on ignorance: Teaching menstrual etiquette in England, c. 1920s to 1960s." *Social History of Medicine* 14:2 (2001): 247–65.

Summerfield, Penny. *Reconstructing women's wartime lives: Discourse and subjectivity in oral histories of the Second World War.* Manchester and New York: Manchester University Press, 1998.

Sutton, Maureen. *"We didn't know aught": A study of sexuality, superstition and death in women's lives in Lincolnshire during the 1930s, '40s, and '50s.* Stamford: Watkinds, 1992.

Szreter, Simon. *Fertility, class and gender in Britain, 1860–1940.* Cambridge: Cambridge University Press, 1996.

———. "The importance of social intervention in Britain's mortality decline c. 1850–1914: A re-interpretation of the role of public health." *Social History of Medicine* 1:1 (1988): 1–37.

Tait, Ian and Susanna Graham-Jones. "General practice, its patients, and the public." In Irvine Loudon, John Horder, and Charles Webster, eds., *General practice under the National Health Service 1948–1997.* London: Clarendon Press, 1998. 224–46.

Tanner, Andrea. "Come all, cure few: The diseases of the in-patients at Great Ormond Street Hospital, 1852–1900." Unpublished paper delivered at the Social Science History Association Conference, November 2005, Portland, Oregon.

Tebbutt, Melanie. *Women's Talk? A social history of "gossip" in working-class neighborhoods, 1880–1960.* Aldershot, Hants: Scolar Press; Brookfield, VT: Ashgate Publishing Co., 1995.

Thomas, James and A. Susan Williams. "Women and abortion in 1930s Britain: A survey and its data." *Social History of Medicine* 11 (1998): 283–309.

Thompson, E. P. *The making of the English working class.* New York: Vintage Books, 1966.

Thompson, Paul. *The voice of the past: Oral history.* 2nd ed. Oxford: Oxford University Press, 1988.

Tinkler, Penny. *Constructing girlhood: Popular magazines for girls growing up in England, 1920–1950.* London: Taylor and Francis, 1995.

Turner, Bryan S. *Medical power and social knowledge.* 2nd ed. London and Thousand Oaks, CA: Sage Publications, 1995.

Turow, Joseph. *Playing doctor: Television, storytelling, and medical power.* Oxford and New York: Oxford University Press, 1989.

Waddington, Ivan. *The medical profession in the Industrial Revolution.* Dublin, Ireland: Gill and Macmillan Humanities Press, 1984.

Walton, John K. *The British seaside: Holidays and resorts in the twentieth century.* Manchester and New York: Manchester University Press, 2000.

———. *Lancashire social history, 1558–1939.* Manchester: Manchester University Press, 1987.

Warner, John Harley. "Grand narrative and its discontents: Medical history and the social transformation of American medicine." *Journal of Health Politics, Policy and Law* 29:4–5 (2004): 757–80.

———. *The therapeutic perspective: Medical practice, knowledge, and identity in America, 1820–1885.* 2nd ed. Princeton: Princeton University Press, 1997.

Watkin, Brian. *The National Health Service: The first phase, 1948–1974 and after.* London: George Allen and Unwin, 1978.

Webster, Charles. "The health of the school child during the Depression." In Nicholas Parry and David McNair, eds., *The fitness of the nation: Physical and health education in the nineteenth and twentieth centuries.* Leicester: History of Education Society of Great Britain, 1982. 70–99.

———. "Healthy or hungry thirties?" *History Workshop* 13 (1982): 110–29.

———. *The National Health Service: A political history.* 2nd ed. Oxford: Oxford University Press, 2002.

Weeks, Jeffrey. *Sex, politics and society: The regulation of sexuality since 1800.* London and New York: Longman, 1981.

Welshman, John. "Dental health as a neglected issue in medical history: The school dental service in England and Wales, 1900–40." *Medical History* 42 (1998): 306–27.

———. "In search of the 'problem family': Public health and social work in England and Wales, 1940–70." *Social History of Medicine* 9:3 (1996): 447–65.

———. *Municipal medicine: Public health in twentieth-century Britain.* Oxford: Peter Lang, 2000.

Whitaker, Elizabeth D. "The idea of health: History, medical pluralism, and the management of the body in Emilia-Romagna, Italy." *Medical Anthropology Quarterly* 17:3 (2003): 348–75.

White, Cynthia L. *Women's magazines 1693–1968.* London: Michael Joseph, 1970.

Whitelegg, John. *Inequalities in health care: Problems of access and provision.* Retford, Nottinghamshire: Straw Barnes, 1982.

Whorton, James C. *Inner hygiene: Constipation and the pursuit of health in modern society.* Oxford and New York: Oxford University Press, 2000.

Wilkinson, John. *Preston's Royal Infirmary: A history of health care in Preston 1809–1986.* Preston: Carnegie Press, 1987.

Williams, Jan. "The controlling power of childbirth in Britain." In Hilary Marland and Anne Marie Rafferty, eds., *Midwives, society and childbirth: Debates and controversies in the modern period.* London: Routledge, 1997. 232–47.

Williamson, Peter. *From confinement to community: The moving story of "The Moor," Lancaster's county lunatic asylum.* Publisher unclear, 2000[?].

Wilson, Adrian. "Participant or patient? Seventeenth-century childbirth from the mother's point of view." In Roy Porter, ed., *Patients and practitioners: Lay perceptions of medicine in pre-industrial society.* Cambridge: Cambridge University Press, 1985. 129–44.

Winstanley, Michael. "The town transformed 1815–1914." In Andrew White, ed., *A history of Lancaster 1193–1993.* Keele, Staffordshire: Ryburn Publishing, Keele University Press, 1993. 145–98.

Witz, Anne. *Professions and patriarchy.* London and New York: Routledge, 1992.

Wohl, Anthony S. *Endangered lives: Public health in Victorian Britain.* Cambridge, MA: Harvard University Press, 1983.

Woods, R. I., P. A. Watterson, and J. H. Woodward. "The causes of rapid infant mortality decline in England and Wales, 1861–1921," Part 1. *Population Studies* 42:3 (1988): 343–66.

———. "The causes of rapid infant mortality decline in England and Wales, 1861–1921," Part 2. *Population Studies* 43: 1 (1989): 113–32.

Woods, Robert and John Woodward, eds. *Urban disease and mortality in nineteenth-century England.* New York: St. Martin's Press, 1984.

Woolf, Stuart. "Order, class and the urban poor." In M. L. Bush, ed., *Social orders and social classes in Europe since 1500: Studies in social stratification.* London and New York: Longman, 1992. 185–98.

Worboys, Michael. *Spreading germs: Disease theories and medical practice in Britain, 1865–1900.* Cambridge: Cambridge University Press, 2000.

Index

≋

Abel, Emily, 5

abortion, 253n; by abortionists, 249–51, 252, 262, 349n2; awareness of, 210; as birth control, 244, 245–47; herbalists/druggists/doctors assisting with, 251; illegal, 97, 209, 245, 246n192, 248–51; influenza-induced, 157; legal, 251, 252–53, 252n214, 253n219, 262; in Preston, 245n189; and reputation/respectability, 247–48, 249, 262; self-induced, 246–49, 246n192, 252; substances to cause, 97–98

Abortion Law Reform Association, 333–34

AIDS, 363–64

All Fours, 97, 97n33

ambulances, 195–96, 200

American Medical Association, 342

Anderson, Michael, 28, 29–30, 47

antibacterials, 26, 355

antibiotics, 80, 100, 200

antiphlogistic treatment, 95, 95n27

anti-Semitism, 301

"The Archers," 337

Armstrong, David, 24

Arrowsmith, 341

babies. *See entries starting with "infant"*

backyards. *See* yards

bacteriology, 147, 172, 172n112

Ballaster, Ros, 318

Barrow-in-Furness: babies delivered by midwives vs. doctors, 283; birth rate in, 243–44; bronchitis in, 159; cottage hospital in, 130n181; diarrhea mortality rate in, 153; diphtheria immunization of children in, 184; economy of, 32; employment in, 32, 46n41, 358; family planning services in, 261; formal health care in (*see* formal health care in Barrow, Lancaster, and Preston); harbor of, 31; health culture of (*see* health culture, working-class, generally); hospital births in, 286, 291; hospital in, 129; housing conditions in, 31–32, 39n12, 42–43; illegitimate births in, 226, 226n95; infant mortality in, 81, 269; influenza in, 157 (table); measles in, 155–56; MOH and annual reports in, 20, 21; neighborhoods/streets in, 44–45; notification system for infectious diseases, 107n80; open-air school in, 181, 291; oral history informants from, 365–70; oral history infor-

D1475863